Handbook Positive Health in Primary Care

Machteld Huber
Hans Peter Jung
Karolien van den Brekel-Dijkstra

Handbook Positive Health in Primary Care

The Dutch Example

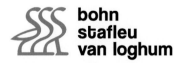

Houten 2022

Machteld Huber, MD, PhD.
Driebergen-Rijsenburg, The Netherlands

Hans Peter Jung, MD, PhD.
Afferden L, The Netherlands

Karolien van den Brekel-Dijkstra, MD, PhD.
Utrecht, The Netherlands

ISBN 978-90-368-2728-7   ISBN 978-90-368-2729-4   (eBook)
https://doi.org/10.1007/978-90-368-2729-4

Our thanks go to the Institute for Positive Health and to All about Health, who supported us to write this handbook.
Editor: Tirza van Hengstum
Translation: Annemieke Righart, Dunfield Editing

NUR 863
Cover Design: AgraphicsDesign, Apeldoornn
Cover template: Studio Bassa, Culemborg
Automatic layout: Scientific Publishing Services (P) Ltd., Chennai, India
Photographs Hippocratic Oath: Gideon van Voornveld
Photographs authors: Thomas Jung

Bohn Stafleu van Loghum
Walmolen 1
Postbus 246
3990 GA Houten
The Netherlands

www.bsl.nl

'If you want to build a ship, don't drum up the men to gather wood, divide the work and give orders. Instead, teach them to yearn for the vast and endless sea.'

Antoine de Saint-Exupéry

Foreword

General practitioners and other primary care providers are very close to those who ask them for help. Consequently, the appeal made to them is not limited to medically defined problems and conditions, but very often also includes issues such as daily functioning, psychosocial problems, and work-related challenges. For primary care, the WHO definition of health seems therefore well-suited, as it describes health not merely as the absence of disease, but as 'a state of complete physical, mental and social well-being and not merely the absence of disease or infirmity'.[1] However, this definition falls short on essential points, as argued by Huber et al. in 2011[2] and further discussed in this handbook.

First, the well-intentioned requirement of complete well-being – to quote Richard Smith, former editor of the BMJ: 'would leave most of us unhealthy most of the time.'[3] And second, this requirement should not guide health care as this may lead to overdiagnosis and overtreatment, doing more harm than good, and wasting many scarce resources. Moreover, because life evolves over time and presents constant physical, social and environmental challenges, we should see health not as a 'state' but rather as a dynamic concept. This should include 'the ability to adapt and self-manage' in the face of social, physical and emotional challenges. This is also a much more inclusive approach, especially at a time of increasing numbers of people with chronic conditions and disabilities. Instead of being declared definitively ill, people with such conditions should remain participants in our collective pursuit of better health, with or without the support of health care. This approach fits very well with the mission of general practice: taking responsibility for continuous, integrated and personal care for the health of individual people and their families, and to respect patient autonomy in a context of shared decision-making.

The concept of Positive Health, the logical next step in the work of Huber et al. and now increasingly substantiated in practice and research, is equally in line with general practice.[4] Health care should focus far more on what patients want to change, on their personal preferences rather than on standard outcome measures, and on opportunities instead of limitations. This provides a fruitful basis for shared decision-making in health care. All this is elaborated in this innovative and comprehensive book. After describing the theoretical and historical backgrounds of Positive Health, it focuses on its relevance and application in general practice. This is accompanied by a wealth of practical tools and approaches to health care and health promotion, multidisciplinary

---

1 About WHO/Who we are/Constitution. ► www.who.int/about/who-we-are/constitution.

2 Huber, M., Knottnerus, J. A., Green, L., et al. (2011). How should we define health? *BMJ, 343*, d4163. ► https://doi.org/10.1136/bmj.d4163.

3 Smith, R. The end of disease and the beginning of health. ► https://tinyurl.com/end-of-disease.

4 Huber, M., Van Vliet, M., Giezenberg, M., et al. (2016). Towards a 'patient-oriented' operationalisation of the new dynamic concept of health: A mixed methods study. *BMJ Open, 6*(1), e010091. ► https://doi.org/10.1136/bmjopen-2015-010091. PMID: 26758267.

cooperation, and preventive care in local communities. It also outlines opportunities for further research and vocational education, to increasingly embed Positive Health in evidence-based health care and the training of primary care professionals.

The authors also address the predominant public health and social context at the time of publication of this book: the COVID-19 pandemic and its massive impact on health care and social well-being. In doing so, they convincingly illustrate the enormous societal importance of resilience and adaptation, core elements of Positive Health.

I recommend this important book to all professionals, students and educators in the field of primary care. It is also useful to public health officials and policymakers who want to promote community health and integrated care. I expect that using this book will lead to better outcomes for patients and more job satisfaction for health care providers. That is a double positive for health.

André Knottnerus MD PhD
Clinical Epidemiologist, Professor emeritus of General Practice, Maastricht University, The Netherlands
Former President of the Health Council of the Netherlands
Former director and chair of the Netherlands School of Public Health and Care Research

Reader

After graduating from medical school, future physicians promise or swear to work according to the values as described in *the – somewhat modernised – Hippocratic Oath*. On entering the Domus Medica in Utrecht, the central office of Dutch medical organisations, this oath is immediately visible, displayed in large format on the wall. As a physician, you promise or swear to promote health, amongst other things. As is the case with all other values described in the oath, this also is perfectly in line with the objectives of Positive Health. These values from the past are still so relevant today that they form the leitmotif of this book. The future of primary care is also central to this book. The Dutch general practitioners of today are under pressure – it is time for a *wake-up call*. Positive Health can be an effective answer to today's challenges in health care.

In writing this handbook, the cooperation between the three authors has meant that Positive Health and its implementation is considered from various perspectives and fields of expertise. Machteld Huber is a former general practitioner, researcher and the founder of Positive Health. Hans Peter Jung and Karolien van den Brekel-Dijkstra are both practicing physicians and actively involved in innovation and application of Positive Health in primary care. Despite perhaps some differences in style, we have tried to give the book coherence. We are well aware of the diversity amongst our readers; a group likely to consist of primary care professionals, young and old, male and female, working in different types of practices, practice staff members, primary care managers, care providers in care groups and facilities, medical students and GP trainees. We hope that this handbook addresses all your fields and needs. The handbook (or digital e-book) can be read from cover to cover, or independently per chapter – readers can focus on specific themes or on the level of implementing Positive Health in primary care, in the local community or network, on regional or national levels. The final chapter discusses the broader international perspective in more detail.

For the structure of the book, we were inspired by *'Start with Why'*, a book by Simon Sinek about successful and sustainable behavioural change (Sinek 2009). According to Sinek, people will only really start doing things differently if they can be convinced that those changes are in line with a deeply felt desire for things to be different. For example, when change could lead to a more meaningful life or work. He calls this the *Why*, but you could also call it de Saint-Exupéry's 'yearn for the vast and endless sea' (see the motto at the beginning of this handbook). Sinek also emphasises that it is very important to first properly explain this *'why'*.

We, the authors, have noticed, each in our own way, what Positive Health has contributed both to our work and our lives. Our pioneering work with implementation of Positive Health has shown us its added value in the primary care practice for professionals themselves, as well as within the health care system as a whole. We have a clear vision of the transformation that is needed in health care, today. We would like to share this vision with health care professionals in and around primary care practices, both in the Netherlands and abroad, as with future professionals and all other interested parties. In Sinek's view, after talking about the '*why*', it makes perfect sense to start explaining the '*how*'. In our case, this is how a new understanding of health could contribute to the desired, essential change. And not until answering the 'how' question is recognised to actually lead to the desired substantial change, does it make sense to start explaining the '*what*' – what exactly would be needed to achieve that change.

Part I of our Positive Health handbook, therefore, first discusses the *why* and *how* of Positive Health, and Part II (from ▶ Chap. 5 onwards) subsequently describes the *what*. Part I aims to take the reader along in a more narrative style, to inspire them to look at health and the challenges for the future of the general practitioner's profession from a different perspective.

▶ Chapter 1 discusses *why* we believe that things really need to change in primary care. ▶ Chapter 2 explains *how* Positive Health, as a new health concept, could contribute to this change. ▶ Chapter 3 explains the characteristics of the Dutch health care system. ▶ Chapter 4, subsequently, elaborates on *how* to apply Positive Health, based on recently updated *core values and tasks of primary care in the Netherlands*.

Part II (▶ Chap. 5 to 8) describes the *what*, the practical tools needed to get started with Positive Health. These chapters show the levels at which Positive Health can be applied, which are linked to the different colours of the *nano, micro, meso and macro levels* of the pyramid (see ▢ fig. 1).

▶ Chapter 5 explains Positive Health at nano level (i.e., person-to-person level). These are the conversations that take place in the consulting room. In a personal conversation, the spider web is used to discuss what the patient considers important. The essence of this 'alternative dialogue' is for the physician or other care provider to listen intently and give the other person insight into what is of value to them. Together, they discuss what the patient would like to change and what he or she needs in order to do so.

▶ Chapter 6 deals with the implementation of Positive Health at micro level, the organisational level. One of the tasks of general practitioners should be to promote health. The mission, vision and strategy of the general medical practice, together with the individual role of the care provider, determine which aspects of Positive Health are the first to be implemented. The process distinguishes between the introduction, implementation and embedding of Positive Health in your primary care practice. Ample attention should be paid to each of these three steps.

▶ Chapter 7 starts with citizens themselves. The pyramid based on De Maeseneer shows that the meso level of Positive Health is that of municipalities, districts and neighbourhoods. Gaining insight into what citizens want and are able to do is essential. Citizen initiatives, informal care and other community initiatives can mean far more to the general practitioners than is currently seen. In their municipality, general practitioners also have the task of promoting the health and well-being of the residents.

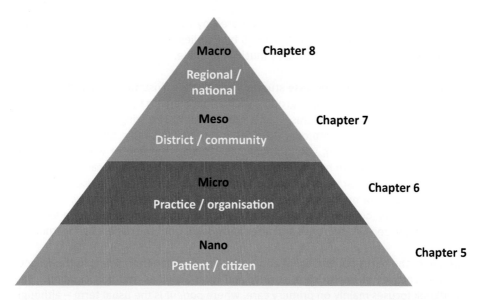

Figure 1 Pyramid of the implementation of Positive Health at different levels; classification based on health care levels by Professor Jan De Maeseneer, University of Ghent, 2017. (Source: De Maeseneer 2017)

If cooperation around citizens is to function properly, it is important that general practitioners are aware of local care and lifestyle counselling services and of social activities available within the district or municipality. Examples of integrated cooperation between primary health care and the social domain include Positive Health Networks. Here, Positive Health is the catalyst of such cooperation.

▶ Chapter 8 provides a broader perspective of Positive Health and insights into consequences and challenges on regional and national levels (the macro level). For the successful organisation and cooperation around patients, Positive Health requires good interaction between various levels of the pyramid. The chapter first describes the challenges of health care innovation in general, followed by more specific, organisational and pre-conditional aspects of implementing Positive Health. These aspects, for instance, include agreements on implementation and funding. The Institute of Positive Health (iPH) stimulates further development of Positive Health in Dutch policy, research and education.

The handbook concludes with ▶ Chap. 9 reflecting on the lessons learned from the Dutch example. Positive Health implementation follows the three phases of inspiration, implementation and embedment. There are many universal aspects to the implementation of Positive Health. Therefore – although there will be culture and country-specific themes – wherever in the world you are, after having read this book, you will be ready to start working with Positive Health.

► Chapters 1, 3, 4 and 6 were mainly authored by Hans Peter Jung; ► Chap. 2 and 5 by Machteld Huber and ► Chap. 7, 8 and 9 by Karolien van den Brekel-Dijkstra, while complementing each other's work, as much as possible.

Using practical examples and case studies, the chapters illustrate how Positive Health can be applied to various target groups, such as people with social problems, chronic diseases, mental health problems, lifestyle challenges or recurring somatic complaints (medically unexplained symptoms (MUPS)), including vulnerable target groups, children (from 8 years of age), young people, the elderly, and people with poor health skills. Positive Health can be applied in all phases of people's lives. It can also be used in first personal contacts, or in cooperation with colleagues in, for example, case study discussions or multidisciplinary consultations. For reasons of privacy, all patient names have been omitted from the examples in this publication, except for a few case discussions, in consultation with and after permission from the patients concerned.

The use of the terms *patient*, *client* and *citizen/resident* generally refers to the respective perspectives of health care, society and local activities and participation. The handbook focuses mainly on primary care, where *patient* is the usual term – although we do realise that its connotation is disease-oriented while it refers to citizens registered at a general medical practice, most of whom are not ill.

However, because of the general use of the term patient, in practice, as well as for the sake of readability, we have opted for this term anyway – with the added comment that this should be read as representing both patients, clients, citizens and residents. Although the handbook focuses primarily on the general medical practice, it is equally applicable to the entire domain of primary care and all future medical professionals. The term *general practitioner* is used as a generic term and also includes *general practice staff, practice assistants, practice nurses, and other primary care professionals.*

Over time, good examples, videos and guides have been produced that show what Positive Health can mean and how it is used in practice. Because we did not want to fill these pages with URLs, at the end of each chapter there is a QR code that can be scanned (using a smartphone) which will direct you to useful links, tools and materials related to the chapter.

An index is provided at the back of the book to trace definitions to the chapters in which they are described. The book concludes with practical tips, which can be put into practice straight away.

We wish everyone lots of reading pleasure. Positive Health is aimed to be in line with what people consider to be of value. We hope that people will be able to take the next step towards a broader approach to their own health, using the practical tools that Positive Health offers. Hopefully this handbook will prove valuable for your own health and provide job satisfaction as well as meaningfulness and health for your patients.

Machteld Huber
Hans Peter Jung
Karolien van den Brekel-Dijkstra

References Reader

De Maeseneer, J. (2017). *Family medicine and primary care. At the crossroads of societal change.* Lannoo Campus.

De Saint Exupery, A. (2012). Citadelle, posthum, 1948. In A. Van der Kaap (Red.), *Het eindeloze verlangen naar de zee.* Histoforum didactiek. Het online tijdschrift voor geschiedenisdidactiek. Accessed in Juni 2021 of ▶ http://histoforum.net/columns/column14.html.

Sinek, S. (2009). *Start with why.* New York: Penguin Books Ltd.

Contents

About the authors

Machteld Huber (1951) obtained her medical degree in Utrecht, in 1977. After a medical internship of two and a half years, she did a bachelor's degree in philosophy, followed by the general practitioner's training at VU Amsterdam. The beginning of her career was overshadowed by several periods of illness. In order to tolerate these experiences better, she decided to study what it meant to be a patient, and investigated whether and, if so, how a certain lifestyle and other factors had any effect. This led her to the realisation that broadening the medical thinking to include resilience, lifestyle and meaningfulness would enrich the profession. After her recovery, around the age of 35, Machteld decided to make use of her experiences and to apply them in practice. She became a researcher and worked with 'damaged' people, such as addicts and people with war traumas. Her research into the promotion of resilience ultimately led to a new perception on health and its elaboration into the Positive Health concept. In 2012, she was awarded the *ZonMw-Parel* award. In 2014, she obtained her PhD in Maastricht, after which she founded the Institute for Positive Health in 2015. In the current phase of her work, she feels particularly grateful that the difficult years of illness of the past have led to such fruitful results.

Hans Peter Jung (1963) studied medicine in Nijmegen and has been working as a general practitioner since 1995. He works in the general practice of Afferden in North Limburg. In 1999, he obtained his doctorate with a thesis on the quality of primary care, seen from the perspective of the patient. Hans Peter is married and had three children. The middle child, a daughter, died in 2010 at the age of 14. During the difficult period after her death, he realised that if he wanted his life to be meaningful again, he had to occupy himself as much as possible with things that gave him energy. This also included his work – in the general practice that had become increasingly busy, over the years, and demanded rather than gave him more and more energy. He therefore opted for making some radical changes: i.e., he reduced the size of his practice and implemented 15-minute consultations in order to have more time for his patients, for real human interactions – the reason why he had wanted to become a general practitioner in the first place. Applying the concept of Positive Health turned out to be key in regaining the pleasure in his work. In 2017, he received the Dutch compassion award (*Compassieprijs*) with the theme: 'Who cares for the care provider?' In 2020, he received the international Value-Based Health Care Primary Care Excellence Award for his 'Afferden initiative on Positive Health'.

Karolien van den Brekel-Dijkstra (1968) studied in Groningen, did her internship at the VUmc in Amsterdam, and completed her general practitioner's training in Utrecht (2001). Because of the international career of her husband, who facilitated the locations, she created opportunities to do research, study and work abroad. Karolien did her doctoral research at New York University, on which she obtained her doctorate in gynaecology and general practice in Utrecht (Prediction of Preterm Delivery 2002). She worked in general practices in Germany (Munich) and Ireland, and followed international coaching training while living in Japan with her family. This time abroad gave her not only wonderful new life experiences but also resilience and a broad perspective on health. Back in the Netherlands, since 2010, Karolien has been working as a general practitioner at the *Leidsche Rijn Julius health care centres*. Her work there as a general practitioner gives her great pleasure and she applies Positive Health in practice on a daily basis. She is also active in community-based prevention and person-oriented care. In the 2016–2018 period, Karolien worked for the Dutch College of General Practitioners (NHG) on a community project on prevention (*Preventie in de buurt*) and followed the Innovating Health for Tomorrow programme at INSEAD (The Business School for the World). Her ambition is to contribute to innovation and health transformation in the Netherlands and abroad by giving lectures, webinars, workshops and trainings for general practitioners and GP trainees and colleagues in the field of health care, in her role as advisor and certified trainer at iPH.

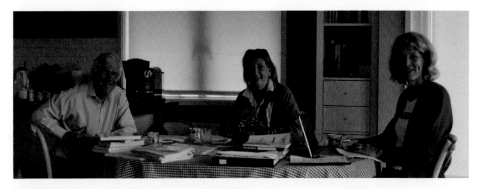

Authors: Hans Peter Jung, Machteld Huber and Karolien van den Brekel-Dijkstra

I swear/promise to practise the art of medicine to the best of my ability for the benefit of my fellow man. I will care for the sick, promote health and relieve suffering.

I will put the patient's interests first and respect his/her views. I will do no harm to the patient. I will listen and inform him/her well. I will keep secret what has been entrusted to me.

I will advance the medical knowledge of myself and others. I will recognise the limits of my possibilities.

I will maintain an open and verifiable attitude,
and I am aware of my responsibility towards society.
I will promote the availability and accessibility of
health care. I will not misuse my medical knowledge,
not even under pressure.

Thus, I will uphold the profession of physician.

This I promise

or
So help me God Almighty

Dutch physician's oath, based on the Hippocratic Oath. (Source: Domus Medica Utrecht)

Part 1 Background and inception of Positive Health in the Netherlands in relation to the future of primary care

Contents

I swear/promise to practise the art of medicine to the best of my ability for the benefit of my fellow man. I will care for the sick, promote health and relieve suffering.

I will put the patient's interests first and respect his/her views. I will do no harm to the patient. I will listen and inform him/her well. I will keep secret what has been entrusted to me.

I will advance the medical knowledge of myself and others. I will recognise the limits of my possibilities.

Introduction

© Bohn Stafleu van Loghum is an imprint of Springer Media B.V., part of Springer Nature 2022
M. Huber et al., *Handbook Positive Health in Primary Care*,
https://doi.org/10.1007/978-90-368-2729-4_1

1

> **Main messages**

- Under the Hippocratic Oath, we pledge to adhere to important values – to ourselves, the patients entrusted to us and the community. Can such a pledge continue to be honoured with the challenges that will present themselves in the near future?
- Health care really can and needs to change
- Positive Health could be an important catalyst, in this respect
- We are shifting from *surviving* to *living as long as possible*, to *leading a meaningful life*
- The general practitioner's role in the Netherlands may change from gatekeeper to guide/coach

---

Case no.1: A meaningful life

A 30-year-old man went to see his general practitioner with complaints of feeling down. He was working in a warehouse, driving a forklift truck. He was not happy doing what he considered to be mind-numbing work. Life generally felt like he was in a rut and he lacked purpose. He also found it difficult to fit in with his colleagues at work – particularly, because conversations were usually rather superficial. With each weekend that followed, he tended to stay in bed longer and longer. He asked his general practitioner if there was some medication that would make him feel better. The general practitioner said he could hear how many things were not going well in the man's life and asked him what he would like to change, how he would like his life to be. After thinking for a moment, the man started to explain that, due to a lack of money, he had never been able to get a proper education, but that he would have liked to. Then, perhaps, he could have found a different job – one that involved using his brain more often.

He also talked about his passion: playing darts, and that he was good at that and would not mind pursuing it as a professional career. The general practitioner noticed how the man's facial expression and posture changed while talking about this subject. From being sombre and sad-faced, to sitting up straight and having a twinkle in his eye. When the general practitioner remarked on this, the man also confided in him that he enjoyed writing poems and other texts. Few people knew this about him – as he feared they might think it strange. The general practitioner told him about how important it is to have a purpose in life, something that makes you want to get up in the morning, and also how good it was to hear that the man could say what would be meaningful to him. The general practitioner briefly talked about the importance of life having meaning and how he hoped there would be opportunities for the man to follow his heart. During the conversation, Positive Health was mentioned and the man asked about the exact meaning of the term. The general practitioner explained. As their conversation was coming to an end, the practitioner returned to the question of possible medication. But the man said he was very happy about their talk; it had made him think about things and gave him the idea that perhaps he would not need any medication. He also thought that even a follow-up appointment was unnecessary. This pleasantly surprised the general practitioner and, when they were saying goodbye, on impulse he asked whether he could perhaps read one of the man's poems, one day. The man thought for a moment and then agreed. 'I will send you a poem that fits our talk.' A few days later, the general practitioner received this poem by email, which has since been hanging on the wall in his waiting room (see ◻ fig. 1.1).

Positive Health

This is the place where the lights turn off
It can be seen, all this nightmare stuff
You've been here before, you recognise it all
It all becomes black, right before you fall
But now it makes sense and your mind is clear
The road ahead, is what you've always feared
Make place for the positive vibes
Let's make something out of this life
No time for standing still anymore
Ask yourself 'Did I even move before?'
You just can't seem to remember
Wake yourself up, because it's almost September
You needed a reason, maybe even two
But all those reasons help you to pull through
Give it some space, give it some room
And I promise, it will all be better soon

J.K, August 2018

◻ **Figure 1.1**   Poem in English, written by a grateful Dutch patient, hanging on the wall of the waiting room in the general practice in Afferden

1.1 Why this book?

At the festive conclusion of their medical studies, new doctors in the Netherlands promise or swear to work according to the values of the – somewhat modernised – Hippocratic Oath. It starts with the words: 'I swear/promise to practice the art of medicine to the best of my ability for the benefit of my fellow man.' How does this relate to the ever-increasing challenges faced by general practitioners? The care we offer and the need for care no longer seem to be properly attuned. Primary care is under pressure because of this. There seems to be a crisis.

The challenges Dutch primary care is facing are not typical of the Netherlands. In other countries, there are similar challenges. The pressure on health care systems is increasing, with respect to access, costs, quality and capacity, due to the universal health challenges each country has to deal with, in one way or another. The International Health Challenges are the ageing population, the increase in unhealthy lifestyles, obesity, chronic and mental diseases, and health inequalities, as well as the crisis the world has recently experienced in the major impact of the COVID-19 pandemic (Kluge et al. 2021).

We believe that Positive Health can be very useful in health transition, and we would like to share the experience and knowledge obtained in the Netherlands, so far, to be able to make a shift from more disease-oriented care to the type of care that is more person-oriented and focuses on health.

1

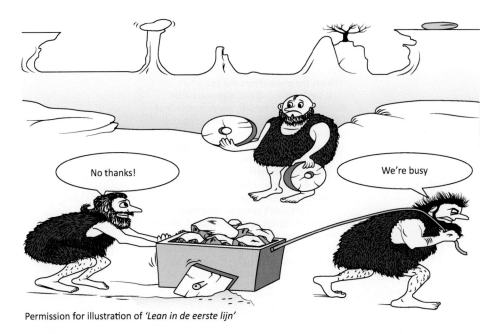

Permission for illustration of *'Lean in de eerste lijn'*

◘ **Figure 1.2**   Sometimes, we are part of the problem, instead of the solution. (Source: variant of square wheels)

The most important organisations in primary care in the Netherlands[1] have already tried to reach politicians with a cry from the heart (Skipr 2019; Kleijne 2020), because, in the words of Machteld Huber, the 'health care system has become unstable' ('Het zorghuis wankelt', Houben 2020). Which is true. But, at the same time, we, as general practitioners, are busy extinguishing so many fires that we lack the time to sufficiently concern ourselves with the underlying causes of the problems and questions of our patients. As a result, it is not always easy to put a person in the most prominent position – which is a missed opportunity, not only for the patient in our consulting room, but also for us, because it means we are perpetuating problems. Sometimes even up to the point of becoming part of the problem instead of the solution. Therefore, it is high time for general practitioners to wake up, too! (◘ fig. 1.2)

The concept of Positive Health, introduced by author Machteld Huber in 2012 (Huber et al. 2011, 2014, 2016), is discussed in detail in ▶ Chap. 2. The concept provides the opportunity to look at health and disease from a different perspective. This handbook describes Positive Health and *what* it could mean in everyday general practice. It provides concrete and practical tools on *how* to implement Positive Health in primary care. The concept may offer a solution for the many general practitioners in the Netherlands

---

1   InEen (association of primary care organisations), IOH (Interfaculty consultative body for general medical practice; Professors of General Medicine), Het Roer Moet Om (manifest of concerned general practitioners 'things need to change'), Huisartsopleiding Nederland (Dutch general practitioner's training), LHV (Dutch National Association of General Practitioners), LOVAH (National organisation of general practitioners in training), Dutch College of General Practitioners, VPH (Association of general practice owners).

who are feeling that things cannot go on like they are and need to change (Het Roer Moet Om 2019). The question is how? Before answering this question, this introductory chapter first explains *why* things really must and can be done differently in health care, and that Positive Health could be an important catalyst, in this respect.

In 2019, the National Association of General Practitioners (LHV), together with the Dutch College of General Practitioners (NHG), the Association of Practicing General Practitioners, InEen (association of primary care organisations) and the members of the medical profession themselves, renewed and delineated the focus of primary care. A few thousand general practitioners participated in conceptual discussions and over 3,500 completed a questionnaire about what is most important to general practitioners. In this way, the Woudschoten Conference formulated the core values and core tasks for the vision on future general medical care (Toekomst Huisartsenzorg 2020a).

The old core values of Dutch primary care from 1959 (person-oriented, generalist and continuous) were found to still hold firm, but with a further clarification and update to suit the challenges of our time. What has changed:

- With respect to the *person-oriented* core value, the input of patients is mentioned more explicitly;
- The term *generalist* has been refined to *medical generalist*. General practitioners have a general medical expertise, with a focus on physical and psychological complaints and the appropriate medical care;
- General practitioners are a constant factor in medical care, with the clarification that *continuity* is important in primary care (but not necessarily by the same individual general practitioner), in that care is always available and provided to address complaints that require immediate medical assessment;
- A new core value has been added: '*together*'. This is a fundamental aspect of implementing the other three core values. General practitioners are team players, seeking a joint approach, together with their patients and others, both within primary care and with other care providers.

This handbook shows the relationship between the concept of Positive Health and these updated core values and core tasks in primary care. ▶ Chapter 4, in particular, goes into further detail on this subject. The handbook also shows how Positive Health can provide an answer to concerns over the currently constricting health care system. An important change in the role of the general practitioner, as advocated here, moves from general practitioners being *gatekeeper* (guarding the access to secondary care) to them taking on the role of *coach, guide or liaison* in health care and support services. This 'guide' function has an important social value, contributes to optimal and efficient care and is highly appreciated by patients (Toekomst Huisartsenzorg 2020b; Brabers et al. 2019).

This handbook describes how Positive Health can offer a common language that facilitates easier cooperation and cooperation between the various disciplines in health care and welfare (for definitions of disciplines of health care and welfare, see the appendix to ▶ Chap. 7) and citizens, and provides an answer to the question of what this means for health care and how it could be organised. This from the context of primary care, written by three general practitioners. It shows how Positive Health can contribute to the health of citizens while also providing greater job satisfaction to general practitioners and the other practice staff. This is an accessible, pragmatic handbook for professionals in general medical practice and can also be used for general medical and paramedical educational purposes.

First, however, a brief history is outlined of developments in general practitioner care in the past, present and future (Jung 2020).

1.2 From merely surviving and living as long as possible to living a meaningful life

1.2.1 Surviving

The first general practitioner in the Dutch village of Afferden (in Limburg, the south-ernmost province of the Netherlands, and currently the practice of author Hans Peter Jung) was Doctor Versélewel de Witt Hamer, who had set up his practice immediately after the Second World War. Because of his very long surname, the people of Afferden used to call him 'Doctor Sniffles', as, in those days, everyone in the village was provided with a nickname. According to legend, he owed his nickname to his forever runny nose (Kreuzer 2008). An illustrative story that some of today's very old patients still recount is about how his pharmacy consisted of two dark brown glass bottles that stood behind him in a cupboard. If you were lucky, his hand would reach back and he would hand out some of the contents of one of them. Either a powder or a tablet; there was not much else in the way of pharmaceutical care in Afferden, at the time.

Did this mean that the role of the general practitioner was insignificant? Far from it. After the war, the village of Afferden was facing many problems. It had no water mains (a situation that lasted up to 1964!) or sewerage system, and living conditions were miserable. The average life expectancy in the early 1950s was 55 years. People used to live in chicken coops, in concrete basements and even in underground caves on the heath, for many years. The general practitioner played an important role in tackling their problems and attracted the attention of the then Bishop of Roermond, Mgr Lemmens. He even paid a visit to Prime Minister Louis Beel (Elsevier's Weekblad 1946). In those days, health care in the Netherlands was not very sophisticated. In the early 1950s, the country had a total of 2,900 medical specialists and 4,500 general practitioners (Eekhof 2017). Health was seen as the absence of disease and the zeitgeist was one of *survival*. Warmth, security and protection in this region (Luyten 2015) was, therefore, not so much offered by the health care system but rather by the Roman Catholic Church, at the peak of its influence in the 1950s (Palm 2012; Mak 1996). Charity and community power played a major role in both the social domain and in health care (hospitals and mental health institutions) and was much more important than the input of the government and the standard provision of care. The fact that 'Doctor Sniffles' was well aware of this is shown by him engaging church and politics for the good of society.

1.2.2 Living as long as possible

Then, on 1 July 1965, the general practice of Afferden came into the hands of Doctor Gerrits. Health care acquired a different connotation, which had already been initiated by the World Health Organization (WHO) in 1948: *Health is a state of complete phys-ical, mental and social well-being and not merely the absence of disease or infirmity*

9

1

1.2 · From merely surviving and living as long as possible to living ...

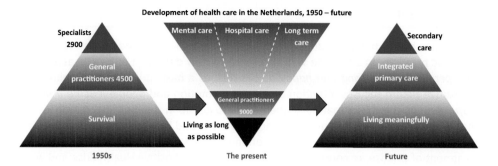

Figure 1.3 Development in health care. (Source: B. Leerink, formerly of Menzis) Blue represents health care costs and pink the costs of health promotion. The numbers of medical specialists and general practitioners in the middle triangle are those from 2010 (Eekhof 2017)

(WHO 2006). Society was no longer merely surviving – above all, people now wanted to *live as long as possible*. Dr Gerrits had a range of medications to prescribe from, a regional hospital was set up, and the financial possibilities seemed unlimited. This also increased the influence of health care in society. A good example is the introduction of the contraceptive pill, symbolising the shift in power, from the church to the health care system. Although the number of medical specialists grew from 2,900 in 1950 to 20,000 by 2010, and general practitioners from 4,500 in 1950 to 9,000 by 2010 (Eekhof 2017; ◘ fig. 1.3), general practitioners in particular, increasingly worked on a part-time basis. This is why the increase in the number of professionals, ultimately, did not mean a real increase in primary care capacity.

Health care did, however, hold considerable sway in society. And with the growing confidence in medicine, life expectancy also increased for the Dutch population: by 2019, this had exponentially increased to 82 years (an increase of 50 %) (RIVM 2020).

1.2.3 What now?

Although primary care had been through an enormous evolution in the years following the Second World War, today's health care still closely resembles that provided in the era of Dr Gerrits. It still focuses on *diagnosing and treating diseases* and *providing the related care*. Health care in the Netherlands still has insufficient attention for the concepts of *health & behaviour* and *people & society* (see ► sect. 1.3 for more details).

The core of ◘ fig. 1.3 shows the evolution of health care, throughout the years. In the 1950s, the focus was on *survival*. People were looking for something to hold on to in religion (pink). Which is why, in those days, religion had the greatest public support. As prosperity increased and the influence of the church and charities declined, the level of support for health care increased. The figure's second triangle shows this transition, with the community's self-reliance being taken over by the government (blue). Society became medicalised. The focus was on treatment and the curing of diseases, in order for people to *live as long as possible*. In the future, the triangle is expected to tilt towards the third variant. Here, the triangle once more stands firm on the broad basis of people *living a meaningful life*. In the future, people's level of health will not be improved by church and charity (as it was in the past) or by government (as it is now), but by citizens themselves.

1.2.4 A meaningful life

In the past, health had been defined simply as the *absence of disease*, with *survival* as the basic principle. In 1948, the WHO presented a new definition of health, associated with *people living as long and happy as possible*, as a basic principle. The philosophy of Positive Health focuses attention on health promotion and people *leading a mean-ingful life* – on the things that make them want to get up in the morning. It emphasises that health is more than the mere absence of disease and living as long as possible. The focus on disease thus shifts to the promotion of resilience – in addition to the proper treatment of disease, of course. How did the concept of Positive Health arise and what is at its core? ▶ Chapter 2 further elaborates on that, but a short introduction is pro-vided below.

1.2.5 Positive Health

When Machteld Huber, one of the authors, fell ill herself several times, in her early thir-ties, she gained first-hand experience in how to contribute to her own recovery. Driven and inspired by this experience, she wanted to broaden the scope of health care. In her opinion, much could be gained by adding the knowledge on how to increase resil-ience to the general medical training of future physicians, which in the Netherlands still focuses mainly on disease rather than health. From the current medical-analytical per-spective, physicians wait until someone is sick and then begin treating the illness to the best of their ability. Adopting a broader perspective, however, may prevent many diseases and ailments – and when they do occur, it may greatly improve people's recovery and how diseases are dealt with. Machteld Huber realised that these find-ings would mean a paradigm shift in medical thinking, which is why she chose to take the path of science. Without a solid foundation, not much would ever change. During her research, she ran into a problem of semantics: she could not refer to *resilience* as *health,* because of the 1948 definition of health by the WHO, which reads: *Health is a state of complete physical, mental and social well-being and not merely the absence of disease or infirmity*.

With this definition, hardly anyone could be called healthy; a state of *complete* well-being can rarely be achieved. Without this being the intention, the definition contributed to medicalisation, due to the elevated objective of the definition in com-bination with the greatly increased diagnostic possibilities. Any symptom that was identified had to be treated immediately. In practice, health was soon being inter-preted as the *absence of disease*. Huber concluded that the idealistic but static defi-nition of the WHO from 1948 bears no relation to something as dynamic as resilience.

The Health Council of the Netherlands and ZonMw (The Netherlands Organisation for Health Research and Development) shared her objection to the definition. In 2009, an international conference was held to present possible alternatives to the static for-mulation. This eventually led to a more dynamic description of *Health as the ability to adapt and self-manage in the face of social, physical and emotional challenges* (Huber et al. 2011).

Commissioned by ZonMw, Huber then investigated the amount of support for this formulation and a step towards its operationalisation. This support turned out to be rather large and the research into its operationalisation led to an elaboration into six dimensions, collectively named *Positive Health* (Huber 2014; Huber et al. 2016). ▶ Chapter 2 discusses this in greater detail.

1.2.6 The spider web

The dimensions of Positive Health are placed in a *spider web* chart, with a numbering from 0 to 10 (in practice 1–10) along its axes (◘ fig. 1.4). People appeared to enjoy assessing themselves on the various dimensions. The method promotes self-reflection.

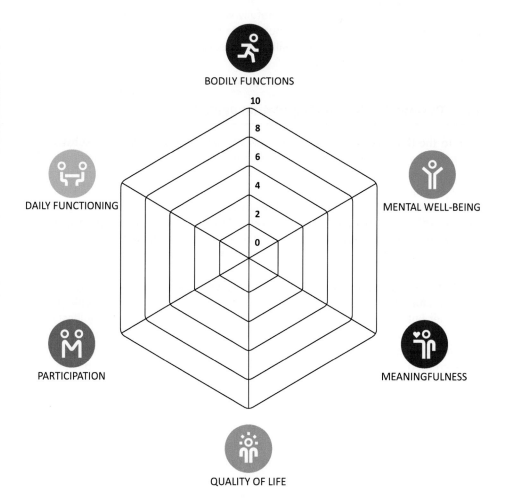

◘ **Figure 1.4**   The six dimensions of the spider web of Positive Health. Source: Huber et al. (2014)

In her ZonMw research, on several occasions, Huber was recommended to take more account of the concept of *meaningfulness*. This led to the practical elaboration whereby patients, after having filled out the list of questions for the spider web, sit down with the care professional for a so-called '*alternative dialogue*' about the results. More information about this type of dialogue is provided in ▶ sect. 1.4 and ▶ Chap. 5. Important element in this alternative method of communication is the way it is conducted; it is important not to focus on the theme or themes on which patients give themselves a low score, but rather to ask open questions. What do you think about the spider web? Would you like to change something? And if so, what and how?

Our experience has shown that people then quite quickly start talking about what is most important to them, at that particular moment. When care professionals hold back on giving advice, but first ask their patients what they think that needs to happen, this often produces surprising answers. It requires that care professionals take on a coaching role and, above all, listen carefully without trying to immediately solve the problem for their patient. As it turns out, under this approach, patients often become active themselves and take responsibility. In essence, they need to move from *having* to do something to *wanting* to do it.

1.2.7 Positive Health and population ageing

Back to the third triangle of ▪ fig. 1.3: How can people give meaningful substance to the additional years of life (in the Netherlands on average 50 %) that they have been given? This in the knowledge that these years of life are added at the end, in the phase of life in which morbidity and reduced quality of life will also be more common. Yes, people are all living longer, but during the last years of their lives they increasingly have to deal with health-related limitations. These limitations lead to less participation in society and, thus, increase loneliness in old age (Dutch National Government 2018). And the number of years with such limitations seems to be increasing (Deeg and Nusselder 2020).

These ailments seem paradoxical, given the success of modern medicine, but they are a residue of the lack of focus on a healthy lifestyle. As a result, people are getting older but also sicker than before. The consequences of an unhealthy lifestyle are being mitigated by medical-technical possibilities, but people are living with these limitations for longer. For the Dutch population, the expected number of unhealthy years has increased by 16 – from 22 years in 1981 to 38 years in 2019. Life expectancy has increased by 6 years over the same period (from 76 to 82 years), but life expectancy *without chronic diseases* has *decreased* by 10 years over the same period (from 54 to 44 years).

In summary, people in the Netherlands, on average, will live 6 years longer than before, but will also spend an average 10 more years living with chronic diseases – thus, becoming chronically ill at a younger age than before. This is expensive, and the burden of disease is also unequally distributed over the population. The difference in healthy life expectancy is even greater for lower educated people, who will also on average live 6 years shorter than those who are higher educated (CBS 2016) (▪ fig. 1.5).

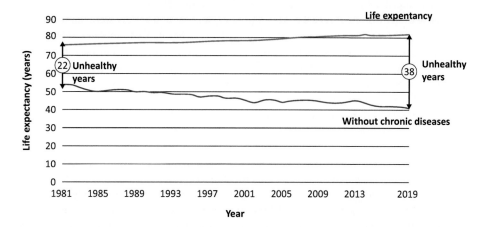

Figure 1.5 Healthy life expectancy for the Dutch population. Source: (CBS 2020)

In our opinion, by adding Positive Health to our highly developed medically and analytically oriented health care, the quality of these additional years of life could actually be increased and thus contribute to meaningful living. The current Dutch health care system is facing a major challenge, which has become starkly clear, partly due to the sudden emergence of the COVID-19 pandemic in 2020. What could Positive Health do to help this situation?

Case no. 2: Things cannot go on like this

An 85-year-old woman complaining of pain in one of her legs was diagnosed by her general practitioner with having bursitis. She had become very demanding of her children, as she felt they should be looking in on her very often. The children indicated that the situation was becoming untenable and that their mother needed to be hospitalised.

The general practitioner organised a family meeting with both the mother and her children. During this conversation, the woman was asked to fill out the spider web questionnaire of Positive Health, to measure her degree of satisfaction with regard to the 6 dimensions of health. After she had done so, the practitioner asked her to talk about the results and what they meant to her. He visualised her scores by drawing lines to connect the score points on the spider web and asked her which of the scores she would like to change, what that change would mean to her and what a first step towards such a change could be. She talked about wanting the pain in her leg to be less severe. This would mean that she could work in the vegetable garden again and ride her bicycle, so that she could be amongst people some more. It became clear that there were important issues of meaningfulness and loneliness. She was visibly pleased that this topic had been brought up for discussion.

1

Because of the open conversation, the patient also felt she had the opportunity to discuss other problems. For example, she appeared to have great anxiety about monthly injections that the ophthalmologist needed to give her into her eye in connection with macular degeneration. She was equally scared of her annual check-up with the surgeon because of her history of breast cancer, earlier in life. Fear and anxiety were dominating her world. She wondered, as a first step, could she stop having these check-ups? In doing so, she would be rid of her fear, while accepting the possibility of living a shorter life. The woman also indicated that she wanted to stop taking tamoxifen (related to the treatment of her breast cancer), because it was making her feel gloomy.

Together, they decided to end the treatment by the ophthalmologist and the check-up by the surgeon and to discontinue the tamoxifen. In consultation with the municipal social team, they agreed to help find some activities for her to fill her days. There was no further discussion about a possible hospitalisation and when she was no longer forcing herself to work in the garden, the pain in her hip no longer took centre stage. Although she was no longer able to ride her bicycle, the purchase of a mobility scooter did increase her mobility and meant she could go to the community day centre a few times a week. This turned out to be a good alternative. Instead of an explicit focus on disease and health care (hip, eye and breast), the emphasis in the family discussion shifted to health and behaviour (her being amongst people and able to move about, without being dependent on others). When the pain in her hip dissipated, the claiming behaviour towards her children also disappeared. Although she would still feel gloomy, from time to time, the general practitioner was no longer consulted for these complaints. As she herself indicated, she found purpose at the day centre, where she took care of a demented neighbour, who was worse off than she was.

Three and a half years later, she discovered a 10-cm hard disk in her armpit – her breast cancer had come back. She remained consistent in her decision not to have any further treatment, although she did want to go to the day centre for one extra day a week. Six months later, her condition worsened rapidly, she entered a phase of acceptance and passed away surrounded by all her children and grandchildren.

Reflection: working from the concept of Positive Health meant that underlying issues, such as fear and loneliness, could openly be discussed. This made it possible to start a conversation about what really mattered to this patient, what could give her life meaning. Leading a meaningful life is a leitmotiv of this handbook.

1.3 Wake-up call

Can the broad focus on health in the Positive Health concept offer a solution for what is going wrong in Dutch health care?

To answer this question, it would be good for general practitioners to heed the wake-up call. It was not without reason that, in the Netherlands, a manifest of concerned general practitioners, titled 'Het Roer Moet Om' (things need to change), was published. From 2015 onwards, this group of concerned general practitioners has been identifying bottlenecks in primary care and advocating that measures be taken to improve coherence within the Dutch health care system. A look at the current system reveals that it is in crisis, when it comes to the system's degree of sustainability. The system was already on the brink of crisis when the COVID-19 outbreak occurred, after which this became more obvious and intense. The term *crisis* can be defined as a serious emergency situation that causes severe disruptions to the functioning of a system (any system). Therefore, it is time to wake up!

The current crisis in Dutch health care is caused by a mismatch between what is offered and what is needed in health care and welfare. This mismatch is widely debated and concrete proposals have been made for how to deal with it (Kaljouw and Van Vliet 2015). However, this discussion seems to be leading attention away from the even greater crisis to come, namely that of the need for health care and the *absence* of supply. The COVID-19 period has revealed the impact of this mismatch on society.

These two crises are further amplified by the current medical-analytical way of thinking and the disregard for the strength and resilience of both individuals and the community, from the perspective of demographic developments in the Netherlands. The next section first discusses these crises, followed by an elaboration of the current medical-analytical way of thinking.

1.3.1 The crisis of the mismatch between the offered and the required type of health care

The Dutch general practitioners' action committee 'Het Roer Moet Om' (things need to change) describes the current mismatch between supply and demand with respect to health care and welfare in the Netherlands as a *silent disaster* that is being caused by a lack of cohesion (Het Roer Moet Om 2019). In recent decades, there has been an enormous increase in the workload of general medical practices (LHV 2017; Van den Brekel et al. 2020). Forty per cent of general practitioners have or have had experienced feelings of burnout (LHV 2018). Long-term sickness absence is on the rise amongst general practitioners as well as for other care professionals (e.g., in nursing and residential care) (Blitterswijk 2020).

There is also the explosive growth in health care bureaucracy, with endless checklists and perverse financial incentives. There is an enormous increase in the number of people with chronic diseases, and the care for these people by hospitals and institutions is increasingly being transferred to primary care practices and local communities – with the emphasis on the disease rather than the patient. Health insurance companies and the Dutch Government have also transferred certain care responsibilities onto municipalities (decentralisation), motivated by the desire to achieve spending cuts and, therefore, not accompanied by the equal transfer of the funds required to take on such additional responsibilities. This has caused budged deficits at municipalities throughout the country, especially with respect to child welfare services. Meanwhile, health care costs are continuing to rise. And an additional problem is that of the benefits of advances in medical-technical medicine, over the last century, not having been equally distributed amongst the population. In the Netherlands, the difference in *healthy* life expectancy between people with low and high levels of education has increased and now stands at 18 years (CBS 2016). Loneliness appears to be a major problem, especially amongst the elderly, people with a disability or health problem, the lower educated, and non-Western migrants (Movisie 2020). International studies show that loneliness even carries a greater mortality risk than smoking (Holt-Lunstad et al. 2010)! Changes made to the health care system in the past seem to have increased the health-related differences within the community. Thus, the care that is on offer

1

is no longer meeting the need – either for health care or welfare. The current lack of cohesion within the Dutch health care system and the mismatch between supply and demand are both blamed largely on the free market and the impact of competition. Or, as *Het Roer Moet Om* puts it: 'Decades of competitive and production-oriented thinking have pushed aside the need for cooperation', with the greatest negative impact on the vulnerable groups in society and health care professionals themselves. This also leads to a large group of care providers being overextended.

It seems obvious that what is currently offered in health care needs to be reassessed. Costs are rising, health care is becoming too expensive and does not meet the need for reducing healthy life expectancy differences between population groups. It also leads to overburdening of an important group of care providers. At the same time, the current health care system does not seem to have an adequate answer to the need to lead a meaningful life in the expected number of years of life that has increased by 50 % since the last century, given the prevalence of loneliness in Dutch society.

The emphasis continues to be on living *as long as possible* and on the WHO's definition of health from 1948, which states that being healthy is a state of complete well-being. This fuels the fire of the medical-analytical approach. Health care still seems to be focused on diagnosing and treating disease and applying care, with too little focus on health and behaviour and people and society (Polder and Van de Lucht 2020; Overgoor et al. 2006).

The Committee Innovation Health Care Professions & Education of the Dutch National Health Care Institute advises care professionals to have a dynamic continuum of competences that is geared to a type of care that enables people to live and function as independently as possible, within their own residential environment. This requires a change in the current provision of health care. This change would put the focus not on diseases and disorders, but rather on the way people function, their resilience and ability to be in control of their lives. The starting point should not be the current supply of care, care professions and education, but the future demand for care, with a focus on what is needed rather than on what is possible (Kaljouw and Van Vliet 2015).

1.3.2   The crisis of not being able to provide the type of health care that is needed

The above-mentioned struggle with the crisis of their being a mismatch between supply and demand in care and welfare is serious. Not only because of the problems described and the current lack of solutions, but also because it threatens to demoralise professionals working in care and welfare and make them more cynical. This leaves no room or energy for them to prepare for an even bigger crisis lying ahead. One that will be far more disruptive to society: the crisis of *not being able to provide* the type of health care that is needed. This would be a true nightmare, the first signs of which can already be seen along the peripheral areas of the Netherlands (in Groningen, Zeeland and Northern Limburg) and has to do with population ageing and shrinking regions.

Here, the Northern Limburg village of Afferden, where co-author Hans Peter Jung has been a general practitioner since 1997, again serves as an example. Located in a region with a shrinking population, it has the strongest shrinkage within the Province of Limburg and is an area that ranks third amongst Dutch regions with respect to having

Pressure of the ageing population

In 2000, the village of Afferden had 5 people working for every person over the age of 65

By 2040, there will be only 1 person working for every person over the age of 65

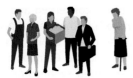

■ **Figure 1.6** Pressure of the ageing population. Source: Lekkerkerker and Pelzer (2017)

an ageing population. Ageing and shrinkage lead to an increase in the so-called old age dependency ratio. In the year 2000, in Afferden, there were five people working for every pensioner, whereas the projection for 2040 is that there will only be 1 person working for every person over the age of 65 (see ■ fig. 1.6).

The number of people in official employment in the Province of Limburg is projected to decrease by 25 %, over the next 20 years. For health care professionals this decrease is expected to be even greater, given the increase in work pressure in primary and residential care. Currently, one in seven people is working in a care profession. By 2040, under continuation of current conditions, this would need to be one in four people. This figure seems unfeasible in Limburg, and in the rest of the Netherlands, according to a report by the Dutch task force on 'the right care in the right place' (Taskforce De juiste zorg op de juiste plek 2017). In addition, the number of people needing care will more than double in Limburg due to population ageing, over that same period. Finding new general practitioners and people working in residential care for the Northern Limburg region is already a problem today (Seuren 2015).

In addition, the cost of health care will continue to rise. Today, the average household in the Netherlands spends a quarter of its income on health care premiums; by 2040 that could increase to between 30 and 45 % (CPB Netherlands Bureau for Economic Policy Analysis 2011). The conclusion here is that, even if we wanted to and even if we had the money, we would not be able to solve this problem. The buildings used as hospitals, nursing homes, care homes and general medical practices will still be standing, but there will be far too few care professionals to populate them, which will have a disruptive impact on society as well as on the remaining professionals.

1.3.3 The COVID-19 crisis

The coronavirus-related lockdown of 2020–2021 may have given us a taste of what is in store for society and health care in the future. The general medical practices largely also were in lockdown. Between 12 March and 10 April 2020, general practitioners in the Netherlands issued an estimated 360,000 fewer referrals to medical specialists than during the same period in previous years (Dutch Healthcare Authority 2020). The coronavirus crisis made it painfully clear that, for a time, there was less primary care

1

and hospital capacity available. The Dutch Healthcare Authority (NZa) is concerned about a backlog in deferred care and care that could not be provided during the crisis. The 'one-and-a-half-metre economy' means that general practitioners and hospitals will have to be organised in such a way that patients can literally be kept at arm's length, wherever possible, until the vast majority of the population is either immune or has been vaccinated.

On the other hand, Dutch general practitioner Barnhoorn is concerned about the use of what he calls 'war language' ('Together against Corona!') in the 'battle' against the coronavirus and is afraid that this will be at the expense of the ability of physicians to have a *'good conversation'* with their patients. According to Barnhoorn, war metaphors cause care offered by physicians often being regarded synonymous with treatment (Barnhoorn 2020). As a result, the focus is on the virus and less on the consequences in other areas of people's lives.

In its outlook study on health care in the future ('Zorg voor de toekomst'), the Social and Economic Council of the Netherlands (SER 2020) stated that the coronavirus crisis above all illustrates the need to make the Dutch health care system more future-proof. The crisis has shown that having enough qualified personnel available to provide high quality care to everyone is not a given. It forces people to think differently about the buffers needed in the health care system. It also shows that certain groups are more vulnerable to health risks, as a result of having had their regular care postponed as well as from the social and mental effects of the lockdown, with the risk that this will lead to further health damage. The coronavirus crisis places an exceptionally heavy burden on all those who work in the health care sector. Sickness absence is already at a high level in this group and has further increased due to the crisis. In addition, internships and training in the health care sector are stagnating, which in turn will have consequences for the influx of new staff in this sector. The SER study also concludes that the coronavirus crisis has greatly accelerated the digital transformation in health care. It expects that the health care sector will develop towards more digital remote care.

As indicated above, the crises have been amplified by the Netherlands' current medical-analytical way of working. Positive Health may provide an answer to the question of how to deal with these crises and make health care more future-proof. It offers a way of working that enables stepping away from the medical-analytical perspective. It strengthens individuals and communities so that they will be more resilient to crises in the future. How then, you ask?

1.4 From a medical-analytical approach to an alternative dialogue

In the Netherlands, medical students, in the basic curriculum, internships and general practitioners are fundamentally trained from the medical-analytical perspective. They learn about the medical symptoms and complaints, which syndromes would fit with those symptoms and complaints and how these should be treated – sometimes called the diagnosis–prescription model. A characteristic example of this method is in the initial contact with patients when they come to the surgery with a medical problem. This can be a patient who wants to get rid of an annoying cough combined with a fever, who is examined and diagnosed with a pneumonia, which subsequently results in the prescription of an antibiotic as treatment, which then leads to their recovery. The problem, however, is that up to 40 % of reported physical complaints (e.g., headaches, abdominal pains) have no discernible physical cause (Olde Hartman et al. 2013; Rosendal et al. 2016; Kroenke 2014). Some clinics in secondary care, such as internal medicine and gynaecology, show even higher percentages (up 60–70 %) (Nimnuan et al. 2001).

If the medical-analytical perspective is maintained when examining these complaints, more analysis will follow and general practitioners will be more likely to refer patients to seek specialist medical care (the fact that the percentage of unexplained medical complaints is even higher at specialists than in general medical practice is an indication that this is precisely what happens). This creates the risk of iatrogenic damage from invasive diagnostics or false positive diagnostic tests. In turn, this results in yet more analysis, which will not lead to an explanatory diagnosis and keeps the patient and the care provider in a stranglehold. In addition, according to the literature, 75 % of these physical complaints disappear again after a certain period of time (from few weeks to months) (Kroenke 2014).

Applying a medical-analytical approach to these self-limiting complaints means further diagnostics to be able to reassure the patient, whereas reassurance from a non-medical perspective may be a much more appropriate option. Of the 25 % of these types of complaints that do last longer, a small proportion (2.5 %) lead to long-term severe medically unexplained physical symptoms (MUPS) (Olde Hartman et al. 2013). Very taxing for the patient and a challenge for the physician, but a medical-analytical approach is not appropriate here.

For a large share of the 60 % of physical complaints for which there is a discernible physical cause, using a medical-analytical approach is perfectly suitable, but some of these complaints relate to a serious chronic disease or the onset of one. We can trace these diseases (e.g., dementia, diabetes), but we cannot solve them using a medical-analytical approach. In the case of dementia, these patients and their carers are more likely to require personal conversations and guidance on how to deal meaningfully with this disease, whereas in the case of diabetes, the role of the patient's lifestyle, behaviour and compliance will be more decisive for the long-term outcome than could be achieved with medical interventions.

For the majority of complaints that patients present to their general practitioner, the medical-analytical approach is therefore not suitable. However, the Dutch disease-oriented health care is primarily designed in favour of this medical-analytical method. Physicians tend to approach most complaints using this model and health care funding is geared towards diagnoses and treatments. Each year, 100 billion euros is being spent on the type of health care in which this medical-analytical method can flourish; only 4 % of that amount is invested in primary care (CBS 2019) and even less in prevention. Precise figures on prevention are not available, but when asked, the Dutch State Secretary for Health, Welfare and Sport, Paul Blokhuis, mentioned an amount of only 2 billion euros, 2 % of the total annual budget spent on health care (Parliamentary document on preventive health care policy (Preventief gezondheidsbeleid 2018; Blokhuis 2020)).

Positive Health could benefit this situation by counterbalancing the compartmentalised way in which the complaints are generally being approached – which you could call the *how-do-I-get-rid-of-something* medicine. Using the Positive Health method means the presented complaints are regarded in a solution-oriented way – the *what-would-you-like-to-achieve* medicine, analogous to the metaphor of the taxi driver.

1

Case no. 3: Taxi drivers and motocross

Solution-oriented approaches are comparable to how taxi drivers work. Patients determine the destination of the ride (i.e., their goal to be achieved) and it is the responsibility of the solution-oriented care provider to get them there safely, via the shortest possible route, as comfortably as possible and at the lowest possible cost. The first question a taxi driver will ask you when you step into his car is usually: 'Where would you like to go?' rather than: 'Where did you come from?' When patients answer: 'Not to the airport' (i.e., 'I don't want this problem' or 'I want to get rid of my headache'), the solution-oriented care provider will ask them what it is that they would like to achieve (i.e., where would you like to go) (Bannink and McCarthy 2014).

The motocross

An 18-year-old man suffered a serious accident at a motocross event three years ago, in which a life-threatening epidural haematoma developed from an impression fracture of the skull and a brain contusion. Successful emergency surgery followed, replacing the damaged part of the skull with a metal plate. After a short period of joy because he survived the accident, it also became clear that he remained very tired and needed extra sleep during the day. He was having difficulty in remembering things and concentrating for long periods. He was also suffering from headaches. A neurocognitive examination revealed problems with stimulus processing and the performance of dual tasks. A non-congenital brain injury was diagnosed and because he was no longer able to keep up with his peers at school, 'suitable education' was sought. What saddened him the most, however, was not being able to pursue his motocross hobby because of the metal plate in his head. Six months after the accident, he visited his general practitioner, complaining of headaches, symptoms of depression, and difficulties related to concentration and sleep.

He struggled with these limitations and what he could no longer do in his life. The general practitioner talked about the metaphor of the taxi driver and asked him if he would like to think about what he was still able to do, given the circumstances, and what he would like to do, if possible. He agreed and the mental health practice nurse helped him consider possible new hobbies and how he could fill his days. Already after two sessions, he indicated that he had sufficient ideas to start from. Two years later, when he was back in the general practitioner's consulting room for an unrelated complaint, he told the general practitioner that he was doing very well. He had started a new hobby: fishing. He was also proud that he quit smoking and had started volunteering at a retirement home.

When the practitioner asked him how he managed to do those things, he said: 'Learn to listen to yourself and what your body is telling you. In addition, don't strive for things that are not feasible; focus on real goals in life, instead. Like that taxi driver story you told me about!', he beamed and concluded with: 'I owe these wise lessons to my accident, I can now accept that, too. And I really suffer less from my lack of concentration and my headaches, I sleep well again and I have purpose in my life!'.

The impact of holding an *alternative dialogue* in the general practice is illustrated by the examples of the taxi driver and the motocross (see text box). With benefits not only for the patient, but also for the general practitioner. This solution-oriented approach can be applied consistently throughout the practice. It offers alternative follow-up steps as well as solutions for the majority of medical complaints. These complaints are largely outside the scope of specialist medical care, but fall within the social domain. Sometimes, they can be solved through self-help or together with others from the community.

The *alternative dialogue* is not new in primary care and not exclusively connected with Positive Health. It connects seamlessly to the core value of *person-oriented care* in the profession of general practitioner, more about which can be found in ▶ Chap. 4. The benefits of the nuances of the broad health-oriented ideas of Positive Health and the *alternative dialogue* are the basis for this handbook. An infographic that sketches the broad applicability of person-oriented care in general and the alternative dialogue in particular can be seen in ◻ fig. 1.7.

Throughout the book, examples and case studies illustrate the added value of holding the alternative dialogue. ▶ Chapter 5 contains many tools for implementing the use of alternative conversations according to the Positive Health concept. It also describes when and with whom a Positive Health conversation could be held. The following section explains what this method means for the role of the professionals in primary care.

1.5 The changing role of care professionals in primary care

What do current developments mean for general practitioners in the future and how does Positive Health relate to this? In view of the challenges faced by society in the Netherlands, in their publication on the future of primary care (Toekomst Huisartsenzorg), Dutch general practitioners have further specified the core value of *generalist* to *medical generalist* (Toekomst Huisartsenzorg 2020a). If for nothing else than to indicate that general practitioners are not the only ones responsible for people living a meaningful life (see the pink section of the triangle on the far right in ◻ fig. 1.3). The concept of Positive Health considers that people see their health as a much broader concept than merely the absence of physical and mental problems, and that they are able to call on their own strength and that of the community, and that they have control over their own lives. Positive Health thus transcends the domain of the health professional. It gives general practitioners the opportunity to allow patients to propose solutions that are lifestyle-related (Sayburn 2018) or that do not exactly fit in with the purely medical-analytical perspective.

Identifying and openly discussing psychosocial and welfare problems is one of the tasks of general practitioners. This task, however, does not include the practical organisation of non-medical follow-up care related to these problems. (Toekomst Huisartsenzorg 2020b), which means that their role of *gatekeeper* to secondary care may change into that of *guide, liaison or coach*. General practitioners in the Netherlands, in certain cases, refer patients onto a specialist for medical diagnostics and treatment. Working within the Positive Health concept, however, means that other solutions may also be sought – far more often than is currently the case. These other solutions, for example, relate to the social domain. In such cases, the focus is on what someone can still do, with emphasis on lifestyle and health promotion and on solutions rather than on limitations. Scientific research has found that the broad view of health is more in line with people's own perspective on health. This is elaborated in ▶ Chap. 2, which also describes the history of the development of the Positive Health concept.

The alternative dialogue

shared-decision making

The core of personalised health care is that care providers do not focus on the symptoms or condition, but on the person presenting the complaint, and on his or her desires and needs.

The alternative dialogue is about giving more time and attention to a patient's personal context. With a greater focus on a personalised approach and taking any functional illiteracy and/or low health skills into consideration. Personalised care is also about actively involving the patient in finding an appropriate solution for care and support.

Why an alternative dialogue?

Personalised care is in keeping with people's need for self-determination. Time and again, research has shown that people want to be independent as much and as long as possible. Even if they are facing medical complaints and disabilities.

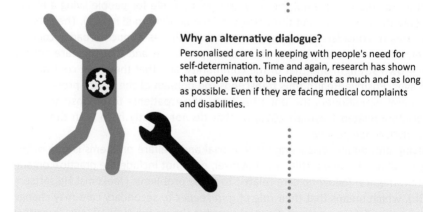

◘ **Figure 1.7**   The alternative dialogue. Infographic Personalised care. Source: InEen (2019)

1.6 Conclusions

General medicine in the Netherlands is under pressure. How long will the currently provided health care remain sustainable? In the future, things will only get worse. With an increasingly ageing population, insufficient numbers of care professionals and costs that are too high. The concept of Positive Health facilitates taking a different look at disease and health. It leads to holding alternative conversations with patients, in a way that is more solution-oriented and stimulates self-management. Positive Health focuses on meaningfulness rather than on today's more dominant medical-analytical approach to patients. The concept offers a solution for things that are currently stagnating in health care in the Netherlands. With more attention being paid to lifestyle, leading a meaningful life, and citizen initiatives that promote community outreach and self-reliance as important elements in the application of Positive Health in general practice.

For more information, background or videos about this chapter scan the QR code.

SCAN ME

References

Bannink, F., & McCarthy, J. (2014). The solution-focussed taxi. *Counseling today*. Accessed in Juni 2021 of ► https://ct.counseling.org/2014/05/the-solution-focused-taxi/.

Barnhoorn, P. (2020). Stop de oorlogstaal en ga het gesprek aan. *Medisch Contact, 75*, 20–21.

Blitterswijk, L. (2020). Ziekteverzuim in zorgsector het hoogst. *Medisch Ondernemen*. Accessed in Juni 2021 of ► https://www.medischondernemen.nl/medisch-ondernemen/ziekteverzuim-inzorgsector-het-hoogst.

Blokhuis, P. (2020). Voorwoord. In M. De Vries, T. De Weijer (Red.), *Handboek leefstijlgeneeskunde. De basis voor iedere praktijk* (p. V). Houten: Bohn Stafleu van Loghum.

Brabers, A., De Wit, N., Meijman, B., & De Jong, J. (2019). Burgers over kernwaarden en kerntaken huisarts. *Huisarts En Wetenschap, 62*(10), 23–28.

Centraal Bureau voor Statistiek (2016). Gezonde levensverwachting naar opleidingsniveau. Accessed in Juni 2021 of ► http://statline.cbs.nl/Statweb/publication/?DM=SLNL&PA=71885ned&D1=0-4&D2=a&D3=0,14&D4=a&D5=0&D6=l&VW=T.

Centraal Bureau voor Statistiek (2019). Zorguitgaven stijgen in 2018 met 3,1 procent. Accessed in Juni 2021 of ► https://www.cbs.nl/nl-nl/nieuws/2019/25/zorguitgaven-stijgen-in-2018-met-3-1-procent.

Centraal Bureau voor Statistiek (2020). Statline. Gezonde levensverwachting; vanaf 1981. Accessed in Juni 2021 of ► https://opendata.cbs.nl/statline/#/CBS/nl/dataset/71950ned/line?ts=1599276583411.

Centraal Plan Bureau (2011). Trends in gezondheid en zorg. Accessed in Juni 2021 of ► https://www.cpb.nl/publicatie/trends-in-gezondheid-en-zorg.

Deeg, D., & Nusselder, W. (2020). Is langer leven ook gezonder leven? *Demos: Bulletin Over Bevolking en Samenleving, 36*(1), 4–7. Accessed in Juni 2021 of ► https://nidi.nl/demos/is-langer-leven-ook-gezonder-leven/.

Eekhof, J. (2017). Het aanzien van de huisarts. *Huisarts En Wetenschap, 60*, 430.

Elseviers Weekblad, Anoniem (1946, 26 oktober). Mgr. Lemmens sprak: "Wij kunnen, wij mogen niet zwijgen" Nood in Noord-Limburg. *Elseviers Weekblad*, 1.

Het Roer Moet Om (2019). Persbericht. Accessed in Juni 2021 of ▶ https://www.hetroermoetom.nu/pdf/Persbericht-HETROERMOETOM-Aanbieding-boekje-enquete-tweede-kamer-20191125.pdf.

Holt-Lunstad, J., Smith, T. B., & Bradley Layton, J. (2010). Social relationships and mortality risk: A meta-analytic review. *PLoS*. ▶ https://doi.org/10.1371/journal.pmed.1000316

Houben, N. (2020). Boodschap huisartsenorganisaties aan politieke partijen. Het Zorghuis Wankelt. *De Eerstelijns, 12*(6), 10–11.

Huber, M. (2014). *Towards a new, dynamic concept of Health. Its operationalisation and use in public health and healthcare, and in evaluating the health effects of food*. Maastricht: Thesis Maastricht University. ISBN 978-94-6259-471-5.

Huber, M., Knottnerus, J. A., Green, L., et al. (2011). How should we define health? *BMJ, 343*(4163), 235–237.

Huber, M., Van Vliet, M., Giezenberg, M., et al. (2016). Towards a 'patient-centred' operationalisation of the new dynamic concept of health: A mixed methods study. *BMJ Open, 2016*(5), e010091.

InEen (2019). Infographic Persoonsgerichte zorg. Accessed in June 2021 of ▶ https://ineen.nl/wp-content/uploads/2020/02/InEen-Nhg-ZO-Infographic-Persoonsgerichte-zorg.pdf.

Jung, H. P. (2020). Overleven, zo lang mogelijk leven, betekenisvol leven. Kantelingen in de zorg aan de hand van de ervaringen van een plattelandsdokter. *Tijdschrift voor Geneeskunde en Ethiek, 30*(4), 118–122.

Kaljouw, M., & Van Vliet, K. (2015). *Naar nieuwe zorg en zorgberoepen: de contouren*. Zorginstituut Nederland: Diemen.

Kamerstuk Preventief Gezondheidsbeleid (2018). Overheid.nl. Staatssecretaris Paul Blokhuis in Kamerstuk 11-06-2018, Tweede Kamer der Staten Generaal 2017–2018, 32793 nr. 312.

Kleijne, I. (2020). Huisartsen geven wake up call in Den Haag. (2020). Accessed in June 2021 of ▶ https://www.medischcontact.nl/nieuws/laatste-nieuws/nieuwsartikel/huisartsen-geven-wake-upcall-in-den-haag.htm.

Kluge, et al. (2021). 'Rethink policy priorities in the light of pandemics', Pan-European Commission on Health and Sustainable Development. Accessed in Juni 2021. ▶ https://www.euro.who.int/__data/assets/pdf_file/0010/495856/Pan-European-Commission-Call-to-action-eng.pdf.

Kreuzer, A. (2008). *Afferdse bijnamen en de verhalen eromheen*. Afferden: Minoprint.

Kroenke, K. (2014). A practical and evidence-based approach to common symptoms: A narrative review. *Annals of Internal Medicine, 161*(8), 579–586.

Landelijke Huisartsen Vereniging (2017). De huisarts kan meer voor minder patiënten betekenen. Factsheet.

Landelijke Huisartsen Vereniging (2018). *Meer tijd voor de patiënt. Uitkomsten onderzoek. LHV 15 maart 2018*. Utrecht: Newcom Research & Consultancy B.V.

Lekkerkerker, J., & Pelzer, P. (2017) Trendverkenning demografische transitie Noord-Limburg. Drukkerij Printvisie, Venlo. Accessed in June 2021 of ▶ https://www.retailinsiders.nl/docs/e364729d-e97b-43a6-8c71-2808ea73a7df.pdf.

Luyten, M. (2015). *Het geluk van Limburg*. De Bezige Bij.

Mak, G. (1996). *Hoe God verdween uit Jorwerd*. Uitgeverij Atlas.

Movisie. Wat werkt bij de aanpak van eenzaamheid. (2020). Accessed in June 2021 of ▶ https://www.movisie.nl/publicaties/wat-werkt-aanpak-eenzaamheid.

Nederlandse Zorg Autoriteit. (2020). Accessed in June 2021 of ▶ https://www.nza.nl/actueel/nieuws/2020/04/20/reguliere-zorg-komt-gefaseerd-weer-op-gang.

Nimnuan, C., Hotopf, M., & Wessely, S. (2001). Medically unexplained symptoms: An epidemiological study in seven specialities. *Journal of Psychosomatic Research, 51,* 361–367. Accessed in June 2021 of ▶ https://doi.org/10.1016/S0022-3999(01)00223-9.

Olde Hartman, T. C., Blankenstein, A. H., Molenaar, A. O., Bentz van den Berg, D., Van der Horst, H. E., Arnold, I. A., et al. (2013). NHG-Standaard Somatisch Onvoldoende verklaarde Lichamelijke Klachten (SOLK). *Huisarts En Wetenschap, 56*(5), 222–230.

Overgoor, L., Aalders, M., & Muller, I. S. (2006). Big! Move, beweging in gedrag van patiënt en huisarts. *Huisarts en Wetenschap, 49*(1), 50–55. Accessed in June 2021 of ▶ https://doi.org/10.1007/BF03084600.

Palm, J. (2012). *De moederkerk. De ondergang van rooms Nederland*. Contact.

Polder, J., & Van der Lucht, F. (2020). Leefstijlgeneeskunde als maatschappelijk medicijn. In M. De Vries, T. De Weijer (Red.), *Handboek leefstijlgeneeskunde. De basis voor iedere praktijk* (pag. 319–325). Houten: Bohn Stafleu van Loghum.

Rapport Taskforce De juiste zorg op de juiste plek (2017). Accessed in June 2021 of ► https://www.rijksoverheid.nl/documenten/rapporten/2018/04/06/rapport-de-juiste-zorg-op-de-juiste-plek.

Rijksoverheid (2018). Aanpak eenzaamheid onder ouderen. Accessed in June 2021 of ► https://www.rijksoverheid.nl/onderwerpen/eenzaamheid/aanpak-eenzaamheid.

RIVM Volksgezondheid en zorg (2020). Accessed in June 2021 of ► https://www.volksgezondheidenzorg.info/onderwerp/levensverwachting.

Rosendal, M., Carlsen, A. H., & Rask, M. T. (2016). Symptoms as the main problem: A cross- sectional study of patient experience in primary care. *BMC Family Practice, 17*(1), 29.

Sayburn, A. (2018). Lifestyle medicine: A new medical speciality? *BMJ, 363*, k4442.

Seuren, E. (2015, 30 oktober). Tekort aan huisartsen dreigt in Noord-Limburg. *Dagblad De Limburger.* Accessed in June 2021 of ► https://www.1limburg.nl/tekort-aan-huisartsen-dreigt-noord-limburg.

Skipr redactie (2019). Huisartsenzorg komt in de knel. Accessed in June 2021 of ► https://www.skipr.nl/nieuws/huisartsenzorg-komt-in-de-knel/.

Sociaal-Economische Raad (SER) (2020). Accessed in June 2021 Zorg voor de toekomst. Over de toekomst-bestendigheid van de zorg. ► https://www.ser.nl/-/media/ser/downloads/adviezen/2020/zorg-voor-de-toekomst.pdf.

Toekomst huisartsenzorg (2020a). Accessed in June 2021 of ► https://toekomsthuisartsenzorg.nl/.

Toekomst huisartsenzorg (2020b). Accessed in June 2021 of ► https://toekomsthuisartsenzorg.nl/kerntak-en-in-de-praktijk/.

Van den Brekel-Dijkstra, K., Cornelissen, M., & Van der Jagt, L. (2020). De dokter gevloerd. Hoe voorkomen we burn-out bij huisartsen? *Huisarts en Wetenschap*, 63(7), 40–43, ► https://doi.org/10.1007/s12445-020-0765-8.

WHO (2006). Constitution of the World Health Organization 2006. Accessed in June 2021 ► https://www.who.int/governance/eb/who_constitution_en.pdf.

2

I swear/promise to practise the art of medicine to the
best of my ability for the benefit of my fellow man.
I will care for the sick, promote health and
relieve suffering.

I will put the patient's interests first and respect
his/her views. I will do no harm to the patient.
I will listen and inform him/her well. I will keep
secret what has been entrusted to me.

I will advance the medical knowledge of myself and
others. I will recognise the limits of my possibilities.

Development of a New Concept of Health

© Bohn Stafleu van Loghum is an imprint of Springer Media B.V., part of Springer Nature 2022
M. Huber et al., *Handbook Positive Health in Primary Care*,
https://doi.org/10.1007/978-90-368-2729-4_2

2

> ❯ Main messages Chapter 2
> - ━ Physicians are committed to enhance health, but what is health, exactly?
> - ━ The medical-analytical conceptual model is only two centuries old
> - ━ The World Health Organization's definition of health is static; a new description is dynamic and is about resilience
> - ━ Patients have a broad view of what constitutes health, and this vision has led to the Positive Health concept
> - ━ The health care professional of the future is professionally qualified and considers the whole person
> - ━ Positive Health involves a paradigm shift in our way of thinking – from disease-oriented to health-oriented

At the festive conclusion of their medical studies, new doctors promise or swear to work according to the values of the – somewhat modernised – Hippocratic Oath. In it, they also promise to 'promote health'.

To be honest, it had been quite a while ago since we, the authors, were truly aware of this phrase – and therefore of this task. At the time of our studies in the Netherlands, we received a maximum of 4 to 6 hours of lectures on nutrition – over the course of our entire study programme. We did not learn much else about *promoting health*. Priority was given to learning about and recognising diseases and how to treat them. Since then, the relationship between knowledge about disease and health promotion has shifted somewhat. The new Dutch Framework Plan 2020 for the medical curriculum even explicitly mentions the importance of education in *prevention and health promotion* (Raamplan NFU 2020) (also see ▶ Chap. 8).

Why is it that medical thinking is so focused on disease? The oath that newly appointed doctors are taking has been derived from Hippocrates, a physician who certainly did not think only about disease. He is credited with saying 'Let thy food be thy medicine and medicine be thy food'. We do appreciate Hippocrates as the father of Western medicine – he closely observed and examined his patients and thought rationally about disease and health – and yet we, generally, look at our predecessors with some pity. With our current state of knowledge, we feel rather superior to them, at times. But is that really justified? Having some knowledge about the history of medicine and how health used to be considered is valuable. The past also held valuable insights that may still serve to inspire us today, in our quest to achieve a greater balance between how we think about disease, on the one hand, and health, on the other. It also helps to better understand the essence of Positive Health. Therefore, this chapter starts by outlining the historical development of medical thinking.

2.1 The concept of health throughout the centuries

Over the years, the approach to health has undergone an enormous transition. From a holistic perspective, to one with a narrow focus on medicalisation. In the current era, we are beginning to see a shift in trend, towards a broader approach again. ◻ Figure 2.1 depicts this change, over the years, as a timeline. The earliest sources of information about humans already describe the difference between disease and a state of 'good health' (Van Veen and Van der Sijs 1997). The word 'health' is believed to find its origins in the Old English 'hælth' which etymologically stands for being 'whole', 'undamaged', as in 'uninjured'. And the origins of 'to heal' and 'healers' is thought to lie in the Germanic 'hailiz', which also stands for wholeness (Lindeboom 1982).

In ancient times, there were various views that considered health as a balance between various 'elements' representing various qualities. In Chinese Taoism (4 BC), these are the five elements and the qualities Yin and Yang. Greek medicine distinguished four humours, related to the four elements. These were based on knowledge from ancient Egypt and Mesopotamia and were further specified by the Greek physician Hippocrates. Hippocrates (460–370 BC) considered nutrition the most powerful lifestyle factor that could restore the balance between the elements. Aristotle, the influential Greek 'father of Western philosophy' who was almost his contemporary (384–322 BC), stated from his vision on mankind that maintaining a good balance – 'the middle' – was a virtue and that extremes should be avoided. He regarded a state of eudaimonia (i.e., well-being) as the ultimate purpose of human existence. Eudaimonia is not a static state but a continuous process of developing one's personal potential and flourishing as a human being. Through such self-actualisation, people will experience happiness and personal well-being, according to Aristotle. Incidentally, in the current movement of positive psychology, the concept of 'eudaimonia' is again described as a goal to be pursued. (Seligman 2012).

Greco-Roman physician Galenus (AD 129–199) refined Hippocrates' lifestyle therapies and even described six lifestyle factors that should be balanced in order to maintain good health. For 15 centuries, these views about the ability of people to create balance and to develop themselves, partly through lifestyle factors, continued to greatly influence the thinking of Western medicine.

From the sixteenth century onwards, a new paradigm in medicine began to emerge. In 1543, Vesalius published his studies on the anatomy of the human body, based on autopsies on the deceased. Thus, he introduced a new research method in medicine, based on empiricism. Around a century later, in 1628, William Harvey described the circulatory system. In 1637, Descartes published (anonymously, at first) his most famous work: *Discours de la méthode*, which laid the foundations for the modern natural scientific approach, also in medicine (Descartes 2021). According to Descartes, body and mind are separate entities and the body can be regarded as a mechanism that should be examined using a mathematical, numerical approach. Descartes, like no other, endorsed the mechanisation of the worldview and the view on human beings (Dijksterhuis 1980). In 1847, Semmelweis discovered the power of disinfection; in 1858, Virchow published on cellular pathology, and, in 1860, Pasteur described the existence of bacteria which he could see under his microscope. With these discoveries, the doctrine of the balance of humours fully disappeared from medical thinking, and the paradigm of cell physiology, microbiology and pathological anatomy became the dominant view in medicine. Diseases were no longer seen as disrupting a balance but were understood on a physical basis and treated accordingly. Health became the absence of disease. Public health care also emerged at this time, in the fast-growing cities during the industrial revolution. Better nutrition, clean drinking water, sewerage systems, waste collection and disposal and the first vaccination programmes caused infectious diseases, such as cholera, typhoid and smallpox, to be reduced and eventually eradicated.

Knowledge has become analytical and scientific (termed *medical-analytical* in the remainder of this book) and with this, high levels of medical knowledge have been achieved. What has gradually become lost, with this paradigm, is our ability to still

2

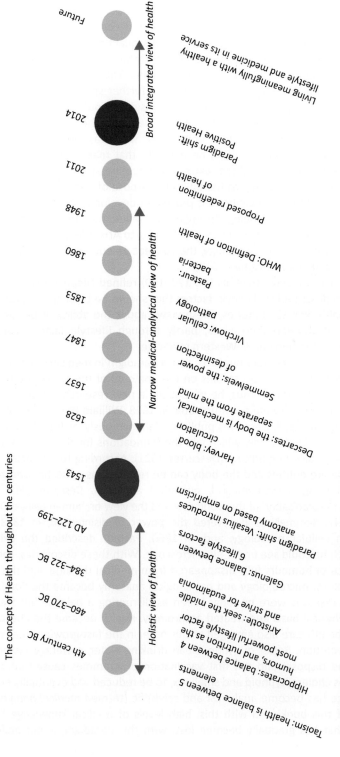

Figure 2.1   The concept of health throughout the centuries

consider *the whole person* and their *health as a situation of balance*, as our prede-cessors in Western medicine used to do. Nevertheless, when we take the Hippocratic Oath, we promise to promote health as well. It is the goal of Positive Health to contrib-ute to this aspect again, in a modern form. In part, because patients do consider them-selves as a whole person and would like to be seen as such (see ▶ Sect. 2.4).

2.2   The foundation of the WHO and the definition of health

After World War I, some initiatives had already been developed to achieve interna-tional cooperation in the field of health care, which was given a further boost by World War II. In 1945, when 50 countries met in San Francisco to establish cooperation that would promote world peace (resulting in the establishment of the United Nations (UN), amongst those present were three doctors, from Norway, Brazil and China. They decided to try to use the international platform to establish, parallel to the UN, one global medical organisation. They succeeded in the word 'health' being included in the UN Charter and in having the UN Assembly recommend the creation of an international health organisation (i.e., the *World Health Organization WHO*). It took from 1945 to 1948 for consensus to be reached on all the rules, formulations and the official estab-lishment of the WHO. On 7 April 1948, the first World Health Assembly was held in Geneva and the WHO Constitution came into force. This constitution begins with the principles on which the WHO is based.

Right at the beginning of *the Constitution*, the *WHO presents its definition of health*:

> Health is a state of complete physical, mental and social well-being and not merely the absence of disease or infirmity.

There were also a few psychiatrists involved in the formulation who had insisted on making the definition broader than 'health as the absence of disease'. The minutes of the preparatory meeting state that: 'micro-organisms are no longer man's greatest ene-mies ...' – after all, antibiotics had been available since WWII – 'but man's inability to live in harmony with himself is the greatest cause of disease.' (WHO 1946).

It is what the WHO wanted to focus on and is the background to this broad and very idealistic definition.

2.2.1   Operationalising the WHO definition

The WHO considers it one of its tasks to present an overview of the health of the global population. At the same time, the organisation also recognises that its definition can-not be easily operationalised. Since 1948, various monitoring systems have been devel-oped, which are collectively called the WHO Family of International Classifications (WHO-FIC) (WHO update 2012, ICPC-International Classification of Health Problem in Primary Care (ICHPPC-2-d) (1976, 1983), Lamberts and Wood 1993, Lamberts and Wood 2002, WHO-FIC 2020). Initially, the focus was on mortality, diagnosis and mor-bidity, but gradually the need arose to also include other aspects in relation to health.

This is reflected in the International Classification of Functioning, Disability and Health (ICF). The ICF distinguishes six domains:
- Health condition
- Bodily functions & Body structure
- Activities
- Participation
- Environmental factors
- Personal factors

The *International Classification of Functioning, Disability and Health (ICF)* is one that provides a standard terminology for functioning and environmental factors and a schematic representing the conceptual model of health. Approximately 1,500 categories have been developed for *Bodily functions & Body structure, Activities, Participation* and *Environmental factors*. As yet, *Personal factors*, have not been classified. The ICF has a certain relationship with Positive Health; the similarities and differences between the two are discussed in ▶ Chap. 7.

The various classifications, described with their defined units, may serve as a basis for research. In addition, the WHO has also developed questionnaires measuring, for example, Quality of Life and Well-being and Health-related Quality of Life, as well as instruments for measuring Quality Adjusted Life Years (QALY) (i.e., 1 QALY represents one year in perfect health), and Disability Adjusted Life Years (DALY) (i.e., the number of years lost due to ill-health, disability or premature death).

2.3   The initiative for a new dynamic concept of health

A number of things were not taken into account by the WHO when it formulated its definition of health. First of all, a *definition* is a *demarcation*, a delimitation. In this case, it means that anyone who does not fit this definition is unhealthy. Secondly, at the time the definition was introduced, the knowledge of physicians mainly concerned infectious diseases. These infectious diseases were believed to be eradicated by administering antibiotics, which had just become available. At the time, there was no indication of humankind, a few decades later, facing mostly non-communicable diseases (NCD), i.e., the chronic diseases.

Since 1948, many thinkers – from both inside and outside the medical profession – have been working on definitions and concepts of health, in addition to that of the WHO (Huber 2014). Despite these efforts, the WHO definition has remained unchanged and is still the standard, today. The WHO definition is mainly criticised for the word *complete* as the state of well-being in the three domains of life, which is virtually unattainable for any person. With the increase in chronic diseases, combined with the ongoing development of medical technology and diagnostics, practically no one could be considered healthy, from a perspective of health as 'a state of complete well-being'. Under this formulation, nearly everyone is a patient who requires continuous treatment or medication. This therefore has the unintentional side-effect of promoting medicalisation, and, in practice, means that health is still seen as 'the absence of disease'.

In 2008, in the *British Medical Journal*, Alex Jadad from Toronto called for a worldwide discussion on how health should be defined (Jadad & O'Grady 2008). In the Netherlands, André Knottnerus (Chair of the Health Council of the Netherlands) and Henk Smid (Director of the Netherlands Organisation for Health Research and Development (ZonMw)) recognised the problems connected to the WHO definition. Earlier, both had – independently of each other – pointed out the importance of a broader view of disease and health than that based on measurable medical-biological parameters alone. They furthermore indicated the significance of the role that professionals should have in helping patients to increase their independence and self-reliance, also in cases of chronic diseases (Gezondheidsraad 2005; De Neeling et al. 2005). Smid and Knottnerus took the initiative to organise an international invitational conference in 2009, in the Netherlands, to discuss 'the definition of health'. The aim was to move from a static definition to one that would be more dynamic and functional. At the end of 2009, 38 experts from various backgrounds met for two days at the conference, which was titled 'Is health a state or an ability? Towards a new dynamic concept of health'. Many points of view were included in the discussions and subsequently described in a report (Health Council of the Netherlands & ZonMw 2010).

Ultimately, a new dynamic concept of health was proposed:

> Health as the ability to adapt and self-manage in the face of social, physical and emotional challenges.
> (Huber et al. 2011).

The new description, based on the conference, follows the three domains of the WHO definition: physical, psychological and social. For the *physical domain*, it is about the ability of the organism to maintain homeostasis, or to reach a new balance under changing conditions and physiological stress (provided those are not too great) through allostasis. For the *psychological domain*, Antonovsky was followed, who describes the *sense of coherence (SOC)* as the foundation of mental resilience (Antonovsky 1979). For the *social domain*, it was emphasised that despite impaired physical functioning, people can successfully learn to manage their lives themselves and experience a high quality of life. This *ability* is, of course, meant to be age-related. Infants cannot realise this in the same way that adults can and, for someone in their final phase of life, this will take on a different form. Nevertheless, from this point of view, it is possible to live as 'healthily' as possible at any age, and therefore even to 'die healthily', in a way that best suits the person.

At the time, the aim of the conference was to formulate a new definition, but it was sociologist Paul Schnabel, who pointed out the limitations of the term *definition*, in that this is a *demarcation* – whereas the conference intended not to provide a demarcation, but rather to indicate a *practical direction* (Health Council of the Netherlands & ZonMw 2010). On the basis of this advice, those involved now speak of a new 'concept of health', intended as a *characterisation*, as is the convention in sociology since Blumer (Blumer 1969).

2.4 The scientific basis of Positive Health

The formulation of the dynamic concept of *health as the ability to adapt and self-manage in the face of social, physical and emotional challenges* was a first step. This concept is often already referred to as Positive Health, but that is not correct. *Positive Health* as a term emerged later, as a result of follow-up research, and represents one of the possible elaborations of the 'concept of health'.

2

After the concept was published in 2011, ZonMw commissioned a study to investigate the support for the concept and to give an impetus to its operationalisation. For this purpose, a *qualitative* and *quantitative* multimethod study was conducted amongst seven groups of stakeholders: patients with various chronic conditions, care providers (medical specialists and general practitioners, physical therapists and nurses and caregivers), policymakers, health insurance companies, health educators, citizens and researchers. The first, *qualitative part* of the study consisted of 50 interviews with a total of 140 people, individually or in focus groups. The interviews revealed a high level of support for the concept.

The interviewees had a *positive opinion* about the focus being on the individual rather than on the disease. Patients indicated that this would address their strengths rather than their weaknesses. Health, as it is described in the new concept, also offers an opportunity to strengthen that health. Spontaneously, several respondents said that health should *not be an end in itself*, but *a means to* live a meaningful life. This is what it should be about in this day and age, now that chronic diseases are often easy to treat and people often live with them for years. On the *negative* side, interviewees indicated that being able to live with chronic disease asks a lot of people: 'Is everyone able to do this successfully?' This is a point of attention. Customised advice is therefore needed. People also remarked that the term 'disease' was not mentioned in the new concept. This raised the question of whether that was no longer relevant. That is not the case. The authors of this book explicitly state that disease needs to be treated well. Disease is considered 'a physical or mental challenge in life'. It is up to patients themselves to determine what they consider to be important, and any treatment should be in line with that, as much as possible (see ▶ Sect. 2.6 and ▶ Chap. 5).

The survey also included questions about what people considered to be *indicators of health* ('How do you judge health?'), and whether the interviewees considered their own indicators to *fit the concept*? The first question resulted in 556 *indicators* of health with widely varying content. Within the group of patients, unlike amongst the other interviewees, people considered concepts related to quality of life to be very important elements of health. The researchers categorised those 556 indicators of health, and on the basis of consensus between two research institutes, these categories were further arranged into *six main dimensions* with *32 underlying aspects*. These main dimensions were initially identified as: Bodily functions, mental functions and perception, spiritual (or spiritual-existential) dimension, quality of life, social participation, and daily functioning. Later, the names of the dimensions were changed into: *bodily functions, daily functioning, mental well-being, meaningfulness, quality of life* and *participation*, as these terms are easier to understand.

For the second question about whether people's indicators would fit the concept, the answers were quite remarkable. Although people mentioned a wide variety of indicators, the vast majority thought that their indicators did fit the concept, and it therefore operationalised them.

In the second, *quantitative part* of the study, the results described above were incorporated into a questionnaire and presented to a much larger representation of the seven target groups for review. A total of 1938 respondents took part. The positive and negative views described above were fully confirmed, so there was a lot of support, and the negative views were taken into account as warnings. The respondents also had to indicate, on a scale of 1 to 9, to what extent they considered the 32 aspects under

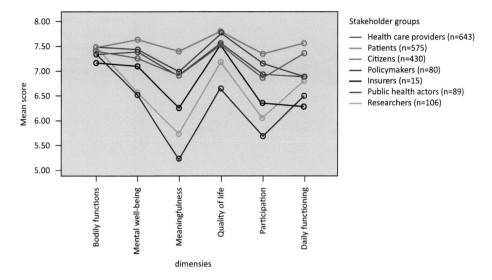

Figure 2.2 Mean scores per target group on a nine-point scale, indicating the importance assigned by respondents to a dimension as being part of 'health'. (Source: Huber et al. 2016)

the 6 main dimensions to apply to 'health'. The groups appeared to widely differ in their opinions, in this respect (■ fig. 2.2).

For the dimension *'bodily functions'*, all agreed that this belonged to health. Opinions were divided on the other dimensions. The patients scored high on all dimensions, demonstrating *a broad view* of how health should be interpreted. Policymakers and researchers, on the other hand, scored high only on the dimension of *bodily functions* and somewhat on *quality of life*; they appeared to have a narrow, mainly *medical-analytical view* and largely followed the opinion of health being 'the absence of disease'. Further subdivision of the care providers into physicians (medical specialists and general practitioners), physical therapists and nurses (and caregivers), in addition to patients, yielded the result shown in ■ fig. 2.3. The answers of the nurses (represented in green) appeared to be very close to those of the patients (purple). The physical therapists (beige) were significantly different from the patients, and the physicians (blue) were again significantly different from the physical therapists. Subdividing the physicians into medical specialists (50 %) and general practitioners (50 %) revealed an identical score between these groups.

University education appeared to be of major influence on the scores, largely leading to a narrow view. For those who had or had had a disease themselves – also university educated respondents – this led to a broader opinion of what constitutes health. Physical therapists formed an exception, for whom this effect of personal experience of disease was not found, something that the researchers could not explain. Age also appeared to be a factor; the older the respondent, the broader their view of health.

2.4.1 Positive Health

The research showed that the new concept of health was widely embraced. However, its *operationalisation* using indicators proved problematic. There were contradictions

2

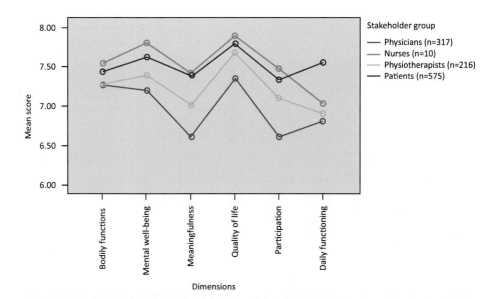

■ Figure 2.3   Mean scores per group of health care providers and patients on a nine-point scale, indicating the importance assigned by respondents to a dimension as being part of 'health'. (Source: Huber et al. 2016)

between the views of various groups, with a narrow or a broad interpretation. The differences in interpretation were so substantial that, when using the word *health*, it was necessary to ask: 'What kind of health do you mean?'

The way out of this dilemma was the decision to follow the trend that is generally recognised in health care today, namely that of *putting the patient first*.

With respect to this objective, the way patients generally think should be recognised – namely that they, as shown above, have a broad view of health. It was decided to follow this broad view. In order to avoid any confusion of terms, the term '*Positive Health*' was chosen as a provisional term in the comprehensive elaboration of the concept. This term was chosen for two reasons. First, the broad content has much in common with positive psychology (Bohlmeijer et al. 2015), and, second, the minutes of the WHO's preparatory meeting revealed that '*positive health*' had been considered as a name for the concept of health. This did not happen, in the end, but after discovering its previous consideration, the term Positive Health was chosen this time, because it appeared to be in line with the intentions of the WHO. Inevitably, the term 'positive' health begs the question of whether there is also such a thing as '*negative health*'. This name can be seen as an indication of '*health through exclusion*', something that will be familiar to the older generations of physicians amongst us.

The term 'positive health' was not used for the concept of 'Health as the ability to adapt and self-manage in the face of social, physical and emotional challenges' because this concept can also be elaborated in a different way than in Huber et al. (2016). An example of this is the work by Alex Jadad in Canada, who elaborated the concept with respect to forms of cooperation aiming to promote health, under the term Trusted Networks (Jadad et al. 2018). Where Positive Health at the individual level has *meaningfulness* as a central concept, Jadad's elaboration at community level uses *trust*. Both elaborations complement each other.

The term positive health has been used before in the literature, but with differing interpretations (Seligman 2008; Walburg 2016). In our current interpretation, Positive Health is the name of the concept of health in the six dimensions, as mentioned above (Huber et al. 2013, 2016; iPH 2020). So, what is Positive Health? *It is the broad elaboration into six dimensions of the concept of 'Health as the ability to adapt and self-manage in the face of social, physical and emotional challenges'.* When this approach was met by a large degree of enthusiasm, the 'Institute for Positive Health' (iPH) was established in 2015, which has been actively contributing from 2016 onwards, to implement Positive Health in practice. The six dimensions were developed into the Positive Health *spider web*. For more information, also visit ▶ www.iph.nl/en.

2.5 Health-based resilience

All these research activities and subsequent development of the various instruments are directed towards effectuating a change of focus in the health care system, to shift the emphasis from disease and health as the absence of disease to people's own resilience and the strengthening of that resilience. What are the general views of resilience and which of these perspectives can we connect to?

The name Antonovsky is very important in relation to resilience. As an Israeli-American medical sociologist, he was interested to discover what makes people healthy. He developed the concept of *salutogenesis*, the origins of health and the factors supporting human health and well-being, which he placed next to *pathogenesis*, the factors that cause disease. Antonovsky worked as a researcher in a hospital in Tel Aviv. There, he saw many patients who had been survivors of concentration camps in WWII and who had subsequently emigrated to Israel. Many of these people were traumatised, but what struck him was that a small group of people amongst these survivors were not traumatised, although they had lived through the same thing. He wondered if these people had some traits in common that had made them more resilient and thus able to survive those terrible circumstances so well. He found three characteristics: comprehensibility, manageability and meaningfulness, which he collectively called the *Sence of Coherence (SOC)*.

— *Comprehensibility* means understanding one's own situation; to a certain extent of course. Fully understanding everything is perhaps impossible, but the point is not to be confused.
— *Manageability* is about being able to take action and make choices in life. It is about not feeling completely powerless or victimised.
— *Meaningfulness* is about having found some form of personal meaning in life. According to Antonovsky, meaningfulness is the most powerful of these three characteristics (Antonovsky 1979).

Another source of knowledge about health is the data on the world's *Blue Zones*. These Blue Zones are areas in various parts of the world where people live to a very ripe old age, often over 100 years, largely without chronic diseases or mental decline. When people die, this is usually without having suffered a long or terrible illness. The term *Blue Zones* was coined by Dan Buettner (Buettner 2012), a journalist from National Geographic (who used to circle the healthy areas on a world map using a blue felt-tip

2

pen). Together with others, he made an overview of lifestyle factors of the people living in these areas. In total, seven of such regions were identified: in southern Japan, several islands in the Mediterranean, in southern Sweden and in Central America and the western United States.

These are the four most important lifestyle factors that these regions have in common:

— *Nutrition*: People in these regions follow a largely plant-based diet with only few animal proteins. In addition, they tend to stop eating when they 'feel full', rather than to continue eating beyond this point.
— *Exercise*: These people lead physically active daily lives, until a ripe old age, without going to gyms or using pedometers.
— *Meaningfulness*: They feel their lives and activities are meaningful and they remain active well into old age. Concepts as retirement and not working anymore are largely absent, although people do take it slow, after a certain age.
— *Social embeddedness*: All people are part of the local community. This can be a village, an extended family or a spiritual community, but most importantly, they are not lonely. Loneliness is a factor known to be very detrimental to health (Holt-Lunstad et al. 2010).

The Sense of Coherence and the Blue Zones strikingly have meaningfulness in common as an important factor. The importance of meaning has also been stressed by psychiatrist Viktor Frankl, who himself survived three years of concentration camps (Frankl 2006). From this experience, Frankl was convinced of the fact that people's deepest need and driving force was that of finding meaning in life, and that this sense of purpose is also the greatest source of inner strength that a person can draw from to endure difficult circumstances. He describes this as: 'When people find a reason to live, they can cope with almost anything'. He developed the concept of Logotherapy – a therapy specifically on this subject, to help people find personal meaning. An accessible description of this theme is provided in Edith Eger's book, *The Choice* (Eger 2017).

The information above, in part, also served to inspire during the development of Positive Health and the spider web. In the method of working with Positive Health, the three elements of the *Sence of Coherence* are incorporated, in a slightly different order:

— The first step is to help people achieve an overall view of their lives and, subsequently, gain the related insight by filling out the spider web, as described in ▶ Chap. 5. In this way, *comprehensibility* is achieved.
— The conversational aspect of this method is primarily intended to motivate people to ask themselves what they would like to change, what they hope for or dream about. A question about their personal sense of meaning (i.e., *meaningfulness*) is also included.
— And looking for a possible first, small step in the direction of achieving their objectives, people discover what they could do themselves. Irrespective of whether the support of others is also still needed, things look more feasible – the *manageability* is activated.

▶ Chapter 5 describes the practical applications.

This form of conversation, therefore, reflects the elements that were described by Antonovsky as resilience-building. In addition, the lifestyle factors, as present in the *Blue Zones*, are all also included in the spider web and can be brought up during the conversation, if needed.

2.6 The T-shaped professional: professional of the future

In the Netherlands, the demographic composition of the population, with baby boomers causing a 'silver tsunami' in the coming years, calls for reorganisation of the current health care system. When the majority of elderly citizens start to suffer from chronic diseases and end up needing help, this will lead to certain practical problems, as the younger generation that needs to care for them is far fewer in number (see ▶ Chap. 1). The Dutch Government is paying attention to this issue, and two reports have been produced by an advisory committee on innovation in health care and training (Adviescommissie Innovatie Zorgberoepen & Opleidingen 2015, 2016, Zorginstituut 2021a, Zorginstituut 2021b). These reports describe the 'professional of the future' – the so-called *T-shaped professional*. Because this description so clearly reflects the impact of the position and possible role of Positive Health for health professionals, this section briefly discusses the *T-shaped professional* (see ◻ fig. 2.4).

The vertical bar of the T represents the profession-specific and disease-oriented expertise of, for example, physicians, nurses and physiotherapists. The horizontal bar contains the knowledge and skills that are not profession-specific, but will be shared by all health care professionals of the future. This concerns the general person-oriented approach to patients and the promotion of health in a broad sense, even when diseases are involved. This is generally about promoting resilience, which is what Positive Health is all about. Currently, the curricula of health care educational programmes are gradually being adapted to this perspective.

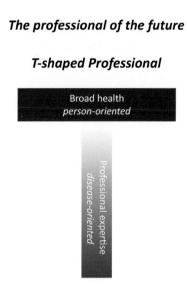

The professional of the future

T-shaped Professional

Broad health
person-oriented

Professional expertise
disease-oriented

◻ **Figure 2.4** Health professionals of the future. They will require two types of skills, with profession- and disease-specific capabilities on the one hand, and person-oriented and health-promoting skills, on the other. (Source: Care Institute 2017; adaptation)

2.7 Health as the starting point: a paradigm shift in a disease-oriented system

When the promotion of health becomes the basis of medical practice, it calls for con-siderable changes in our medical thinking as well as our health care system. The image of the inverted triangle in ▶ Chap. 1 (◘ fig. 1.3) illustrates this change in the system. ◘ Figure 2.5 is an illustration of the necessary change in our way of thinking.

These images originate from ecology and depict two types of equilibrium, brought about in very different ways. Martin Scheffer (Wageningen University & Research) has developed mathematical models that can be used to calculate the stability of a cer-tain equilibrium and to determine the conditions under which the stability of a system reaches a tipping point after which a breakdown occurs (Scheffer 2009). In the illus-tration on the left, the system is unstable. It must be kept under control by external measures; this is a static equilibrium. In the right-hand illustration, the system is stable because of its intrinsic design, which is multifactorial by definition; this is a dynamic equilibrium. The situation on the right involves resilience. It is a case of having adaptive capacity.

General medical education, today, mainly trains students to think along the lines of the left-hand image of ◘ fig. 2.5. The use of medication allows physicians to respond to certain health situations in a very targeted way and keep those situations under control. This is the result of a highly developed medical-analytical science that has produced many good things. The type of thinking according to the illustration on the right is also scientific, but is still in the early phases of development. It is, by the way, already being applied within the medical domain (Gijzel 2020). To promote resilience in patients, physicians will have to think in a broader, multifactorial way, which is per-fectly in line with the Positive Health concept, and the related lifestyle medical science with its many perspectives on treatment. This does, however, require a paradigm shift that is already under way.

Towards 'resilient systems', according to the adaptation model

Control model	**Adaptation model**
traditional approach	*'resilient' approach*

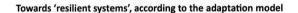

– Focus on problem	– Focus on system
– Avoid variation	– Utilising variation
– Continuous monitoring	– Stimulate self-regulation
– Direct intervention	– Indirect guidance
– Static balance	– Dynamic balance

◘ **Figure 2.5**   Two conceptual models about *health* brought into focus. (Source: Ten Napel et al. 2006)

2.7 · Health as the starting point: a paradigm shift in a ...

41

2

The next chapter deals with the relationship between Positive Health and the recently established core values of primary care.

Case no. 4: Regained life energy because of a camera

Theo Hermsen had been employed for 25 years at the same employer who gave him an anniversary bonus with which he decided to buy a camera. It had been a rather difficult time; 25 years of changing schedules and the many night shifts had taken their toll. Now, at age 67, he was sleeping badly, waking up early, with pain in his shoulders and back and worries about work, as well as having a seriously handicapped grandchild. He often went to his general practitioner for his problems. Having filled out his Positive Health spider web resulted in only two satisfactory scores: a 6 for 'my contact with other people is good' and a 7 for 'I am very capable of looking after myself'. Antidepressants were considered, and Theo made use of the option to retire early, in consultation with his employer. His sleeping pattern did not recover. Turning a necessity into a virtue, Theo decided that instead of staying in bed worrying, he would simply get up at 4 am. each day and head into the countryside with his camera. He recounted the time when he felt really happy walking around the Quin nature reserve, located in the Maasduinen National Park near the village of Afferden when the sun came up through the trees and the fog (◼ fig. 2.6). This became a turning point for him; he learned that each time he looked through the eye of the camera, he would experience a small moment of happiness. The camera showed him how nice it was to be able to enjoy the little things in life.

'My camera helps me to see the beautiful things better,' he said. The first thing he would do after getting up was to check whether there was any dew on the car. If so, this already would make him happy, because it meant a chance of fog and of a beautiful sunrise. The initial problem of not being able to sleep had become an advantage! He and his partner noticed that his new hobby made him much calmer. 'Walking in nature gives me peace of mind, and that feeling stays with me all day. When I see deer, I have no problem watching them for 45 minutes or more. I never used to be able to do that. Now, I no longer watch the news or read newspapers, I prefer to see the world through my own lens', he said. He often would go out again in the afternoons, joined by his wife, who had also started to look at nature differently because of his hobby. And she knew Theo so well that she could tell from the photographs what kind of mood he was in when he took them.

She could follow how his moods would improve by following her husband's photographs. He was no longer on anti-depressants and he tended to visit the surgery much less often. He stated, 'I feel good, so why should I go to the doctor's office? My back pain has gone completely, I no longer walk with a hunched back. When I'm outside, I only think of beautiful things. I enjoy the silence, the peace. It has really changed my view of the world. I have become milder.' A new spider web filled out for 2020 no longer showed any negatives, with even a 9 for 'I am enjoying my life' and a 9 for 'My contact with other people is good'. The latter still calls for an explanation.

He had great reactions to his photographs from the people around him and they advised him to share his photos on the Internet. He did so and to great effect; his photographs can be seen on YouPic. He has 26,000 followers, and his photographs have been liked on YouTube 1.2 million times, and Facebook and YouPic add up to 25 million views.

2

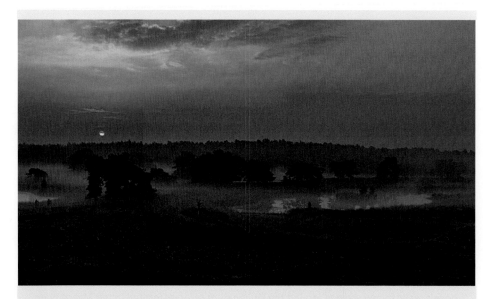

◨ Figure 2.6   Feeling of happiness when the sun appeared above the trees and the fog. (Source: Hermsen, ▸ www.youpic.com 2020)

Reactions show that he is particularly appreciated for the warmth and atmosphere that his photographs evoke. People from all over the world turn out to go on holiday to North Limburg to see the Quin nature reserve because of his photographs. Top photographers are also visiting his site and compliment him on his work. 'That does something with you, I am quite proud of that. People come up to me in the street to speak to me, they recognise me. They are happy with what I'm doing,' he said. He told about another moment of pride when, at one of the Netherlands' largest consumer and business fairs (the Hiltho in Horst), he presented a 150-metre-long photo collage of his photographs, which visitors could cycle past to become acquainted with the Maasduinen National Park. Here, we show one of the photographs Theo took at the Quin on that first morning that made such an impression on him and, looking back, proved to be the start of his regained life energy.

2.8   Conclusions

This chapter sketches the historical development of the thinking on health. Where people, in the past, thought about health in terms of balance, this was subsequently replaced by medical-analytical thinking. Since then, this perspective has been broadening again, as expressed, for example, in the World Health Organization's definition of health from 1948. However, the WHO definition is formulated in a static way. Over the past decade, a Dutch initiative led to a proposal for a new description of health, based on resilience and personal control. This formulation has been further elaborated into the Positive Health concept, with six dimensions that are in line with how patients perceive their own health. At its core is a meaningful life. The chapter discusses how the care provider of the future will be trained as a T-shaped professional.

These professionals combine knowledge on disease (vertical bar of the T) with a broad health-oriented vision of humankind (horizontal bar of the T). A paradigm shift is taking place in the thinking on health care: from thinking in terms of disease-control to thinking in terms of resilience.

For more information, background or videos about this chapter scan the QR code.

SCAN ME

References

Antonovsky, A. (1979). *Health, stress and coping*. Jossey-Bass Publishers.

Blumer, H. (1969). *Symbolic interactionism: Perspective and method*. Prentice Hall.

Bohlmeijer, E., et al. (2015). *Handboek positieve psychologie. Theorie, onderzoek en toepassingen*. Boom Uitgevers.

Buettner, D. (2012). *The Blue Zones. 9 Lessons for living longer from the people who've lived the longest*. National-Geographic-Society.

De Neeling, J. N. D., Sterk, A. H. J. M., & Knottnerus, J. A. (2005). Beoordelen, behandelen, begeleiden: de Gezondheidsraad over medisch handelen bij ziekteverzuim en arbeidsongeschiktheid. *TBV – Tijdschrift voor Bedrijfs- en Verzekeringsgeneeskunde*, 11/200.

Dijksterhuis, E. J. (1980). *De mechanisering van het wereldbeeld*. Meulenhoff.

Descartes, R. (2021). Accessed in April 2021 of ► https://nl.wikipedia.org/wiki/Ren%C3%A9_Descartes.

Eger, E. E. (2017). *De keuze*. Leven in vrijheid.

Frankl, V. (2006) *Man's search for meaning. Part one, experiences in a concentration camp*. Pocket Books.

Gezondheidsraad & ZonMw (2010). *Invitational conference 'Is health a state or an ability? Towards a dynamic concept of health'*. Report of the meeting of December 10-11-2009.

Gezondheidsraad (2005). *Beoordelen, behandelen, begeleiden. Medisch handelen bij ziekteverzuim en arbeidsongeschiktheid*. Gezondheidsraad, 2005; publication nr 2005/10 ► http://www.mediprudentie. steungroep.nl/images/pdf/Gezondheidsraad_beoordelen_behandelen_begeleiden.pdf.

Gijzel, S. (2020). *Bouncing back. Using a complex dynamical systems approach to measure physical resilience in older adults*. Thesis Radboud Universiteit. ISBN 978-94-028-1891-8.

Hermsen, T. (2020). Photo accessed on June 2021 of ► www.youpic.com (► https://youpic.com/photographer/theohermsen3/).

Holt-Lunstad, J. et al. (2010). Social relationships and mortality risk: A meta-analytic Review. *PLoS*. ► https://doi.org/10.1371/journal.pmed.1000316.

Huber, M. (2014). *Towards a new, dynamic concept of health. Its operationalisation and use in public health and healthcare, and in evaluating health effects of food*. Thesis Maastricht University. ISBN 978-94-6259-471-5.

Huber, M., Knottnerus, J. A., Green, L., et al. (2011). How should we define health? *BMJ, 343*(4163), 235–237.

Huber, M., Van Vliet, M., Giezenberg, M., & Knottnerus, A. (2013). *Towards a conceptual framework relating to 'Health as the ability to adapt and to self manage'. Operationalisering gezondheidsconcept*. Louis Bolk Instituut, Rapport 2013-001 VG.

Huber, M., Van Vliet, M., Giezenberg, M., et al. (2016). Towards a 'patient-centred' operationalisation of the new dynamic concept of health: A mixed methods study. *British Medical Journal Open, 5,* e010091.

iPH (2020). Accessed on June 2021 of ► https://iph.nl.

ICPC-International Classification of Health Problem in Primary Care (ICHPPC-2-d) (1976, 1983). Accessed on June 2021 of ▶ http://www.ph3c.org/PH3C/docs/27/000150/0000103.pdf.

Jadad, A. R., & O'Grady, L. (2008). How should health be defined? Join a global conversation at blogs.bmj.com/bmj. *BMJ, 337*, a2900, 1361–1364.

Jadad, A. R., et al. (2018). *Trusted networks: The key to achieve world-class health outcomes on a shoestring*. Beati Inc.

Lamberts, H., & Wood, M. (1993). *ICPC in the European Community*. University Press.

Lamberts, H., & Wood, M. (2002). The birth of the International Classification of Primary Care (ICPC). Serendipity at the border of Lac Léman. *Family Practice, 19*, 433–435.

Lindeboom, G. (1982). *Begrippen in de Geneeskunde* (pp. 33–41). Editions Rodopi.

Raamplan (2020). Accessed June 2021 of ▶ https://www.nfu.nl/sites/default/files/2020-08/20.1577_Raamplan_Artsenopleiding_-_maart_2020.pdf.

Scheffer, M. (2009). *Critical transitions in nature and society*. Princeton-university-press.

Seligman, M. (2008). *Positive health*. Accessed June 2021 of ▶ https://doi.org/10.1111/j.1464-0597.2008.00351.x.

Seligman, M. E. P. (2012). *Flourish: A visionary new understanding of happiness and well-being. The practical guide to using positive psychology to make you happier and healthier*. Atria Books.

Ten Napel, J., Bianchi, F. J. J. A., & Bestman, M. W. P. (2006). Utilising intrinsic robustness in agricultural production systems. *Invention for a sustainable development of agriculture* (pp. 32–54). TransForum.

Van Veen, P., & Van der Sijs, N. (1997). *Etymologisch woordenboek: De herkomst van onze woorden* (2nd ed.). Van Dale Lexicografie.

Walburg, J. A. (2016). *Positieve gezondheid. Naar een bloeiende samenleving*. Bohn Stafleu van Loghum.

World Health Organisation. (1946). *Minutes of the technical preparatory committee for the international health conference*. Official Records of the World Health Organization.

WHO-FIC (2020). Accessed June 2021 of ▶ https://www.who.int/standards/classifications/international-classification-of-functioning-disability-and-health.

Zorginstituut (2021a). Accessed June 2021 of ▶ https://www.zorginstituutnederland.nl/publicaties/adviezen/2015/04/10/naar-nieuwe-zorg-en-zorgberoepen-de-contouren.

Zorginstituut (2021b). Accessed June 2021 of ▶ https://www.zorginstituutnederland.nl/publicaties/adviezen/2016/11/17/anders-kijken-anders-leren-anders-doen-grensoverstijgend-leren-en-opleiden-in-zorg-en-welzijn-in-het-digitale-tijdperk.

3

I swear/promise to practise the art of medicine to the best of my ability for the benefit of my fellow man. I will care for the sick, promote health and relieve suffering.

I will put the patient's interests first and respect his/her views. I will do no harm to the patient. I will listen and inform him/her well. I will keep secret what has been entrusted to me.

I will advance the medical knowledge of myself and others. I will recognise the limits of my possibilities.

The Dutch health care system

© Bohn Stafleu van Loghum is an imprint of Springer Media B.V., part of Springer Nature 2022
M. Huber et al., *Handbook Positive Health in Primary Care*,
https://doi.org/10.1007/978-90-368-2729-4_3

> **Main messages**
> — For people in the Netherlands, general practitioners are the first point of contact with the health care system.
> — In the Netherlands, general practitioners have a strong position within the health care system, compared to those in other countries.
> — The gatekeeper function in referrals to secondary care, the patient enrolment system, and the involvement of general practitioners in out-of-hours services all play an important role in this.
> — Dutch general practitioners provide a wide range of care and are in a key position as coordinators of patient care.
> — Compared to other countries, the average time per consultation is short, while the number of registered patients per general practice is relatively large.

3.1 Introduction

This handbook describes the importance of Positive Health from the context of primary care in the Netherlands (*The Dutch Example*). This chapter describes the organisation of general medical care in the Netherlands, the services provided by general medical practices and how those are financed. Countries all have their own way of organising their health care system. This means that a certain degree of caution is in order when considering the pointers and tips provided throughout this handbook. What works in one health care system may not be feasible in another. In addition, other health care systems may offer different opportunities for working with the Positive Health concept; possibilities that may be less obvious under the Dutch health care system. It is, furthermore, also complicated to compare health care systems. This starts with the lack of a standard and unambiguous description of the role of general practitioners – also known as family doctors, primary care physicians or ambulatory care physicians – and differences per country in the tasks they perform.

A number of review studies were recently published in which an attempt nevertheless was made to compare primary care and the related financing systems, in a large number of countries, both within and outside Europe (e.g., Australia, Canada and New Zealand) (Groenewegen 2020; Scaioli et al. 2020; Schäfer et al. 2016a, 2016b, 2019; Van Den Berg et al. 2016; Van Kemenade 2018; Van Kemenade 2019). We used these studies to derive an overall picture of the things that are typical to the Dutch type of primary care, which are subsequently described in the following sections: (2) Organisation of primary care in the Netherlands; (3) The task of general medical practices in the Netherlands; (4) Financing primary care in the Netherlands.

3.2 Organisation of primary care in the Netherlands

In the Netherlands, general practitioners are *people's first point of contact* with the health care system. An important feature of primary care in the Netherlands is that almost every Dutch person is *registered* at a local general medical practice (Nielen 2021). These practices provide general practitioner care to those people. People are free to change practices, but cannot be registered at two or more practices at the same time. A general medical practice can reject the application of new patients if they live at too great a distance from the practice, or if the practice has reached its maximum number of patients.

Research shows that it is easier for general medical practices to feel responsible for assessing the needs within a community if they work with a patient enrolment system. These practices are more strongly community-oriented, more likely to use their patients' medical records to obtain an overview of the practice population, and offer a wider range of services, particularly those related to prevention (Vermeulen et al. 2018). Vulnerable and disadvantaged patients seem to have easier access to health care when they are registered at a general medical practice. A characteristic of general practices with a patient enrolment system is the equal availability of care for all their registered patients, continuity of care over time, and the ability to coordinate different types of care. It helps to organise people's care around individual needs rather than according to type of disease.

3.2.1 Other characteristics of primary care in the Netherlands

In 2019, the size of the Dutch population was over 17.4 million (CBS 2020). In total, 12,766 general practitioners were working in the Netherlands at that time, divided over 5,000 general medical practices, which is equivalent to about 9500 FTEs. Of those general practitioners, in 2019, 58 % were women (Batenburg 2019). There are about 2200 registered patients to each full-time general practitioner (Van Kemenade 2018). Dutch people, on average, can choose from 9.6 general medical practices within a 3-kilometre radius around their place of residence (Volksgezondheidenzorg.info 2021). Compared to those in other countries, Dutch general practitioners have a larger number of patients and a long working week (Schäfer et al. 2016b), and consultation times are short, with an average of 11 min per consultation. In a survey of 34 countries, the Netherlands ranked 25th on a list from long to short consultation times, near the United Kingdom and Austria. Consultation times are generally longer in Scandinavian countries, with the exception of Denmark. In the Netherlands (as in Scandinavian countries), keeping an electronic health record, per patient, including electronic prescription of medication, is part of the daily routine. This is far less the case in Eastern European countries and in some countries in Southern Europe (Groenwegen et al. 2020).

Less than a quarter of Dutch general practitioners has a solo practice, 40 % work in a practice with one other general practitioner, and 39 % work in a group practice of 3 to 7 general practitioners (Van Kemenade 2018). This means that Dutch general medical practices are relatively small. In almost two thirds of the 34 countries surveyed, fewer GPs work by themselves; in Sweden and Norway, there are almost no practitioners with a solo practice (Groenewegen 2020), see ◘ fig. 3.1. In the Netherlands, in addition to general practitioners themselves, usually, three other disciplines are also represented in general medical practices (i.e., nursing assistant, practice nurse, mental health practice nurse; for an explanation of the related tasks, see ► sect. 3.2). In half the countries surveyed, the number of other disciplines is lower. In Belgium, it is not unusual for a general practitioner to work without any support at all. At the other end of the spectrum, there are Finnish and Lithuanian health centres where 50 % have more than six other disciplines present (Groenewegen et al. 2015). Compared to other countries, patients in the Netherlands have relatively fast access to their general practitioner.

3

Around 70 % of Dutch patients are able to secure an appointment on the day they contact the practice, or on the next day (Groenewegen 2016). Dutch general medical practices are open for an average of 10 hours per weekday. In the evenings and on weekends, practices are generally closed, in the Netherlands. The country does distinguish itself by the large degree of involvement of general practitioners in out-of-hours services, which in the Netherlands are operated from nearby hospitals and organised on a municipal level (out-of-hours cooperatives of general practitioners). At these out-of-hours services, specially trained nursing assistants both man the phones and perform triage. The general practitioners on duty determine whether a patient needs to go to hospital. The practices at which these patients are registered receive a message from the out-of-hours service about their patient's visit to the clinic. The general practitioners work in rotation at the hospital clinic and receive an hourly reimbursement for their work.

In most other countries where out-of-hours services are available, general practitioners usually do not participate in working shifts at these services, but have arranged for these services to be provided by other organisations (Schäfer et al. 2016b).

Accessibility and continuity of primary care have been shown to influence the use of care by patients. An easily accessible general practice where continuous care is offered appears to go hand in hand with fewer visits to hospital emergency rooms. In countries where patients are registered at 'their own' general medical practice, visits to the hospital emergency room also occur less often. The survey showed that the Netherlands was the country with the second lowest number of visits to hospital emergency rooms (18 % in one year, compared with over 29 %, on average, in all 34 countries surveyed) (Van Den Berg et al. 2016), see ◘ fig. 3.2.

3.3   The task of general medical practices in the Netherlands

3.3.1   The role of gatekeeper

The *'gatekeeping'* principle, together with the patient enrolment system, is one of the most important characteristics of the Dutch health care system and means that hospital and specialist care (with the exception of emergency care) is only reimbursed if patients are *referred by a general practitioner* (or other primary care provider, such as midwife or dentist). It is common practice for Dutch general practitioners to give the referral letter directly to their patients to take to their specialist appointment themselves. Over 90 % of Dutch general practitioners works in this way (Groenewegen et al. 2020), as do their UK colleagues. In Italy and Germany, this is less than 10 %. In countries where general practitioners have a gatekeeper role, they more frequently receive feedback from the specialist they referred their patient to (Scaioli et al. 2020). In those countries, it is also more common for general practitioners to take their patient's preference into account when choosing a secondary health care provider. More than in any other of the 34 countries, Dutch general practitioners (92 %) say that they take a referral decision together with their patient (Rotar et al. 2018), see ◘ fig. 3.3.

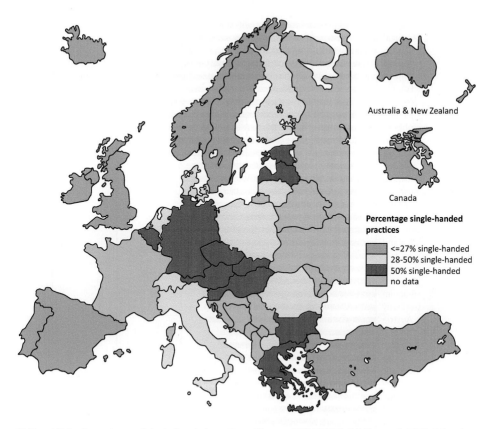

Australia & New Zealand

Canada

Percentage single-handed practices

<=27% single-handed
28-50% single-handed
50% single-handed
no data

Figure 3.1 Percentages of single-handed practices. (Source: QUALICOPC, Schäfer et al. 2019. Printed with permission)

3.3.2 Dutch general practitioners play a central role in care coordination

The core task of *care coordination*, with general practitioners in a central role, provides practitioners with an overview of their patients' health care and treatment process. They know which care providers are involved and are aware of their tasks and responsibilities. General practitioners coordinate primary care, general medical care and, thus, have a signalling function for the patients registered at their practice. Dutch general practitioners are not responsible for coordinating secondary care – specialist and follow-up care – nor for the daily care or support of patients at home (Toekomst Huisartsenzorg 2019). The practitioners carry out their tasks supported by other members of the general practice team, such as practice assistants, practice nurses and mental health practice nurses.

Practice nurses play a crucial role in the organisation of the general practice. In particular, they plan the surgery hours largely on the basis of triage. Triage is the dynamic process of determining urgency and follow-up action. Patients and their health-related issues are at the core of this process (Dutch triage standard 2014 (*Nederlandse Triage Standaard*)). Most questions first arrive at the practice by telephone. Nursing assistants

3

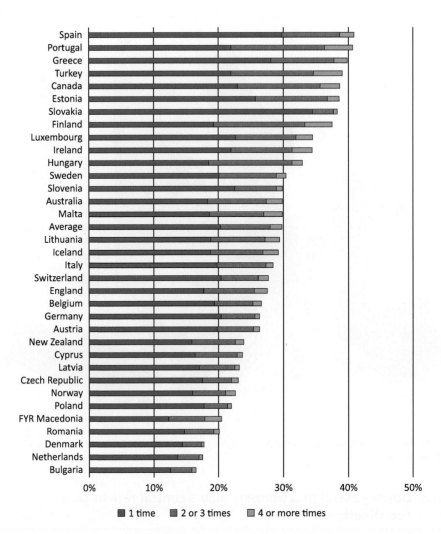

Figure 3.2   Patient-reported visits tot he Emergency Department during the past year bij country. (Source: QUALICOPC, based on Van den Berg et al. 2016, Scháfer et al. 2019. Printed with permission)

must process the questions to the best of their ability, often under high time pressure. The largest share of these questions is subsequently passed on to the general practitioner, with the exception of repeat prescriptions. The degree of urgency of health-related questions varies. Some patients require to be seen by the general practitioner immediately, while others do not need a same-day appointment. Some patient questions may be solved by another care provider, such as the practice assistant or physiotherapist. Nursing assistants answer some of the questions themselves, on the telephone, giving certain self-care advice, referring patients to the website (► https://gpinfo.nl), or arrange an appointment for a patient at the practice assistant's surgery hour for certain simple procedures (e.g., checking blood pressure, unblocking ears and measuring glucose). Remaining health care questions are passed on to the general practitioner and other care providers.

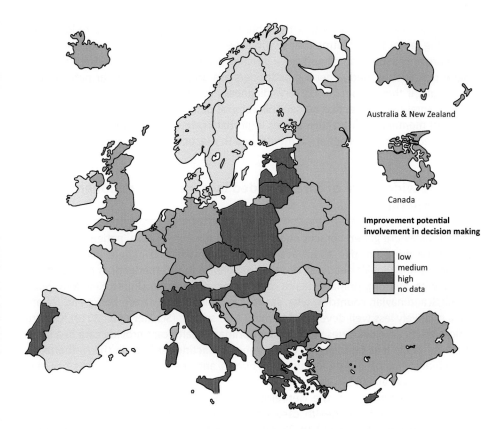

Australia & New Zealand

Canada

Improvement potential involvement in decision making

- low
- medium
- high
- no data

◧ **Figure 3.3**   Patient-reported improvement potential for shared involvement in decision-making, per country. (Source: QUALICOPC, based on Schäfer et al. 2015, 2019. Printed with perimision)

Practice nurses support general practitioners in treating patients who have a chronic physical condition. In most cases, this concerns diabetes, asthma, COPD (bronchitis and emphysema) or cardiovascular disease. The position of practice nurse was created at the beginning of this century to support general practitioners. This support consists of providing structural care (i.e., chain care) for people with such chronic conditions and is very successful! Today, 85 % of patients with type 2 diabetes, for example, receive care that complies with the guidelines and standards. At the beginning of this century, this was around 66 % (Den Klomp et al. 2020; Outer 2019).

The position of *mental health practice nurse* was created in 2007, to alleviate the increasing demand for psychological and psychosocial care and reduce costs in the relatively more expensive secondary care sector. Mental health practice nurses share responsibility with general practitioners and supervise patients independently. In principle, they see patients with psychological complaints for whom there is no suspicion of a psychiatric disorder (i.e., a disorder classified under the Diagnostic and Statistical Manual of Mental Disorders (DSM)). In certain cases of DSM disorders or a suspected DSM disorder, the mental health practice nurses can also see these types of patients with low functional limitation, symptoms with a limited impact, and who are at low risk of serious neglect, violence, suicide or self-mutilation. In addition, mental health

3

practice nurses also see patients with stable chronic problems, who require long-term monitoring rather than treatment and who have a support system in place. Since 2014, people are only allowed to go and see a psychologist if they have been referred by their general practitioner. And general practitioners are only allowed to refer patients to a psychologist if they suspect a 'DSM-IV' diagnosis. In all other cases, patients are seen by the mental health practice nurse. This referral policy has led to a large increase in the use of mental health practice nurses in primary care – today, almost 90 % of Dutch general medical practices employ a mental health practice nurse.

3.3.3 The wide range of care provided by general practitioners in the Netherlands

In countries where general practitioners offer a wide range of care, patients have been found to be more positive about accessibility, continuity and patient involvement in decision-making (Schäfer et al. 2018). Internationally, the Netherlands is regarded as a country with a strong primary health care system, as are the United Kingdom, Spain and the Scandinavian countries, whereas for example Cyprus, Luxembourg and Iceland have a relatively less well-developed primary care system (Schäfer et al. 2019). General medical practices in countries with stronger primary health care provide care in a larger number of disciplines besides that of the general practitioner (e.g., in the Netherlands, this includes nursing assistants, practice nurses and mental health practice nurses) (Groenewegen et al. 2015).

General practitioners in the Netherlands have a strong position as people's first point of contact with the health care system. This is also true for their Danish and Swedish colleagues. Compared to 27 other European countries, Dutch general prac-titioners are more involved particularly in medical problems related to children and women. In a number of – mainly Eastern European – countries, these problems are addressed by gynaecologists, obstetricians and paediatricians. Furthermore, Dutch general practitioners are slightly more than average involved in the treatment and care of patients with chronic diseases – comparable to the level of involvement on this sub-ject of general practitioners in Hungary and Italy. General practitioners in Slovenia are most actively involved in this area and those in Slovakia the least. There are major dif-ferences between general practitioners in Europe, with respect to the performance of minor technical and surgical procedures. Compared to those in the Netherlands, only Finnish general practitioners perform a higher number of such procedures. In Lithuania, general practitioners perform the lowest number of such procedures. For example, most general practitioners in the Netherlands place IUDs and remove warts. Further-more, in most countries, general practitioners are less active in prevention, whereas in the Netherlands, there was a sharp increase after the introduction of the practice nurse, at the beginning of the century. The strongest increase in preventive activities concerns the more systematic education about the dangers of smoking (Schäfer et al. 2016a). Following the introduction of the practice nurse mental health, the role of Dutch general practitioners in addressing social problems has also increased (Schäfer et al. 2016c). In addition, in 2015, the responsibilities for, amongst other things, youth care, elderly care and those who require long-term care were transferred from the

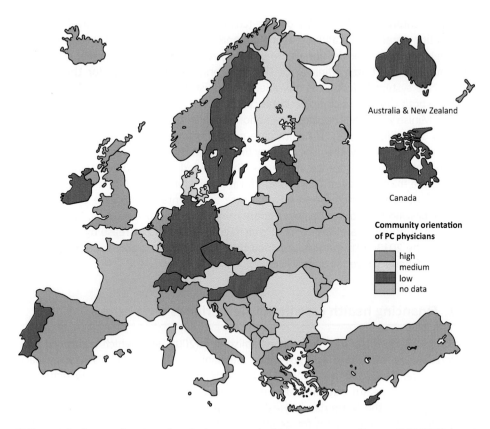

Figure 3.4 Community orientation of primary care physicians, per country. (Source: QUALICOPC, based on Vermeulen et al. 2018, Schäfer et al. 2019. Printed with permission)

national government to municipalities. This decentralisation was accompanied by a sharp decline in the available budget, which in turn led to an increase in social problems, increased reliance on general practitioners and mental health practice nurse support, and to more cooperation between municipalities and general medical practices, in regard to social problems (see ◘ fig. 3.4).

3.4 Financing primary care in the Netherlands

In Europe, reimbursement of health care costs is still a national affair. Health care expenditure in Europe differs from country to country (Van Kemenade 2018, 2019; Stichting Beroepseer 2019). This section provides a brief introduction to how health care is organised and financed in the Netherlands.

The Dutch Government and the Ministry of Health, Welfare and Sport (VWS) reaches political decisions with the aim of ensuring the health and welfare of the Dutch population as well as promoting a healthy lifestyle. The Dutch Government has formulated three goals for the health care system: (1) *quality of care* (effective, safe and patient-oriented); (2) *accessibility of care* (costs for individual citizens, travel distances and waiting times should all be reasonable) and (3) *affordability of care* (cost control). Although health care professionals are primarily responsible for the quality of the care they provide, the Dutch Minister of Health is primarily responsible for the way the health care system functions as a whole. The Ministry of VWS and municipal authorities have both similar but complementary roles.

The Ministry of VWS decides the national health care budget (in 2020, this was close to 100 billion euros). If health care providers and health insurance companies spend too much money, the ministry may decide that they, respectively, must pay back this amount or lower insurance premiums. This is called the Macro Control Instrument. In 2013, the ministry, together with health care providers, agreed on a voluntary maximum for the annual increase in hospital care and mental health care costs. If costs increase beyond this point, the government may implement budget cuts. This with the exception of primary care, the costs of which were allowed to increase by 1.5 %, annually, over the 2013–2017 period, provided this would demonstrably contribute to substituting secondary care for primary care.

3.4.1 Financing health care in the Netherlands

The Dutch Health Insurance Act was established in 2006, with which *controlled market forces* were introduced as a governing mechanism in health care. Previously, basic health insurance was partly organised by the state, whereas under this new legislation, taking out basic health insurance at a private insurance company became mandatory for all citizens in the Netherlands. Health insurance companies, in turn, are obligated to accept anyone who applies for health insurance (i.e., no exceptions for pre-existing conditions), and policyholders are all free to change insurance companies at the start of each calendar year. The stakeholders in the health care sector (insurance companies, care providers and the insured) are active on three markets: that of health insurance, that of care providers and that of the insured.

Thus, in 2006, basic health insurance was delegated to private health insurance companies. These insurance companies are financed for 50 % through the premiums they collect from the insured (e.g., in 2017, the annual nominal premium was 1,308 euros per person) and the other 50 % comes from the Dutch Health Insurance Fund, which collects income-dependent employer's contributions (45 %) and state contributions (5 %). The distribution of these funds depends on the health risk profile of the citizens insured with that insurer. The government has determined that health care must be accessible to all, including people on low incomes – this last group of people is therefore compensated for part of their health care premiums under the Care Allowance Act, with an income-dependent contribution (care allowance) being paid by the government. There is a deductible for incurred health care costs per year (in 2017, this was 385 euros), with the exception of the costs of general practitioner care and health care for children, which are always fully covered.

3.4.2 Financing general practitioner care in the Netherlands

The financing of primary care in the Netherlands is divided into three segments.
- The first segment concerns *basic primary care*. This is the type of care for which general practitioners are the first point of contact and where they have the role of gatekeeper for specialist care. There are three payments in this segment. Firstly, there is a capitation fee for each patient registered at the practice, differentiated according to age (younger than 65, 65 to 75, 75 to 85, 85 and older) and residential postcode area (type of neighbourhood). In addition, each consultation and home visit performed by general practitioner, practice assistant, practice nurse and mental health practice nurse can be declared. The Dutch Healthcare Authority (NZa) determines the rates in this segment.
- The second segment relates to the provision of *integrated care*. A bundled payment system was introduced for this type of care. Integrated care concerns care for people with type 2 diabetes, COPD, asthma and people with a high risk of cardiovascular disease. What is considered appropriate care for these groups of people is described in official care standards. A care group organises all care required for patients with one of these four conditions and the group receives financing according to a system of bundled payments, i.e., a fixed amount per patient per year. Usually, general practitioners in a particular region are themselves the owners of such a care group, which varies in size from 4 to 200 general practitioners. The care group organises the care and pays the participating general practitioners for the patients whom they treat in accordance with the guidelines. A contract with a health insurance company is a precondition for providing this integrated care under these conditions. This payment is in addition to the capitation fee obtained for basic care. Consultations and visits that relate to this integrated care form part of this bundled payment. Consultations relating to requests for help that do not fall under the four chronic conditions can be claimed separately from the health insurance company.
- The third segment refers to *pay-for-performance and innovation*. This also requires a contract with a health insurance company. The pay-for-performance payment relates to the accessibility of the practice (by telephone or in person), efficient prescription of medicines, and efficient referral to secondary care, and practice accreditation.

Research on primary care in 35 countries shows that patients of general medical practices in countries with capitation systems were more positive about their general practitioner than in cases where general practitioners were reimbursed through other means (Murante 2017; Schäfer et al. 2019).

3.4.3 Financing hospitals in the Netherlands

Hospitals in the Netherlands have both inpatient and outpatient departments and 24-hour emergency care departments. There are different types of hospitals: (1) General hospitals, providing practically all inpatient and outpatient care as well as emergency care. With the exception of the last category, all patient appointments require a referral from the general practitioner; (2) University hospitals (the Netherlands has 8 university hospitals, each with their own university medical centre which is connected

3

to the faculty of medicine. This is for tertiary specialist care; (3) Private, independently run hospitals for particular conditions in the so-called free segment, also called focus clinics (e.g., ophthalmology, and orthopaedic surgery centres), for day hospitalisations in an outpatient setting and 4 trauma centres. There are 85 general hospitals and 8 university hospitals in the Netherlands. Hospitals are required by law to be non-profit institutions. Hospitals are financed via a modified diagnosis-related group system (DRG): Diagnosis Treatment Combinations (DBC). Pharmaceutical care is part of these DBCs. Almost all specialists work at a hospital. They are either independent professionals who have organised themselves into hospital partnerships (60 %) or are on the hospital's payroll (40 %, especially at the university hospitals). At most hospitals, the independent specialists have organised themselves in Medical Specialist Companies to enable them to negotiate their remunerations with the hospital.

The following chapter will look more closely at *the core values and tasks of primary care* in the Netherlands. In addition, trends in changes in primary care are discussed that are relevant, not only for the Netherlands, but also for the rest of Europe and beyond.

3.5 Conclusions

This chapter briefly describes the organisation of primary care in the Netherlands, the tasks of general medical practices and the way those are financed. For the Dutch population, general practitioners are, generally, the first point of contact with the health care system. General practitioners in the Netherlands have a strong position in the health care system. The gatekeeper function in referrals to secondary care, patient enrolment at general medical practices, and the involvement of general practitioners in out-of-hours services all play an important role in this respect. Dutch general practitioners provide a wide range of care and are in a key position as care coordinators. Compared to other countries, the average time per consultation at the surgery hour is short, in the Netherlands, while the number of registered patients per practice is relatively large.

For more information, background or videos about this chapter scan the QR code.

SCAN ME

References

Batenburg, R., Van Der Velden, L., Vis, E., & Kenens, R. (2019). *Cijfers uit de registratie van huisartsen – een update van de werkzaamheidscijfers voor 2018 en 2019*. Nivel.

CBS (2020). Bevolking groeit naar ruim 17,4 miljoen inwoners. Accessed in April 2021 of ► https://www.cbs.nl/nl-nl/nieuws/2020/01/bevolking-groeit-naar-ruim-17-4-miljoen-inwoners.

Den Outer, B. (2019). Ketenzorg vraagt om een persoonsgerichte, geïntegreerde benadering. De eerste lijns platform voor strategie en innovatie. Accessed in in april 2021 van ► https://www.de-eerstelijns.nl/2019/10/ketenzorg-vraagt-om-een-persoonsgerichte-geintegreerde-benadering/.

Groenewegen, P. P., Heinemann, S., Greß, S., & Schäfer, W. (2015). Primary care practice composition in 34 countries. *Health Policy, 119*, 1576–1583.

Groenewegen, P., Schäfer, W. L. A., Schellevis, F. G., & Boerma, W. G. W. (2020). Kernwaarden van Nederlandse huisartsen in internationaal perspectief. *Huisarts en Wetenschap*, 63. ► https://ur.booksc.eu/book/83459723/e6c0db. (English abstract).

Klomp, M., Mutsaerts, J. F., Rempe, J., Neumann, R., & Vogelzang, F. (2020). *Denkraam integratie zorgprogramma's voor chronische aandoeningen*. InEen.

Murante, A. M., Seghieri, C., Vainieri, M., & Schäfer, W. L. A. (2017). Patient-perceived responsiveness of primary care systems across Europe and the relationship with the health expenditure and remuneration systems of primary care doctors. *Social Science and Medicine, 186*, 139–147.

Nederlandse Triage Standaard (2014). Nederlandse Triage Standaard, ketenstandaard voor triage in de acute zorg. Accessed in Juni 2021 of ► https://de-nts.nl/.

Nielen, M., Hek, K., Korevaar, J., Van Dijk, L., Weesie, Y. (2021). Cijfers zorgverlening huisartsen – Nivel Zorgregistraties Eerste Lijn. Accessed in Juni 2021 of ► www.nivel.nl ► https://www.nivel.nl/nl/nivel-zorgregistraties-eerste-lijn/cijfers-zorgverlening-huisartsen.

Rotar, A. M., Van Den Berg, M. J., Schäfer, W., Kringos, D. S., Klazinga, N. S. (2018). Shared decision making between patient and general practitioner about referrals from primary care: does gatekeeping make a difference? *PLos ONE* 13, e0198729.

Scaioli, G., Schäfer, W., Boerma, W. G. W., Spreeuwenberg, P., Schellevis, F. G., & Groenewegen, P. P. (2020). Communication between general practitioners and medical specialists in the referral process: A survey in 34 countries. *BMC Family Practice, 21*, 54.

Schäfer, W., Boerma, W. G. W., Schellevis, F. G., & Groenewegen, P. P. (2018). general practitioner practices as a one-stop shop: How do patients perceive the quality of care. A cross-sectional study in thirty-four countries. *Health Services Research, 53*, 2047–2063.

Schäfer, W. L. A., Boerma, W. G. W., Van den Berg, M. J., De Maeseneer, J., De Rosis, S., Detollenaere, J., et al. (2019). Are people's health care needs better met when primary care is strong? A synthesis of the results of the QUALICOPC study in 34 countries. *Primary Health Care Research & Development, 20*, e104.

Schäfer, W. L. A., Van Den Berg, M. J., Boerma, W. G. W., Schellevis, F. G., & Groenewegen, P. P. (2016a). Two decades of change in European general practice service profiles: Conditions associated with the developments in 28 countries between 1993 and 2012. *Scan J Primary Health Care, 34*(1), 97–110.

Schäfer, W. L. A., Van den Berg, M. J., Boerma, W. G. W., Schellevis, F. G., & Groenewegen, P. P. (2016c). Taakprofielen van huisartsen in Nederland en Europa. *Huisarts en Wetenschap, 59*(7), 286–291.

Schäfer, W. L. A., Van Den Berg, M. J., & Groenewegen, P. P. (2016b). De werkbelasting van huisartsen in internationaal perspectief. *Huisarts en Wetenschap, 59*(3), 94–101. (English abstract).

Stichting Beroepseer. (2019). Accessed in April 2021 of ► https://beroepseer.nl/blogs/trends-van-twintig-jaar-gezondheidszorg-in-22-europese-landen-deel-1/.

Toekomst Huisartsenzorg (2019). Accessed in Juni 2021 of ► https://toekomsthuisartsenzorg.nl/kerntak-en-in-de-praktijk/#zorg-coordinatie.

Van den Berg, M. J., Van Loenen, T., & Westert, G. P. (2016). Accessible and continuous primary care may help reduce rates of emergency department use. An international survey in 34 countries. *Family Practice, 33*, 42–50.

Van Kemenade, Y. W. (2018). *Health Care in Europe 2018. The finance and reimbursement systems of 11 European countries. EIT Health 2018*. Amsterdam: De boekdrukker.

Van Kemenade, Y. W. (2019). *Health Care in Europe 2019. The finance and reimbursement systems of 11 European countries. EIT Health 2019*. Amsterdam: De boekdrukker.

Vermeulen, L., Schäfer, W., Pavlic, D. R., & Groenewegen, P. (2018). Community orientation of general practitioners in 34 countries. *Health Policy, 122*, 1070–1077.

Volksgezondheidenzorg.info (2021). Accessed in April 2021 of ► https://www.volksgezondheidenzorg.info/onderwerp/eerstelijnszorg/regionaal-internationaal/huisartsenzorg.

4

I swear/promise to practise the art of medicine to the
best of my ability for the benefit of my fellow man.
I will care for the sick, promote health and
relieve suffering.

I will put the patient's interests first and respect
his/her views. I will do no harm to the patient.
I will listen and inform him/her well. I will keep
secret what has been entrusted to me.

I will advance the medical knowledge of myself and
others. I will recognise the limits of my possibilities.

Positive Health and the core values of Dutch primary care

© Bohn Stafleu van Loghum is an imprint of Springer Media B.V., part of Springer Nature 2022
M. Huber et al., *Handbook Positive Health in Primary Care*,
https://doi.org/10.1007/978-90-368-2729-4_4

4

> **Main messages**
>
> — In their project on the future of primary care in the Netherlands (Toekomst Huisartsenzorg), the group of professionals has formulated its four core values: person-oriented, medical generalist, continuous and together;
> — Positive Health is able to make a real contribution to all these core values;
> — Positive Health fits well with the trends and factors in primary care as described by the project *Toekomst Huisartsenzorg*.

Case no. 5: The core values of primary care and Hepatitis C

The re-evaluated core values of primary health care in the Netherlands, as formulated by the project on the future of primary care in the Netherlands (Toekomst Huisartsenzorg), are: **continuous, medical generalist, together and person-oriented (Toekomsthuisartsenzorg.nl** 2019a).

A vital 73-year-old woman, who had been registered **continuously** since birth at the same general practice, which she visited only sporadically but was familiar with, was also insured in Germany because of her work history. She visited the practice to obtain a referral to a Dutch internist. Her internist in Germany had advised her to undergo an expensive treatment with ledipasvir and sofosbuvir against hepatitis C that she probably contracted in 1970 after a blood transfusion. This treatment, however, was not reimbursed under her German insurance, but the Dutch insurance did cover such treatment. The costs involved would be more than EUR 50,000. The general practitioner remarked that he had not seen her for a long time and that he would like to know how she was doing before he would give her the requested referral letter. He asked her if she would like to fill out a questionnaire that would measure her level of satisfaction with respect to 6 dimensions of health.

This surprised her, but she did agree. After filling out the questionnaire, the general practitioner asked her to talk about her scores and what they meant to her. He visualised the overview of her health by writing her scores on the Positive Health spider web and drawing lines to connect them. He then asked her which score she would perhaps like to change, what that change would bring her and what a first step towards achieving this could be. She turned out to live a very meaningful life (in her opinion) and was very satisfied with the things she was able to do. She was even still working in her husband's company. She had no physical complaints and would not like to change anything. Therefore, she was not looking to receive any additional treatments. During the conversation, it became clear that the internist had been making her afraid of the consequences of not taking the treatment (cirrhosis of the liver, liver cancer). She herself was afraid of the possible side effects of treatment; she was doing well at that moment, and if she suffered because of the treatment, she would be worse off, in her eyes. During an extensive conversation where she felt supported in maintaining the status quo, she decided to refrain from treatment and the referral.

On a second visit to the same German internist, he said that she was doing herself an injustice; the likelihood of any side effects from the hepatitis C treatment was low (< 10 %) and the chances of being cured were high (> 90 %). This made her doubt again and she made a new appointment at the Dutch general practice. During this second visit, it became clear again that she was not experiencing any limitations herself, but that the medical advice from the German internist was making her doubt her decision

('He doesn't say that for nothing, does he? What should I do now?'). In order for the patient to be able to take control of her life, to consider the various choices carefully and to make decisions on the basis of facts, the necessity of treatment had to be better investigated.

The Dutch general practitioner explained in simple terms that he was a **medical generalist**. That he therefore was very capable of clarifying, together with the patient, exactly which answers she would need to find in order to make an informed choice for either treatment or non-treatment. But he also said that he had insufficient knowledge about hepatitis C to provide the answers to these questions himself. That the advice of a medical specialist was needed. **Together**, they decided that he would consult a Dutch gastroenterologist at the university hospital. This specialist confirmed the opinion of the German internist, but indicated that, given the duration of the chronic infection (which had started almost 50 years ago), an examination using a fibroscan should first determine whether there was liver fibrosis (Grintjes-Huisman and Tjwa 2018). Then, should there be no evidence of liver fibrosis, the risk of cirrhosis and the subsequent possibility of liver cancer would be negligible, in which case the patient could hold off on the procedure if she would want to, without putting her liver at risk. Based on this information, the patient decided to have a fibroscan done, which showed no evidence of fibrosis. This reassured the patient, her general practitioner and the gastroenterologist to such an extent that treatment with ledipasvir/sofosbuvir was abandoned. Two **personal** consultations with attention paid to the 6 dimensions of Positive Health, one consultation by telephone with the gastroenterologist and one fibroscan, together, prevented an expensive follow-up treatment of over EUR 50,000.

4.1 The project on the future of primary care

What does the future of general medical practice look like? What do general practitioners do and what not, and what are the values on which they base their profession? What can patients expect from their general practitioners and their practice? What do these values mean for the daily practice and how does the Positive Health philosophy relate to this? This chapter provides answers to this question. To have a better understanding of how Positive Health can be applied in primary care, it is important to zoom in on the core values and core tasks of general practitioners. These were developed as far back as in 1959 and were recalibrated in 2019. This chapter discusses how Positive Health plays a role in each core value of the general practitioner.

In January 1959, at a conference centre Woudschoten, the very first core values of Dutch primary care were formulated. At the time, there were three of such values: *person-oriented, generalist and continuous*. In 2012, the vision of the future of primary care *was elaborated* (Dutch College of General Practitioners and the Dutch National Association of General Practitioners 2012). The core values remained the same and concrete objectives were formulated for the period up to the year 2022. In 2019, another conference was organised in Woudschoten as part of the project on the future of primary care (Toekomst Huisartsenzorg), a cooperation between eight parties in primary care (Dutch National Association of General Practitioners, Dutch College of General Practitioners, InEen (association of primary care organisations), Het Roer Moet Om (manifest of concerned general practitioners, 'things need to change'), Landelijke

4

> ▣ **Table 4.1** Twelve themes that determine core values and core tasks for the profession of general practitioner (the project on the future of primary care: Toekomst Huisartsenzorg)
>
> | themes of the *Toekomst Huisartsenzorg* project |
> | --- |
> | 1. basic primary care |
> | 2. out-of-hours services |
> | 3. palliative care |
> | 4. gatekeeper role |
> | 5. prevention |
> | 6. practitioner–patient relationship |
> | 7. network care |
> | 8. education and training |
> | 9. research |
> | 10. innovation |
> | 11. final responsibility |
> | 12. contract type |

Organisatie van Aspirant Huisartsen (Dutch national organisation of general practitioners in training), Interfacultair Overleg Huisartsen (interfaculty consultative body for general medical practice), Landelijke Huisartsen Opleiders Vereniging (Dutch national association of general practitioner trainers) and the Vereniging Praktijkhoudende Huisartsen (Dutch association of general practice owners). The objective was *to reassess* the core values and tasks of general practitioners. In the run-up to this conference, 70 think tank sessions were held during which 1,300 general practitioners and GP trainees were able to express their views on 12 themes that were used for determining the core values (values that, in conjunction, would form the basis for the working methods of general practitioners) and core tasks of the profession (tasks that were indisputably part of the general practitioner's profession and would be essential for achieving the objectives) (▣ tab. 4.1). These were drawn up in advance by a committee of general practitioners (Toekomsthuisartsenzorg.nl 2019a).

During the think tank sessions, for each of the 12 themes, the participating general practitioners were asked: 'What are the options for general practitioners to contribute to this theme?' For each question, the response options were formulated on three levels, A, B and C (▣ fig. 4.1). Option A described the more traditional approach to the tasks of the general practitioner and primary care. Option B broadly described the vision as expressed in the project on future general medical care (Toekomstvisie Huisartsenzorg) by the Dutch College of General Practitioners and the Dutch National Association of General Practitioners (2012), and Option C described an alternative in which a conscious effort was made to follow the trends and factors visible in general practice. The coordinate system in ▣ fig. 4.1 shows, at a glance, what the answer options A, B and C entail. The x-axis shows for whom general practitioners and primary care are working, i.e., for their own patients or for the entire population. The y-axis shows by whom the task is performed; by general practitioners themselves or by care providers in the socio-medical network, of which general practitioners are a member.

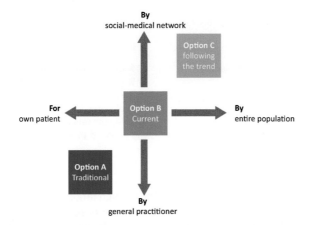

Figure 4.1   What options do general practitioners have to organise a task? Source: De Argumentenfabriek (2019a)

Now that the set-up of the project on the future of primary care has been described, it is interesting to see which answer option (A, B or C) is most in line with the ideas of Positive Health. For this purpose, first the trends and factors need to be elaborated.

4.2   Trends in primary care

What will be the challenges, trends and factors of primary care in the future? An important starting point is the fact that almost all people in the Netherlands are registered with a general medical practice. In addition, the committee of the project on the future of primary care (Toekomst Huisartsenzorg) has described over 40 trends and effects that are relevant to how the future of primary care is considered. These trends and effects are described in the appendix to this chapter. The trends and effects, from our perspective, can be summarised in two main developments that influence the content of general practitioner work and patient contact. The first development concerns changes in the continuity and person-oriented approach in primary care, and the second is about the increase in the primary care workload.

4.2.1   Changes in continuity and person-oriented care

Table 4.2 shows that, in the 1970–1990 period, general practitioners were predominately male, independently established in solo practices and worked fulltime. In 2019, the majority of general practitioners consisted of women (58 %), only 61 % of general practitioners were self-employed and only 15 % were working in solo practices. Over time, the average number of FTEs that general practitioners were working decreased from fulltime to 0.67 FTE. At the same time, the number of other practice staff members and the number of functions in the practice increased. Until the end of the previous century, it was common for small groups of general practitioners to share taking shifts (evenings, nights and weekends) for a small patient population (5,000–15,000); nowadays, 95 % of Dutch general practitioners are affiliated with

4

▢ **Table 4.2** Developments in primary care, in the Netherlands	
1970–1990	**2015–2020**
the majority of general practitioners consists of men; the majority of general practitioners has a solo practice; the vast majority works fulltime; all evening, night and weekend shifts are shared between small groups of practices	58 % of general practitioners are women (2019); 17 % have a solo practice (2017); on average, each represents 0.67 FTE; 95 % of general practitioners are connected to out-of-hours services which cover evening, night and weekend shifts

so-called out-of-hours services for all care for a much larger patient population (up to more than 150,000) included in so-called 'out-of-hours services' (primary emergency care) (Van Hien 2008). The amount of contact people are having with their *own* general practitioner has decreased, over time. Continuity is largely a task of the primary care practice and primary care as a whole.

Agreements about working methods and ICT currently play an important role in this respect. It is clear that the continuity and a person-oriented approach in primary care are less shaped by the contact patients have with their own general practitioner. When it comes to the person-oriented approach, the physician–patient relationship has also changed to a patient–physician relationship. The dominant working method of general practitioners over the past century could be called paternalistic (the doctor was the expert), whereas nowadays, patients are far more often regarded as equal partners in discussions and the emphasis is more on shared decision-making processes (Zorginstituut Nederland 2013). The patient is often better informed about the possibilities and is also more assertive (Jung et al. 2001; Broersen 2011).

4.2.2 Increase in workload

It almost seems like a paradox: on average, Dutch general practitioners work fewer hours today than they did in the past, but the workload has undeniably increased (also see ► Chap. 1). Two thirds of all general practitioners in the Netherlands consider the workload to be too large (Landelijke Huisartsen Vereniging 2018; Van den Brekel-Dijkstra et al. 2020). There are a number of reasons for this situation:

— The consumption of care is increasing. The number of patient contacts in the general medical practice is increasing. This also has a number of causes:
  — Increased ageing of the patient population;
  — Enormous increase in diagnostic possibilities, medical knowledge and treatment options;
  — Substitution of care (amongst other things, to curb health care costs) from the hospital and mental health care system to primary care;
  — The elderly remain living in their residential environment for longer (fewer residential and nursing homes, and other forms of extramural care, for example, mental health care and for people with an intellectual disability).
— The increased administrative burden in primary care plays a role in the increased workload (on average, general practitioners in the Netherlands spend almost 20 % of their time on non-patient-related activities) (Maes 2019).

— A shortage of health care professionals is starting to emerge. At the moment, this occurs mainly during holiday seasons, when insufficient capacity is available in residential care, but some regions are already showing general practitioner shortages, succession problems and a shortage of general practice staff.

The increase in the workload is noticeable in the level of sickness absence in health care. In the Netherlands, sickness absence amongst care providers has increased to a record high of 6.2 % (Barometer Nederlandse Gezondheidszorg 2020). In 2019, sickness absence in the health care sector was the highest of all sectors, with a Dutch national average of 4.4 % (Volksgezondheidenzorg.info 2020). The high level of sickness absence and staff shortages are due to ageing of both the general population and the labour force of the Dutch health care sector. There is a double impact. On the one hand, there is a greater demand for care while, on the other, the health care labour force is decreasing. This certainly applies to labour-intensive care sectors such as elderly care, mental health care, care for the disabled and child welfare. This also increases the workload for general practitioners. In addition, and also because of this, there is a rapidly changing supply of care providers due to changing contracts with municipalities and rapid personnel changes at municipal and societal organisations. General practitioners in the Netherlands experience almost daily that primary care is having to make up for care shortage in certain other areas of health care. (Het Roer Moet Om 2019 (i.e., manifest of concerned general practitioners)).

Requests for care addressed at general practitioners are also becoming increasingly complex as a result of substitution and people living at home for longer. In addition, the Dutch Government is asking for the population to be more self-reliant (participation society) and has implemented cutbacks in the decentralisation of health care and welfare from the national level to the municipal level. However, one in three people in the Netherlands has limited health skills, which means they find it difficult to obtain, understand and apply health care information. Part of this group is functional illiterate (in the Netherlands, this concerns around 15 % of the population, or 2.5 million people). Many citizens are thus less able to be self-reliant and, for them, the general practitioner is often also the first point of contact (Pharos 2020).

4.3 · New core values

In relation to the trends and factors identified in the project on the future of primary care, the committee asked the participants in the 70 think tank sessions to formulate, for each of the above 12 themes, which developments they would most like to see in primary care. They were asked which of the options A, B or C mentioned in ◨ fig. 4.1 were the most attractive, and to answer these questions: Why have you chosen this particular option? What arguments support this choice? Why do you find these arguments important? And what underlying values play a role in this? Further elaborations of response options A, B and C are shown in ◨ fig. 4.2.

These think tank sessions produced a set of wishes, arguments and points for discussion, which formed the input for a survey on the future of primary care in the Netherlands. All general practitioners and GP trainees subsequently received an invitation to voice their personal (but anonymous) opinion on the future of their profession

	Option A Traditional	Option B Current	Option C following the trend
Organisation	O The general practitioner provides primary care O The organisation is small in scale and consists of a general practitioner plus support team	O The general practitioner is part of a primary care facility O It is a medium-scale organisation	O The general practitioner is part of a social-medical network O The primary care facility and community teams are part of the social-medical network O It is a large-scale organisation
Role definition	O The general practitioner is ultimately responsible for a small support team O The general practitioner is gatekeeper	O The general practitioner is part of a team of general practitioners O The general practitioner is ultimately responsible for all health care provided by the primary care facility O The general practitioner may be jointly responsible for the organisation of the primary care facility	O The general practitioner is part of a multi-disciplinary team O The general practitioner is jointly responsible for the provision of care
Service provision	O The primary care focuses on medical questions O Only indicated and care-related prevention are part of the primary care	O The primary care facility is focused on medical and health issues	O The social-medical network is focused on medical, health and social issues
Domain definition	O The primary care is focused on its own patients	O The primary care facility is focused on patients in the district or village	O The social-medical network is focused on the entire population

Figure 4.2 Three options for the development of primary care: traditional, current and following trends. Source: De Argumentenfabriek (2019b)

through a survey. They were given two weeks to respond, during which time 3,109 general practitioners (out of more than 11,000) and 345 general practitioners in training (out of more than 700) completed the survey. The results showed that general practitioners were unanimous about the values and tasks that they consider important for the future of their profession.

The results from the survey showed that the original core values of general medical care from 1959 (*person-oriented, generalist and continuous)* were still rock solid, according to the committee of the project on the future of primary care (Toekomst Huisartsenzorg). They did, however, make them more specific, because *generalist* became *medical generalist*. According to the committee: 'It is precisely the broad medical knowledge of the general practitioner that is needed when deciding, together with the patient, what constitutes optimal care within a health care system that has become increasingly complex and fragmented, amongst other things due to super-specialisms. The strength of general medicine lies in medical generalism'. And for the *person-oriented* core value, the committee explicitly named the input of the patient. Also, a fourth core value was added: *together*. General practitioners can only provide optimal care if they do so together with others: their patient, their direct colleagues and other care providers.

4.4 New core tasks

In the relation to the core tasks, the committee also describes the essence of primary care: 'General practitioners are the medical generalists of the Dutch health care system. They offer general medical care to their patients during weekdays and make sure that, in medically urgent situations and for patients in the terminal phase, primary care is available 24 hours a day. General practitioners consider prevention to be of great importance and greatly contribute to this aspect, from their area of expertise, through indicated and care-related prevention. They also play an important role in coordinating the various types of care received by their patients. In addition to being ultimately responsible for the care provided by their own team, general practitioners are also often the liaison in the care chain and the first point of contact for other care providers who have medical questions about their patients'. The reassessed *four core values* and the *five core tasks* are illustrated in ◘ fig. 4.3. How Positive Health may contribute to the core values is discussed in ▶ sect. 4.5, and the contribution to the core tasks is addressed in ▶ Chap. 5.

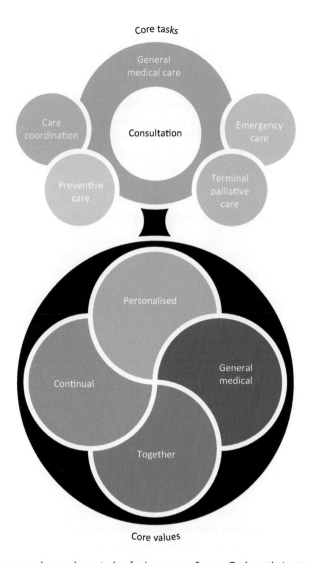

◘ **Figure 4.3**   The core values and core tasks of primary care. Source: Toekomsthuisartsenzorg.nl (2019b)

4

4.5 Positive Health's contribution to the core values

The four core values of *person-oriented*, *medical generalist*, *continuous* and *together* have been further elaborated by the committee with respect to the way general practitioners practice their profession in ◘ fig. 4.4. The remainder of this chapter provides a point-by-point elaboration and describes the relationship with Positive Health. The most important question here is about what the concept of Positive Health may contribute to the realisation of the core values.

Core tasks are covered by subsequent chapters. ► Chapter 5 discusses *general medical care during consultation*; ► Chapter 6 addresses *emergency and terminal palliative care*, and ► Chapter 7 looks at *care coordination* and *preventive care.*

The core value: person-oriented

> ▬ *General practitioners focus on the person rather than only on their disease or disabilities (Source: Project Toekomst Huisartsenzorg)*

Positive Health is particularly focused on making people feel that they are more than their disease or disability. ► Chapter 2 describes the development of the Positive Health concept and how it centres around the whole person. Practitioner and patient looking together at the six dimensions of Positive Health quickly reveals that there is more than the patient's disease or disability. ► Chapter 5 explains how this can be applied at the time of consultation; for example, by using a dialogue tool such as the 'spiders web'. The solution-oriented method ('what would you like to achieve', rather than 'what would you like to get rid of') also provides many tools and tips for how to do this.

> ▬ *General practitioners take the individual characteristics, needs and context of their patients into account (Source: Project Toekomst Huisartsenzorg)*

General practitioners are particularly capable of considering the whole person, from the individual characteristics, needs and context of their patients. The way of conducting consultations, under the Positive Health method, provides a wealth of possibilities for taking a fresh look at 'what it is that makes this particular person want to get up in the morning'. The method focuses on possibilities rather than on limitations. It encourages people to talk about what they hope for, what difference that would make in their lives, what would be effective, and what could be the first sign of progress, in this respect (see ► Chapter 5).

> ▬ *Together with their patients, general practitioners consider the type of care that is needed and suitable. (Source: Project Toekomst Huisartsenzorg)*

General practitioners have been trained to apply a medical-analytical model of thinking to determine the type of care that is needed. The most commonly used approach is the diagnosis–prescription model. Working with the person-oriented approach reveals that only a small number of the questions patients ask their general practitioner can be addressed in this way. Positive Health provides opportunities for general practitioners

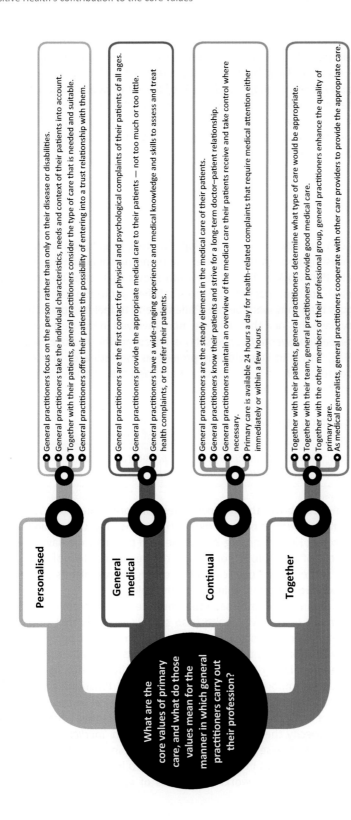

Personalised

- General practitioners focus on the person rather than only on their disease or disabilities.
- General practitioners take the individual characteristics, needs and context of their patients into account.
- Together with their patients, general practitioners consider the type of care that is needed and suitable.
- General practitioners offer their patients the possibility of entering into a trust relationship with them.

General medical

- General practitioners are the first contact for physical and psychological complaints of their patients of all ages.
- General practitioners provide the appropriate medical care to their patients — not too much or too little.
- General practitioners have a wide-ranging experience and medical knowledge and skills to assess and treat health complaints, or to refer their patients.

Continual

- General practitioners are the steady element in the medical care of their patients.
- General practitioners know their patients and strive for a long-term doctor–patient relationship.
- General practitioners maintain an overview of the medical care their patients receive and take control where necessary.
- Primary care is available 24 hours a day for health-related complaints that require medical attention either immediately or within a few hours.

Together

- Together with their patients, general practitioners determine what type of care would be appropriate.
- Together with their team, general practitioners provide good medical care.
- Together with the other members of their professional group, general practitioners enhance the quality of primary care.
- As medical generalists, general practitioners cooperate with other care providers to provide the appropriate care.

What are the core values of primary care, and what do those values mean for the manner in which general practitioners carry out their profession?

□ **Figure 4.4**   Elaboration of the core values. Source: Toekomsthuisartsenzorg.nl (2019b) to consider other appropriate solutions to the physical, mental, emotional and social challenges their patients are facing. Often, such solutions are found in the social domain (see ► Chap. 7). Using Positive Health, means general practitioners can change from being a *gatekeeper* to adopting the *role of liaison or coach*. Gatekeepers defend gates; they determine who may or may not enter through the gate, which in this case is secondary care. A coach or liaison, however, is someone who gives professional advice, showing people the options and discussing them so that, subsequently, patients can decide which path is the most suitable for them. This is an essential difference.

> — *General practitioners offer their patients the possibility of entering into a trust relationship with them(Source: Project Toekomst Huisartsenzorg)*

A relationship of trust takes time to develop, for trust to grow on both sides, which also requires investing enough time in interaction and personal contact. Research into general practices that work with Positive Health shows that, after the introduction of the Positive Health concept, patients are more satisfied about the primary care offered by these practices than they were before. Patients tend to feel heard and better understood, and they have the idea that they are more involved in the decision-making process during the *person-oriented* conversations based on the *Positive Health concept* (Jung et al. 2019). This is in line with the project on the future of primary care (Toekomst Huisartsenzorg), where the input of patients and the *person-oriented* core value is explicitly mentioned as an important element.

The core value: *medical generalist*

> — *General practitioners are the first contact for physical and psychological complaints of their patients of all ages(Source: Toekomst Huisartsenzorg)*

As already mentioned above, the original *generalist* core value from 1959 has been made more specific. *Generalist* became *medical generalist*. It is understandable that, in this project (Toekomst Huisartsenzorg 2019a), general practitioners have unequivocally stated that the core of their professional expertise lies in the field of general medical care and, thus, is related to the physical and psychological complaints of their patients. Within this context, two important things must be realised.

In the first place, an important lesson that must be learned from scientific research into the development of Positive Health (also see ► Chap. 2) is that physicians (and, therefore, also general practitioners), mostly, have a far narrower perception of health, compared to how their patients think about this. Patients, generally, consider for example meaningfulness, quality of life, participation and daily functioning as elements of health that are just as important as physical and mental functioning. General practitioners place a greater emphasis on physical than psychological complaints when defining health (Huber et al. 2016). It is therefore understandable that general practitioners wanted to further specify the core value of 'generalist' to 'medical generalist'. At the same time, it is good to realise that patients and people in general consider a broader context in defining health. This means there appears to be a discrepancy between the needs of the patients and the working methods of general practitioners. However, because patients, with their more general view of health, are the ones determining when and why they contact their general practitioner, consultations will continue to include many patient questions that are not strictly of a *general medical* nature. General practitioners will have to relate to this fact, whether they like it or not.

Secondly, many physical and even more psychological complaints have no *general medical* explanation. Studies show that, for almost 50 % of the physical complaints presented at the general practice, no physical explanation can be found (Olde Hartman et al. 2013). Because general practitioners nevertheless have to deal with these complaints, the Positive Health concept offers an excellent opportunity to explore the extent to which meaningfulness, quality of life, participation and daily functioning are being affected by the presented complaints (Wijergangs et al. 2017). Solution-oriented primary care may offer opportunities for patients to look at their physical and psychological complaints from a different perspective, and to explore how they might deal with those complaints differently, or consider being referred to a more appropriate care service (also see ▶ Chap. 5).

> ▬ *General practitioners provide the appropriate medical care to their patients — not too much or too little (Source: Toekomst Huisartsenzorg)*

Positive Health can deliver substantial added value, in this respect. An important role of general practitioners under the Dutch health care system is that of *gatekeeper*. Patient are only able to go see medical specialists if they are referred by their general practitioner. In this way, general practitioners prevent any unnecessary use of the often-expensive specialist care. However, when confronted with a patient requesting an inappropriate referral to secondary care, the *gatekeeper* cannot merely say 'no'. Together with the patient, the general practitioner will need to look at how the patient's question could be answered in a way that is appropriate and who could help to achieve that. General practitioners have a major role and responsibility in the many non-medical questions that are presented to them, not only to prevent any unnecessary use of medical-specialist care, but also to prevent this care from not being offered when needed.

Applying the concept of Positive Health in consultations means that, in such cases of non-medical solutions being needed, general practitioners can find answers outside the traditional medical model to these issues in a solution-oriented way that is appropriate for the situation of the patient concerned. This does not mean that general practitioners should be solving these issues, but rather that they can coach the patient into doing so for themselves or, together with the general practitioner, determine where to go to find the appropriate solution to the problem at hand. This makes the general practitioner not only a *gatekeeper, coach and liaison*, but also fits in well with the new core value of *'together'* and core task of *'care coordination'*.

> ▬ *General practitioners have a wide-ranging ex and skills to assess and treat health complaints, or to refer their patients (Source: Toekomsthuisartsenzorg)*

In this respect, it is essential that general practitioners continually consider whether the medical-analytical model of thinking is appropriate for the patient's needs, or whether the solution-oriented approach could be used from the concept of Positive

4

Table 4.3 Differences between the medical-analytical model and the solution-oriented model. (Source: Bannink and Jansen. Positive Health care. Solution-oriented approach in primary care (2017, p. 45) Included with permission of the publisher)

medical-analytical model	solution-oriented model
paradigm of the analysis	paradigm of the synthesis
cause-and-effect model	functional approach: do what works
examination → diagnosis → treatment = reduction in complaints	start by designing the desired outcome
diagnosis describes the deviation from the standard	value-free. Room for variety
focus on pathology and shortcomings	focus on possibilities and strengths
the practitioner is the expert	the practitioner takes a 'not knowing' perspective: asks questions and sees patient as co-expert
the practitioner is leading, advises	the practitioner invites an alternative way of thinking and taking action
the standard (usually the average of the 'healthy' population) determines the direction	the patient determines the direction: every patient is unique
the theory determines the conversation	the patient determines the conversation
according to protocol, based on averages	in keeping with the circumstances of the patient concerned, at this moment, in this context

Health. Bannink and Jansen (2017) see the solution-oriented model as an extension of Positive Health. The medical-analytical model could also be called the diagnosis–prescription model and is most appropriate for clearly described, diagnosable diseases and ailments, for which a treatment is available that leads to symptom reduction. However, for most requests for help, the medical-analytical model is not suitable and a solution-oriented approach would be far more effective.

Table 4.3 shows the differences between the medical-analytical model and the solution-oriented model. The solution-oriented approach is about promoting health in a broad sense, also when disease is involved, and thus is about promoting resilience. It is important that, in the future, all health care professionals are familiar with this approach. After all, the approach is not profession-specific, nor is the field of Positive Health. The knowledge and skills of the professionals of the future will demand a profession-specific, disease-oriented expertise from, for example, physicians, nurses and physiotherapists, which requires them to have been trained according to the medical-analytical model. In addition, the broad solution-oriented way of thinking will also have to be included in medical training. In this context, in the Netherlands, the advisory committee on innovation in health care professions and training (Adviescommissie Innovatie Zorgberoepen en Opleidingen) refers to the *T-shaped professional* as the professional of the future (Kaljouw and Van Vliet 2014; Van Vliet et al. 2016) (also see ► Chaps. 2 and 8).

The core value: *continuity*

> ▬ *General practitioners are the steady element in the medical care of their patients (Source: Toekomst Huisartsenzorg)*

The above-mentioned role change *from gatekeeper to coach or liaison* shows how general practitioners can be positioned as a consistent factor within Positive Health.

> ▬ *General practitioners know their patients and strive for a long-term doctor patient relationship relationship (Source: Toekomst Huisartsenzorg)*

The person-oriented approach of Positive Health contributes to general practitioners getting to know their patients better, particularly because there is more attention for meaningfulness, quality of life, participation and daily functioning. With Positive Health, both patient and care provider obtain more insight into what is important for the patient, apart from the context of a complaint. Within the network of care providers, one care provider can elaborate on what has already been discussed in a Positive Health conversation with another.

> ▬ *General practitioners maintain an overview of the medical care their patients receive and take control where necessary (Source: Toekomst Huisartsenzorg)*

The control function and the overview of medical care takes on a different meaning if this is looked at from the broad health perspective of Positive Health. After all, in the underlying concept of Positive Health (*the ability to adapt and self-manage in the face of the social, physical and emotional challenges of life*) control is already explicitly mentioned, namely as a skill of patients themselves. Where necessary, general practitioners can help to strengthen patients' ability to adapt and take control *themselves*, such as by injecting medical knowledge that patients do not or not yet have.

> ▬ *Primary care is available 24 hours a day for health-related complaints that require medical attention either immediately or within a few hours (Source: Toekomst Huisartsenzorg)*

Continuity has taken on a different meaning, compared to 1959. In health care in the Netherlands, these days, it is not people's own *general practitioner* but *primary care* (the sector in Dutch health care that relates to this) that is responsible for coordinating care, really knowing the patient, maintaining the overview, and being in control, 24 hours a day. This has undeniably become more complicated with the shift from care by the general practitioner to primary care. Also, with health complaints that need to be assessed either immediately or within a few hours and which particularly need to be approached through a medical-analytical thinking model, meaningful additions can be made from Positive Health and a solution-oriented working method to the policy to be pursued.

4

The question is how to arrange providing care 24 hours a day in the general medical practice – perhaps arrange that everyone has the same basic knowledge about Positive Health; for example, by offering courses and intervision, at the level of the general practice group?

The core value: *together*

> — *Together with their patients, general practitioners determine what type of care would be appropriate (Source: Toekomst Huisartsenzorg)*

Compared to 1959, '*together*' is a new core value of primary care. It is quite understandable that, in the past, general practitioners were the experts in relation to their patients, with a more directive and paternalistic style. Today's patients are supposed to be co-experts, who are much better able to help determine the direction of care and take control themselves. Appropriate care has therefore become the search for a good balance between paternalism and consumerism (Jung et al. 2001), which can only be achieved together.

> — *Together with their team, general practitioners provide good medical care (Source: Toekomst Huisartsenzorg)*

In the 1950s, in the Netherlands, most general medical practices consisted of a solo general practitioner and a colleague/spouse, whereas today the organisation of the general medical practice is much more complex. Positive Health, therefore, becomes a team effort. ▶ Chapter 6 elaborates on how Positive Health can contribute to the provision of good medical care by the general medical practice.

> — *Together with the other members of their professional group, general practitioners enhance the quality of primary care (Source: Toekomst Huisartsenzorg)*

Good quality of primary care based on the '*Quadruple Aim*' principle means: better care, better health, greater affordability, a better-balanced workload and job satisfaction. This goes beyond the use of evidence-based guidelines. The first pilot projects of general medical practices working with Positive Health are indicating that patients are more satisfied with this type of care, as well as showing that care becomes cheaper and that the job satisfaction of general practitioners increases and the workload can decrease (Jung et al. 2019).

> — *As medical generalists, general practitioners cooperate with other care providers to provide the appropriate care (Source: Toekomst Huisartsenzorg)*

When explaining the core tasks of primary care, the committee of the project on the future of primary care (Toekomst Huisartsenzorg) stated: 'General practitioners play an important role in the coordination of the care their patients receive'. General practitioners are not only ultimately responsible for the care provided by their own team, but they are also often the connecting factor in the care chain. They ensure control of the care provided to their patients with complex medical problems. They are also the first point of contact for other care providers with medical questions about their patients. General practitioners and their team help patients with social problems to find the right care. ► Chapter 7 discusses the contribution of Positive Health to the realisation of the core value of 'together', amongst other things by showing how you can work from the concept of Positive Health together with professionals and residents in the medical-social domain, for example by setting up regional Positive Health networks. For general practitioners who want to work with Positive Health, it is helpful if their cooperating partners approach the patients from the same perspective. This means that they train together and develop a common vision and 'language'. A Positive Health network can play an important role in this respect. ► Chapter 7 discusses this in more detail.

4.6 Challenges for the future of primary care

The committee of the project on the future of primary care asked the participants in the 70 think tank sessions in relation to the 44 trends and factors identified to formulate how they themselves would like to see primary care develop. Three options were presented for each of the 44 trends, with the question of which was the most attractive. Option A represented the traditional variant (the general practitioner as practice owner, gatekeeper, for medical questions), option B was called the current variant (the general practitioner as part of a primary care facility, focused on patients in a district or village) and option C was called trend-following (the general practitioner as part of a social medical network, part of a multidisciplinary team, focused on the entire population), see ◻ fig. 4.2. An elaboration on the answer options in ◻ figs. 4.1 and 4.2 shows that, from the concept of Positive Health, primary care is most in line with option C, the option in which the described trends and factors visible in primary care are consciously taken into account.

It is not possible to deduce, from the available data from De Argumentenfabriek (2019a, b), which option general practitioners in the Netherlands at the time of the survey thought would best fit the future of primary care. As authors of this handbook, we were curious to know what Positive Health might mean in relation to the 44 trends and factors described by the committee of the project on the future of primary care (Toekomsthuisartsenzorg.nl 2019a, b). The trends are divided into the following groups: (a) organisation; (b) staffing of care; (c) quality and type of care; (d) training and innovation; and (e) care policy and funding.

To determine the possible impact of these trends on working with Positive Health or conversely what effect Positive Health could have on the trends, a digital focus group was organised in July 2020 with 8 professionals from general medical practices, 5 of them practitioners. The appendix (◘ tab. 4.4) shows the comments made per trend. In summary, the trends to which Positive Health can make an important contribution are:

— *Continuity of health care*
— *Person-oriented health care*
— *Workload*

4

■ **Continuity of health care and Positive Health**

The decreasing continuity of the individual general practitioner in favour of that of the general medical practice, goes hand in hand with the increase in attention for a more person-oriented focus, rather than a more disease-oriented approach. Working from the concept of Positive Health offers optimal opportunities to discuss the *real needs of patients*. Essential, here, is for general practitioners to realise that their work is on the interface between medical and non-medical care and within that framework try to interpret their patients' questions. More than 90 % of the requests for help are solved by general practitioners together with their patient (Cardol et al. 2004). And if something cannot be solved in this way, the general practitioner knows what is being offered in secondary care and is able to discuss the possibilities with the patient involved. General practitioners are expected to be able to assess which medical and diagnostic steps are useful for a particular patient.

■ **Person-oriented health care and Positive Health**

Analogous to the above, general practitioners have an equal level of responsibility for questions outside the medical domain. Positive Health can thus counterbalance the diminished personal continuity of the general practitioner by contributing to the personalisation of general medicine. This requires that primary care not only focuses on the patients in the practice, but also on the local population as a whole (i.e., in the community or village). It is also important that the general medical practice, in consultation with the patient, tries to formulate answers not only to medical questions, but also to health-related and social questions. In order to achieve this, primary care facilities, community teams and civil organisations must be part of a larger care network, so that questions can be directed to the right place. ▶ Chapter 7 elaborates on this in greater detail.

■ **Increased workload and Positive Health**

Positive Health offers hopeful perspectives with regard to the increasing workload. Patients seem to be happier with the type of care they receive when it is organised according to the Positive Health concept. The same applies to the degree of job satisfaction experienced by the health care professionals themselves. In experiments that combine more time for patient and Positive Health, the workload seemed to actually diminish, as well as the costs related to that care (Jung et al. 2019).

4.7 Conclusions

This chapter deals with the relationship of Positive Health with the recently established core values of primary care in the Netherlands and the options general practitioners have for fulfilling their task. The described trends in primary care, from our perspective, can be summarised in two main developments that influence the content of general practitioner work and patient contact. The first development concerns changes in the continuity of primary care, with less personal contact with the same general practitioner, but the care is more person-oriented. The second concerns the primary care workload, which has undeniably increased. This chapter also discusses the contribution of Positive Health to the identified trends and the core values of primary care (*person-oriented, medical generalist, continuous* and *together*).

▪ **Conclusion of Part I**

This concludes Part I, which discusses the *why* question of this handbook. Why do general practitioners want to do things differently in primary care (▶ Chapter 1)? Followed by the question of *how*. How would they like to do things differently, based on the concept of Positive Health (▶ Chaps. 2 and 4)? ▶ Chapter 3 describes the Dutch health care system, and primary care in particular.

Part II is the practical part of the handbook and discusses the *what* question. What does this mean for the patient–physician conversation in the consulting room (▶ Chap. 5), the organisation of the general medical practice (▶ Chap. 6), the cooperation between the practice and the community (▶ Chap. 7), and for medical training and national policy (▶ Chap. 8)?

Appendix 4.1 Trends and factors in primary care and in relation to Positive Health

The committee of the project on the future of primary care (Toekomst Huisartsenzorg, 2019a) describes 44 trends and factors in primary care. These 44 trends are divided into groups of internal and external trends and factors. To determine the possible impact of these trends on applying the Positive Health concept or, vice versa, what effect Positive Health could have on the trends, a number of general practitioners were invited to participate in a survey during a digital focus group meeting. ◻ Table 4.4a shows some of the comments that were made.

4

⬛ Table 4.4a   Internal trends and factors: Organisation of health care in the Netherlands

type of Trend	relation to Positive Health
The Netherlands has out-of-hours services at 120 locations; 95 % of general practitioners are affiliated with such services.	Working via out-of-hours services reduces health care continuity. A larger number of patients are unknown to the treating physician, which can lead to a less person-oriented approach.
Practising general practitioners are increasingly delegating their out-of-hours care to others.	Contributes to the practitioner's own health and reduces the workload.
The number of consultations, both in person and by telephone, and treatments at out-of-hours services is increasing.	This leads to an increase in workload, less job satisfaction, a firefighting mentality, and does not promote patients taking control themselves.
The number of general practitioners (including substitutes) has increased from 8,612 in 2006 to 11,834 in 2016.	A larger number of general practitioners should provide more time for their patients. Working part-time means that general practitioners could pay more attention to their own health.
The number of general medical practices has increased from 4,469 in 2006 to 5,028 in 2016.	The growth in the number of general practitioners is larger than that in the number of practices. This therefore means that there are more practitioners per practice, which in turn will decrease continuity.
Increasing numbers of general practitioners are working in a practice with more than one practitioner.	More general practitioners per practice may also lead to more cooperation and possibly easier cooperation with, for instance, the social domain. This may lead to differentiation between general practitioners, something that is not possible in solo practices.
The number of patients per standard general medical practice is declining, while the number of consultations is rising.	When the real issues remain unsolved, patients will keep coming back to the practice. Because of its person-oriented approach, Positive Health could reverse this trend.
General practitioners work with very diverse forms of cooperation.	This makes it more difficult to provide a blueprint for working with Positive Health. There are multiple perspectives. Positive Health can be the unifying factor in cooperation, with a shared vision and language.
For patients with chronic diseases, general practitioners in the Netherlands are organising multi-disciplinary coordinated care for 115 care groups.[a]	This leads to equal treatment across all disciplines, but is often also disease-oriented rather than person-oriented. There is the risk of ticking boxes of indicators, instead of those of patient needs. There should be more care provided within a health care network, because this includes more disciplines. Multi-disciplinary coordinated care may provide a platform for training general practitioners and informing them about Positive Health.
In the Netherlands, general practitioners spend 18 % of their time on non-patient-related activities, such as in meetings.	The more meetings, the less time for patients. On the other hand, to start working with Positive Health will also require some time to organise, by all those involved. Cooperation is a positive thing. Alternative dialogue, offering another type of care.

[a]A *care group* organises all the care necessary for managing specific chronic conditions (e.g., diabetes). Care groups are mostly organised by general practitioners in a certain region, and vary in size from 4 to 200 physicians. The care group coordinates the care and remunerates the care providers involved.

◼ **Table 4.4b** Internal trends and factors: Staffing health care in the Netherlands

type of Trend	relation to Positive Health
The number of consultations that people have with their own general practitioner has declined.	This may reduce continuity, but may also be a conscious decision by the patient. Shifting tasks can be more efficient, making time for a longer conversation with a patient's own general practitioner, while straightforward issues can be resolved through self-care or by the practice assistant or specialised nurse. It is a good thing that general practitioners do not have to do everything themselves.
Increasingly often, general practitioners work with medical support staff.	If the staff is well trained and enthusiastic about Positive Health, this need not be a disadvantage. In addition, it may also give general practitioners more time to apply the alternative dialogue with their patients.
General medical practices are becoming ever-larger organisations, while the practitioners have not been trained to be entrepreneurs.	This may distract from working with Positive Health; much of general practitioners' time and energy is being spent on tasks they have not been trained to perform. The role of practice manager seems important, in this respect, also for managing Positive Health themes.
Since 2016, women have been in the majority amongst general practitioners, and their share is still increasing.	
General practitioners are increasingly working part-time (4 in 10 men, 8 in 10 women).	It is important to consider the personal balance between private and professional life. However, working part-time may be a disadvantage with respect to continuity and implementation of Positive Health.
The number of general practitioners with an employment contract or who work as substitutes is increasing.	General practice owners may be able to exert more influence when they seek to implement the Positive Health concept. Changes due to substitutes can have a negative impact on continuity. Should experience with Positive Health or the preparedness to train as such be a criterion when choosing an HIDHA[a] or substitute? Discussing Positive Health with regional association of substitute general practitioners → striving for continual offer of training courses (as the inflow of newcomers is continuous).
In certain Dutch regions, there is a shortage of general practitioners, successors and substitutes.	This threatens working with Positive Health, 'the work needs to be done'; possibly an incentive for citizens' initiatives and self-management.

(continued)

4

◨ **Table 4.4b** (continued)

type of Trend	relation to Positive Health
Hardly any young general practitioners are choosing to become general practice owners.	For young general practitioners, working with Positive Health depends on whether the practice at which they are employed does so. They have less influence on shaping the need for working with Positive Health. Practices where Positive Health has been implemented may be more appealing to young general practitioners to apply to work there as HIDHA.
General practitioners are experiencing a heavy workload and, often, look at their profession as a job rather than a calling.	Part of the workload may be caused by the way general practitioners work. Using the Positive Health concept may relieve part of the pressure and increase job satisfaction. Considering the profession a calling may contribute to an effective implementation of Positive Health.

[a]HIDHA = general practitioner employed at a general medical practice.

◨ **Table 4.4c** Internal trends and factors: quality and type of health care offered in the Netherlands

type of Trend	relation to Positive Health
General practitioners are performing increasingly more specialist medical tasks (i.e., substitution of tasks previously performed by medical specialists).	More medical specialisation in general medical practices may lead to less attention for Positive Health, is often disease-oriented, but may also lead to less medicalisation for patients who would otherwise have been referred to a hospital.
General practitioners organise multi-disciplinary coordinated care for their patients with chronic diseases.	Multi-disciplinary coordinated care, often, is disease-oriented rather than aimed at health and the patients themselves. The challenge is to apply Positive Health also in these cases. Positive Health may provide a large incentive for self-management and compliance. For example, in line with the core task of *preventive care*.
Primary care is increasingly locked down in protocols.	It feels like being boxed in and limits the scope for a broader perspective. Positive Health is rather customised and provides scope for professionals to work in a different way.
Increasing numbers of general practitioners are specialising in a particular medical theme.	Training is disease-oriented, it is important to see the whole person, on the other hand, it also provides the opportunity to look at a medical theme through general practitioner's glasses with attention for the person behind the disease.
General practitioners feel obligated to participate in the annual NHG practice accreditation.	Feeling obligated does not release energy. In practice accreditation, the implementation of Positive Health may be chosen as a pathway to improvement.

◻ Table 4.4c (continued)

type of Trend	relation to Positive Health
Internal quality systems, review groups and mutual reviews are demanding on the time and energy of general practitioners.	Introduce the importance of person-oriented care into quality systems, review groups and mutual reviews.
General practitioners' working methods are becoming more defensive due to the ever-louder call for transparency.	This does not contribute to Positive Health. It also seems related to locums and substitutes (who know patients less well, are anxious not to miss any medical matters, and this causes them to be more defensive in their work). Meet with supervisory and financing parties in an effort to achieve acknowledgement for Positive Health.
General practitioners rebel against an increasing administrative burden on their workload.	Less administration, more time for patients.

◻ Table 4.4d Internal trends and factors: training, innovation, and funding of health care in the Netherlands

type of Trend	relation to Positive Health
General practitioners in certain regions are unable to fill their trainee positions for new practitioners.	Threatens continuity.
General practitioners are offering too few internships to support staff, such as practice assistants. The options for digital diagnostics, treatments and communication are increasing in primary care.	The heavy workload offers little room for investing in the future, and threatens continuity in primary care.
Insufficient standardisation and non-communicating ICT systems are hampering the work of general practitioners.	Digital Positive Health questionnaires are not very compatible with HIS software (i.e., the Dutch general practitioners digital information system) which is considered a disadvantage.
The target for 2022, for general practitioners to participate structurally in scientific research, has not yet been achieved.	Good monitoring of what Positive Health can do for both patients and general practitioners is very important for the foundation of the concept.
General practitioners have relatively little influence on the contracting of primary care in their region.	Also creates the feeling of having little influence on including Positive Health in those contracts or, for example, having more time for patients.
General practitioners are organising themselves in care groups for health insurance contracting of multi-disciplinary coordinated care.	Is this more likely to enable the inclusion of Positive Health in contracting? Currently, still too much focus on disease.

4

■ **Table 4.4e** External trends and factors: patients, innovation, type of health care offered, policy and funding of health care in the Netherlands

type of Trend	relation to Positive Health
Virtually all citizens (16.4 million people) are registered at a general medical practice.	Important for working with Positive Health: continuity, with possibilities to address medicalisation and consumerism.
The number of elderly people is rising, three quarters of those over the age of 75 have one or more chronic diseases.	Sense of purpose and learning to cope with limitations, meaningful living, loneliness – all themes that Positive Health deals with, especially in the case of the elderly.
When there are shortcomings in care elsewhere, patients look to their general practitioner as the ultimate provider of care.	Major responsibility for general practitioners, looking closely at what is medical and what is not, general practitioners as final support or waste basket? Role of practitioner as coach and liaison.
Patients expect more from their general practitioners, because they are better informed.	Promote personal control, important to place certain responsibilities with patients themselves, risk of medicalisation.
The diversity of patients is increasing and with it the complexity in the consulting room.	Requires a broad view, Positive Health can help with that, general practitioners will be able to enjoy complex patients more through Positive Health. Having more time for this is important; customised work is required! Are there special concerns about working with Positive Health in people with low socioeconomic status (SES), migration background or low health skills?
Patients live in a 24-hours economy and often want care when it is convenient for them.	Patients must learn to arrange their own care to some extent. Positive Health can help with that.
Technological applications such as e-health and domotics enable remote care.	Remote Positive Health? Should also be possible to do with video calls, real-life meetings remain important; for example, for the non-verbal element of the issue. Because not everyone has to come in for an in-person consultation, there is more time available?
From 2020 onwards, patients are entitled to access their electronic health record (EHR).	Stimulates self-management and insight and can thus contribute to Positive Health.
Care providers must handle privacy-sensitive (digital) data of patients with care.	How to display the spider web in the dossier? May contain personal data. Customisation is required.
Around 2.5 million people (15 % of the Dutch population) have difficulties reading and writing and working with computers.	Spider web form for patients with functional illiteracy helps to have the alternative dialogue with this group.

For more information, background or videos about this chapter scan the QR code.

SCAN ME

References

Bannink, F., & Jansen, P. (2017). Positieve gezondheidszorg. Oplossingsgericht werken in de huisartspraktijk. Amsterdam: Pearson Benelux B.V.

Barometer Nederlandse Gezondheidszorg. (2020). Accessed in September 2021 of. ► https://assets.ey.com/content/dam/ey-sites/ey-com/nl_nl/topics/health/barometer-zorg/2020/ey-barometer-nederlandse-gezondheidszorg-2020.pdf

Broersen, S. (2011). Shared Decision Making voor beginners. *Medisch Contact*. Accessed in April 2021 of ► https://www.medischcontact.nl/nieuws/laatste-nieuws/artikel/shared-decision-making-voor-beginners.htm.

Cardol, M., Van Dijk, L., De Jong, J. D., De Bakker, D. H., & Westert, G. P. (2004). *Tweede nationale studie naar ziekten en verrichtingen in de huisartspraktijk. Huisartsenzorg: wat doet de poortwachter?* Utrecht/Bilthoven: NIVEL/RIVM.

De Argumentenfabriek (2019a). *Toekomst huisartsenzorg. Herijking kernwaarden en kerntaken*. Accessed in April 2021 ► http://toekomsthuisartsenzorg.nl/wp-content/uploads/2019/01/Boek-Herijkte-Kernwaard-en-Kerntaken.pdf.

De Argumentenfabriek (2019b). *Toekomst huisartsenzorg. Gespreksleidraad denksessie*. Accessed in April 2021 of ► https://www.argumentenfabriek.nl/media/2980/gespreksleidraad_toekomsthuisartsenzorg_v18juli2018.pdf.

Grintjes-Huisman, K. J. T., Tjwa, E. (2018). Elastografie van de lever met de Fibroscan®. Bijblijven 34, 541–545. ► https://doi.org/10.1007/s12414-018-0338-y.

Het Roer Moet Om (2019). *Patiënten tussen wal en schip. Hoe gebrek aan samenhang vooral de kwetsbare patiënten treft*. Accessed in April 2021 of ► https://hetroermoetom.nu/pdf/Boekje-HETROERMOETOM-Patient-tussen-wal-en-schip.pdf.

Huber, M., Van Vliet, M., Giezenberg, M., et al. (2016). Towards a 'patient-centred' operationalisation of the new dynamic concept of health: A mixed methods study. *BMJ Open, 5*, e010091.

Jung, H. P., Wensing, M., & Grol, R. (2001). Tussen paternalisme en consumentisme. Het dilemma van de huisarts. *Huisarts en Wetenschap, 44*, 594–600.

Jung, H. P., Liebrand, S., & Van Asten, C. (2019). Uitkomsten van het hanteren van positieve gezondheid in de praktijk. *Bijblijven, 35*, 26–35.

Kaljouw, M., & Van Vliet, K. (2014). *Naar nieuwe zorg en zorgberoepen: De contouren*. Diemen: Zorginstituut Nederland.

Kaljouw, M., & Van Vliet, K. (2015). Naar nieuwe zorg en zorgberoepen: de contouren. Zorginstituut Nederland: Diemen.

Landelijke Huisartsen Vereniging (LHV) (2018). *Meer tijd voor de patiënt. Uitkomsten onderzoek*. Utrecht: Newcom Research & Consultancy B.V.

Maes, A. (2019). *Variabelen bij capaciteit huisartsenzorg bijtijds agenderen*. Accessed in April 2021 of ▶ https://zorgenstelsel.nl/variabelen-bij-capaciteit-huisartsenzorg-bijtijds-agenderen/.

Nederlands Huisartsen Genootschap (NHG), Landelijke Huisartsen Vereniging (LHV). (2012) *Toekomstvisie Huisartsenzorg. Modernisering naar menselijke maat. Huisartsenzorg in 2022*. Utrecht: LHV NHG.

Olde Hartman, T. C., Blankenstein, A. H., Molenaar, A. O., Bentz van den Berg, D., Van der Horst, H. E., Arnold, I. A., et al. (2013). NHG-Standaard Somatisch Onvoldoende verklaarde Lichamelijke Klachten (SOLK). *Huisarts en Wetenschap, 56*(5), 222–230.

Pharos (2020). *Factsheet juni 2020. Laaggeletterdheid en beperkte gezondheidsvaardigheden*. Accessed in April 2021 of ▶ https://www.pharos.nl/factsheets/laaggeletterdheid-en-beperkte-gezondheidsvaardigheden/.

Toekomsthuisartsenzorg.nl. (2019a). Accessed in April 2021 of ▶ https://toekomsthuisartsenzorg.nl/.

Toekomsthuisartsenzorg.nl. (2019b). Accessed in April 2021 of ▶ https://toekomsthuisartsenzorg.nl/downloads/.

Van den Brekel-Dijkstra, K., Cornelissen, M., & Van der Jagt, L. (2020). De dokter gevloerd. Hoe voorkomen we burn-out bij huisartsen? *Huisarts en Wetenschap, 63*(7), 40–43. ▶ https://doi.org/10.1007/s12445-020-0765-8.

Van Hien, A. (2008). *CPB Memorandum. Ontwikkelingen rondom de rol van de Nederlandse huisarts*. Accessed in April 2021 of ▶ https://www.cpb.nl/sites/default/files/publicaties/download/memo202.pdf.

Van Vliet, K., Grotendorst, A., & Roodbol, P. (2016). *Anders kijken, anders leren, anders doen. Grensoverstijgend leren en opleiden in zorg en welzijn in het digitale tijdperk*. Diemen: Zorginstituut Nederland.

Volksgezondheidenzorg.info (2020). Accessed in April 2021 of ▶ https://www.volksgezondheidenzorg.info/onderwerp/ziekteverzuim/cijfers-context/bedrijfssector.

Wijgergangs, L., Ras, T., & Reijmerink, W. (2017). *Signalement Zingeving in zorg*. Den Haag: ZonMw.

Zorginstituut Nederland (2013). *Richtlijnen en shared decision making in de praktijk*. Accessed in April 2021 of ▶ https://www.zorginzicht.nl/ontwikkeltools/ontwikkelen/richtlijnen-en-shared-decision-making-in-de-praktijk.

Part II Applying Positive Health in primary care in the Netherlands & Positive Health from an international perspective

Contents

Chapter 5

Macro
Regional /
national

Meso
District / community

Micro
Practice / organisation

Nano
Patient / citizen

I swear/promise to practise the art of medicine to the
best of my ability for the benefit of my fellow man.
I will care for the sick, promote health and
relieve suffering.

I will put the patient's interests first and respect
his/her views. I will do no harm to the patient.
I will listen and inform him/her well. I will keep
secret what has been entrusted to me.

I will advance the medical knowledge of myself and
others. I will recognise the limits of my possibilities.

Positive Health in the consulting room

© Bohn Stafleu van Loghum is an imprint of Springer Media B.V., part of Springer Nature 2022
M. Huber et al., *Handbook Positive Health in Primary Care*,
https://doi.org/10.1007/978-90-368-2729-4_5

> **Main messages**
> - Positive Health starts with you.
> - The spider web facilitates starting up a conversation.
> - The alternative dialogue means making contact, listening carefully and helping the other person find their own solutions.
> - Who is doing the work? When people find their purpose in life, they will take the reins more easily.
> - Time is not only about the clock; one of the key elements is to slow down. Sometimes it is better to lean back and listen with intent.
> - This chapter discusses with whom you can have a Positive Health conversation, based on the core tasks.

5.1 Positive Health in the consulting room

Part I of this book describes how the concept of Positive Health offers possibilities to look at disease and health differently, in a way that is more solution-oriented and more focused on a meaningful life. This approach may offer a solution to the increasing pressure that general practitioners will be facing in the near future. Paying attention to a meaningful life is a central element of Positive Health and stems from the basis on which the concept was founded. Part 1 contains a description of the relationship between Positive Health and the recently established core values of primary care in the Netherlands and the options general practitioners have for carrying out their core tasks from a connection with Positive Health.

Part II, which starts with this chapter, becomes more practical and describes how Positive Health can be applied to the various areas of your work. Here, we chose the four levels of De Maeseneer's pyramid: nano, micro, meso and macro (De Maeseneer 2017).

This chapter is about Positive Health in relation to one-on-one personal contact – the nano level. It is the level of the patient, the person and you yourself as general practitioner. It describes how you can use Positive Health in the consulting room, but also talks about the impact this may have on your own life. After all, apart from being a professional, you are also a human being.

To get straight to the point of this chapter: we did not accidentally choose Antoine de Saint-Exupéry's quote *'If you want to build a ship, don't drum up the men to gather wood, divide the work and give orders. Instead, teach them to yearn for the vast and endless sea'* as the motto for this book.

This quote (2012) describes a hierarchy of motivations; orders given by a manager or professional are generally not the most effective way of achieving a certain goal. On the contrary, the dreams and motives of the people themselves are what sets them in motion and, in addition, establishes order in their activities. This will ultimately lead to the desired outcome – in the case of Antoine de Saint-Exupéry to the building of a ship. In the context of a general medical practice, this may consist of job satisfaction and cooperation between care providers, and to a healthier lifestyle and/or greater sense of well-being for the patients. Whether we call them dreams, motives or values is not that important – it is about what gives meaning and significance to people's lives, and about what they truly *want* rather than what they feel they *have* to do.

The focus in Positive Health on a meaningful life stems from the foundation on which the concept is based. As discussed in ▶ Chap. 2, according to Huber's research, the interviewees recommended a meaningful life as an addition to the conceptual model of medical-analytical thinking in health care. The literature (▶ sect. 2.5) supports the importance of placing meaningfulness at the centre of people's lives as a guiding principle, and the authors' practical experiences have shown how effective this can be.

However, this type of approach requires something other than what physicians are primarily trained to do. The T-shaped professional of the future, as described in ▶ sect. 2.6 may contribute to putting this new approach into practice. Traditionally, physicians are trained in the vertical bar of the T, expertise and disease-oriented, from a medical-analytical perspective. Working with Positive Health, however, means physicians are actively focusing on the horizontal bar of the T, which has a person-oriented, broad health and solution-oriented fucus. As a physician, you do not think in terms of control, but of promoting adaptation and resilience (◼ fig. 2.5).

The dialogue that is in line with this approach, as also described in Part I, is what in the Positive Health concept is called *the alternative conversation* or *alternative dialogue*. In Positive Health, the *spider web* is the tool that contributes to holding this alternative dialogue. As this approach is currently not, or not yet, included in the medical school curriculum, experience has shown that becoming familiar with this approach does require some training (see ▶ https://www.iph.nl/en/participate/training).

Below, first, a number of tips, tools and materials are introduced. These are discussed to explain how they can be applied when starting to use Positive Health with your patients.

5.2 Tools and materials – My Positive Health

5.2.1 The tools

▪ **Adults tool**

The basic spider web of My Positive Health, together with a list of questions (see ▶ www.mypositivehealth.com, see ▶ https://www.iph.nl/en/participate/free-downloads), has 42 related aspects that are distributed over 6 dimensions. This is an elaboration into more simplified wording of the original spider web from the study by Huber (2016) which contained 32 aspects, as the original, more scientific language was considered too complicated for everyday use. This prompted a panel of content experts to rework the wording into simpler language and to add positively formulated questions. Language experts, subsequently, converted the content to the CEFR B1 language level. This is how version 1.1 was developed (◼ fig. 5.1).

In line with the original research, the various aspects represent indicators of health. A concession was made about two added ones, namely 'Housing circumstances' and 'Having enough money', because, when providing feedback, professionals mentioned that although the spider web worked well, it was also very important to know whether someone might be homeless or in debt. Formally, these are determinants rather than direct indicators of health. They promote health. However, because of their importance, they were included in the new spider web, version 1.1. This brought the number of aspects to 42: 6 × 7.

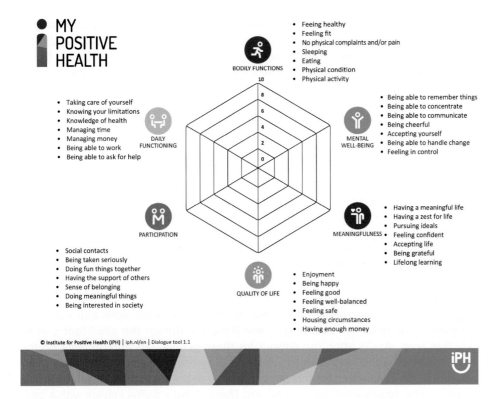

Figure 5.1   The Adults Tool spider web, My Positive Health 1.1. (Source: ▶ www.iph.n/en)

Along the axes of the spider web, the numbers 0 to 10 have been positioned from the centre to the periphery. In practice we work with number 1, representing the least favourable score and 10 the most favourable – a scoring method that is assumed to be familiar to most people.

The idea is for patients to use the spider web to rate their lives and circumstances in the various domains and indicate whether and, if so, where they would like to make changes or improvements.

The questionnaire is available both as a paper printout and digitally, and results in a spider web.

In 2020, the spider web was evaluated and work was started on the 2.0 version. For example, the 1.1 version's questionnaire does not include sexuality or intimacy. In addition, it also lacks the possibility for patients to add a topic themselves. There are different tools available (▶ www.mypositivehealth.com) and in a variety of languages (▶ https://www.iph.nl/en/participate/free-downloads). The 2.0 version will appear soon.

■   Children's tool
Huber's research was conducted amongst adults aged 18 to 80 and resulted in the concept of Positive Health (Huber 2016), as already discussed in ▶ Chap. 2. At the end of 2016, the Dutch Wilhelmina Children's Hospital (WKZ), in the city of Utrecht, enquired whether a spider web could also be developed especially for children. A joint

study was started with WKZ, students from Utrecht University and the University of Groningen, the Youth Health Care Department (JGZ) of the municipality of Utrecht, the foundation Stichting Kind en Ziekenhuis, and the Institute for Positive Health. To this end, 180 children and their parents, the sick and the healthy, were interviewed, which resulted in the development of the *Children's tool*, for children aged 8 to 16. This version of the spider web is available on paper and in digital form, the latter of which has its own questionnaire. ► www.mypositivehealth.com.

- Adolescents and young adults tool

Once the *Children's tool* had been developed, the question arose whether a tool could also be created for older children and young adults, with typical adolescent themes. This question also led to a project in close cooperation with the stakeholder group. This resulted in the *Adolescents and young adults tool* for the 16–25 age group (both a paper and a digital version were created, with questions). Some 17-year-olds may still feel more at ease using the Children's tool – this depends on the individual.

    ► www.mypositivehealth.com.

- Simple tool

As the new tools were being developed, health professionals were also asking for a version to be made for people with low literacy. Although the adult tool is at B1 language level, this is often too difficult for these people. iPH took to work on this issue, together with Pharos, Dutch Centre of Expertise on Health Disparities, which resulted in the *Simple tool* for this target group. A paper version and a guidance document can be downloaded and printed out. There is also a digital version with a 'read aloud' function (still in Dutch). This has also proven to be very useful for people with a visual impairment.

    ► www.mypositivehealth.com.

5.2.2   iPH materials

In addition to the digital tools, there are also tear-off pads in A5 format with a spider web depicted on each page, for the adults, children's, and adolescents and young adults tools. Handy for on your desk.

There is a brochure (A5 format) with information to become acquainted with the ideas and a condensed version of the spider web (◘ fig. 5.3) and a poster (◘ fig. 6.8). There are also tablecloths imprinted with the spider web, for group activities or other purposes.

The various materials (presently still in Dutch) can be ordered from the iPH website: ► https://www.iph.nl/meedoen/materialen-bestellen/ (in Dutch).

5.3   Personal experience

Working with Positive Health is not a trick. The more familiar you become with the concept's essence, the more convincing and effective you will be in conversations with your patients. During the training session (Training *Working with Positive Health*, also see ► Chap. 8), participants first start with their own spider web and the related questions. That is why we start this chapter with an exercise for you to experience filling out the spider web for yourself. Subsequently, you will answer a few questions about your completed version of the spider web. This will provide a moment of reflection. You are invited to participate!

Reflection

How are you doing yourself, at this moment?

What does health mean to you?

Please, fill out the My Positive Health spider web for yourself, for example on paper, as in ◘ fig. 5.1. You can enter an estimated average score on each dimension of the spider web. Then, if you take a pen and connect these scores, your health overview emerges within the spider web.

You can also fill out the digital questionnaire on ▶ www.mypositivehealth.com. The starting screen is shown in ◘ fig. 5.4. In the digital version, you are presented with a statement for each concept and you are asked to answer to what degree you agree with the statements, on a scale of 1 to 10 (1 = completely disagree; 10 = completely agree). After completing the questionnaire, you will immediately be able to see the average scores of your answers per dimension and your health overview, represented within the spider web. If you like, the result can be printed out.

In relation to this action, ask yourself the following questions:

- *What does your completed spider web, your overview of health look like?*
- *What is going well and what are you satisfied with? Is there anything that is going less well?*
- *Regarding the aspects, did any of them trigger or touch you in any particular way?*
- *What are your dreams and what drives you? Are you acting accordingly?*
- *Is there anything that you would like to change or give more attention to, and, if so, what would that be?*
- *Can you think of anything that might be a first step in that direction?*
- *Is this feasible?*
- *Is there something holding you back?*
- *If so, what is it? And what could you do about it?*
- *What will you decide to do?*
- *What would be the first concrete step that you could take?*
- *What or who would you need to make that happen?*

Good luck!

There is also a video with practical instructions for completing the spider web. Scan the QR code at the end of this chapter to take a look at the video and the useful links and tools.

Experiencing for yourself how the spider web works has multiple benefits. Filling it out may provide some eye-opening results. You may come across certain themes which you would not have thought of yourself. Furthermore, you will probably find it is not too difficult to formulate an intention, but putting it into practice and sticking with it is quite another matter. It is therefore not surprising that patients often struggle to really change certain aspects of their lives. As care provider, it is a valuable experience to address a certain theme yourself, looking at what you would like to change in your life and at what happens when you are either very motivated to do so, or not at all. This includes considering whether or not you are on the right track to connect to your dream. During the alternative dialogue, patients will intuitively sense that you know what you are talking about from personal experience.

Another benefit may be that you could be faced with wondering how much balance there is in your own life and to what extent you yourself are a *positively healthy care provider*. It is a fact that general practitioners are not exempt from suffering a burnout – quite the opposite (Van den Brekel-Dijkstra et al. 2020). Perhaps this will stimulate you to pay more attention to yourself and your general health and well-being. That, too, will benefit the quality of your work.

5.4   How to hold the alternative dialogue?

5.4.1   Why an alternative dialogue?

As already mentioned in Part I, general medical education trains students to think about sick people according to the medical-analytical model. In consultations with patients you will learn to explore their request for help – to arrive at a diagnosis if possible and provide information, medication and advice (CRU+ 2019).

These skills are very valuable and fit the expertise in the T's vertical bar of the T-shaped professional (see ► sect. 2.6), with respect to professional knowledge applied to the benefit of the sick person. These are problem-oriented skills and, as a physician, with your knowledge, you are the expert in the conversation with your patient.

In general Dutch medical education, attention is also paid to having difficult conversations that also involve emotions, and you learn to show empathy and respect for patients' opinions and emotions (CRU+ 2019). This is already part of the traits in the horizontal bar of the T.

In your general medical practice, you will see some patients more often than others. This may be because of recurring complaints that just will not get any better. For example, headaches that keep coming back. Based on medical-analytical knowledge, physicians tend to start by alleviating the symptoms, such as by prescribing painkillers. This form of symptom relief is effective in the short term. But what if this person is suffering from headaches because they are worried about something; housing, a difficult relationship, an escalating conflict, loneliness or finances? In such cases, the complaints will not disappear until the underlying problems are solved. Using the method of the *alternative dialogue*, which looks at the whole person rather than just the complaint, will uncover any underlying problems.

Having such an alternative dialogue is about seeing the whole person in addition to their disease or condition (if any). It is an addition to your *medical knowledge* and your *professional intuition* – this sense that there is 'nothing to worry about' or 'something not feeling quite right'. Your intuition helps you to assess whether you could start with a broad health-based approach, or if medical diagnostics must first be applied to exclude or identify a certain disease. The *alternative dialogue* gives your patient the feeling that they are being seen and heard as a human being. The point is also to understand the context that may be important. Although general practitioners often already have a general perception of their patient's circumstances, the alternative dialogue may add more depth and nuance. What is important to this particular person in his or her life? To what extent are they on the right track, and how is the general practitioner meeting the needs of this patient?

Remember, you do not need to be sick to get better!

This is personalised care, in the best sense of the word. It is about motivating patients to take control of their own lives and to give life a more self-determined direction. In addition, personal health levels can often be improved and lead to a greater feeling of well-being. The patient is not pushed into a certain direction that is predetermined, incentivised by the health care professional. The Indian proverb 'The shortest distance between two points may not be a straight line' is particularly applicable here. As is illustrated by a story about two widowers in a village in the south of Limburg.

The story goes that two elderly widowers had each filled out the spider web during a neighbourhood activity and discovered that they wanted more interaction with other people. They both chose to start working in the community garden which is especially for residents from the local community. After having spent an afternoon working in the garden, the two men contentedly looked at their work, while smoking a cigarette. One of them asked the other: 'So you're a smoker, too? I should really stop.' Upon which the man said: 'So should I, shall we stop together?' And they did so successfully!

They both chose to counter their loneliness by working together with others, in the community garden. The loneliness dissipated, which gave them the strength to stop smoking. If health professionals had first began to focus on them quitting their smoking habit, there is a good chance that this would not have succeeded. Now it did. Which goes to show that taking a detour may sometimes prove to be the shortest route.

In the *alternative dialogue* between patient and care professional, the patient is the expert and the one who should have the floor. The professional should mainly listen, only now and then asking an open question. Not easy, when we know that physicians generally interrupt a patient 18 seconds, or even 11 seconds, after the start of a consultation, as recent US research has shown (Mauksch 2017; Ospina et al. 2019). Furthermore, general practitioners are only partially successful in discovering their patient's health-related needs and expectations, and tend to interrupt their patient soon after the 10-minute consultation has started (Campion et al. 2002).

It would be good to realise that all people – more or less consciously – instinctively know what they need and what would be best for them, at any particular time. The method of the alternative dialogue helps patients to bring such insights to the surface. As a health care professional, you can support people to arrive at the right answers to their questions themselves. The idea behind this is that, in this way, people will also experience that they are in control and can choose their own course of action.

During the *evaluation* of a project on holding the alternative dialogue (Voer Eens Het Andere Gesprek) that had been carried out in the general practice of one of the authors, patients indicated that they had gained more insight into their own situation and that they felt more heard. For the professionals, the alternative dialogue also helps to better understand any issues underlying the initial question of their patient (◘ fig. 5.2).

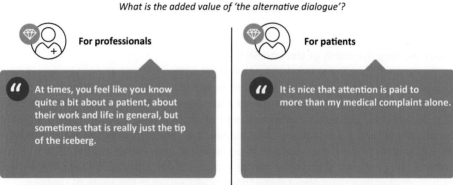

What is the added value of 'the alternative dialogue'?

For professionals

" At times, you feel like you know quite a bit about a patient, about their work and life in general, but sometimes that is really just the tip of the iceberg.

- More knowledge and understanding of patiënts
- Awareness of the other disciplines and what they do.
- Giving the patient more responsibility
- More work enjoyment

For patients

" It is nice that attention is paid to more than my medical complaint alone.

- Insight into the personal situation
- Feeling heard
- Ideas for the first steps

Figure 5.2   Added value of the personalised alternative dialogue in general medical practice. (Oude Weernink 2020) (Source: ▶ www.lrjg.nl/andergesprek 2020)

5.4.2 Introducing the alternative dialogue

Many professionals who start working with Positive Health often ask how they should initiate using the spider web with a patient, and whether there are examples of the questions one could ask to introduce the spider web. We have deliberately not presented one format that would apply to all. Your own style and working methods determine what would suit you best, but of course there are examples of how to connect the particular question of a patient to the Positive Health approach.

- General interest: *'I'm curious to know how you look at your own health. Could you indicate how healthy you feel, on a scale from 1 to 10?'*
- In relation to the request for help or the complaint: *'I have heard that (or: in my practice, I see that) your complaints often have to do with other elements of life. Shall we explore the wider possibilities?'*
- Invite the patient to join you in looking a little more broadly at how they are doing.
- Hanging an image of the spider web on one of the walls of the practice or having one on the table may also help, as it may spark curiosity in patients.
- Animation videos could also be made available to put on display via a digital information system in the waiting room.

The Positive Health spider web can be a good way of starting an alternative dialogue. There are several possibilities for filling out a spider web questionnaire. First, assess the language skills of the patient. The condensed version may serve as an introduction to the method, with only six dimensions and one question per dimension, as is shown in the brochure *'How are you doing?'* (fig. 5.3).

The brochure presents six statements and invites the reader to rate themselves, on a scale from 1 to 10, on each statement: 10 = fully agree; 1 = fully disagree.

The statements are:

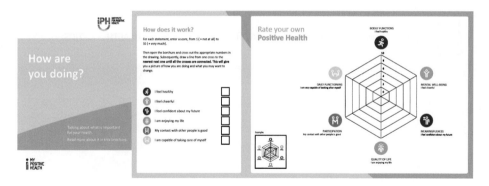

■ **Figure 5.3**   Brochure on Positive Health for the general medical practice. (Source: ▶ www.iph.nl/en)

– I feel healthy	☐
– I feel cheerful	☐
– I feel confident about my future	☐
– I am enjoying my life	☐
– My contact with other people is good	☐
– I am capable of taking care of myself	☐

In the brochure, the scores can be entered onto the picture of the spider web, after which the scores can be connected by drawing a line from one to the next. This creates an overview of someone's perceived health. The questions above were taken from the extensive questionnaire.

The more elaborate form of the spider web, with 42 aspects for each of the 6 dimensions and a QR code, in the Netherlands, is available as a tear-off pad (A5 format), to put on your desk in the consulting room (■ fig. 5.1).

People can also fill out the digital questionnaire with 42 questions at home, via ▶ www.mypositivehealth.com, (■ fig. 5.4; also see the QR code in ■ fig. 5.1) and print out the resulting spider web or take the login details along to the appointment (■ fig. 5.5).

5.4.3 Discussing the spider web

The spider web is a *dialogue tool* (not a measurement tool) to use as a conversation starter. The scores (0 > 2 > 4 > 6 > 8 > 10) along the axes of the spider web are intended to stimulate patients to reflect on their own situation. Connecting the scores on the six axes gives an overview of their health. In this form, the spider web provides insight and a basis for starting the conversation.

Please note that, often, there is a tendency, especially amongst professionals, to talk about the lowest score and how this could be improved. However, this is not the intention here. The aim is to talk about what the patient considers important and what gives them strength or what they would like to change or pay more attention to, when something is bothering them, or because it would bring their dream a little closer.

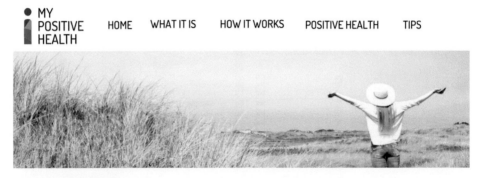

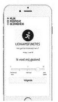

MY POSITIVE HEALTH

Positive Health is a way of looking at health in a broader sense. For example, are you able to manage sufficiently? Do you feel happy or perhaps just lonely? And is there perhaps a need for medical care or support from your surroundings? The point is that you feel healthy and energetic, in the way that suits you.

Why fill out the questionnaire?   How it works

☐ **Figure 5.4**   The login screen of the digital questionnaire on the website

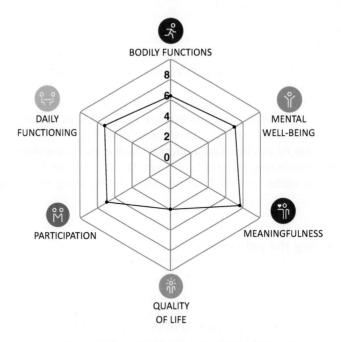

☐ **Figure 5.5**   Example of a filled-out spider web. (Source: ▶ www.iph.nl/en)

Filling out the spider web often generates all kinds of thoughts and associations in people. Allowing these associations can lead the conversation into an unexpected direction and provide unanticipated starting points for taking new steps.

Start the conversation by asking open questions, such as:

- *How do you feel about it?*
- *How did you feel when filling out the questionnaire?*
- *Would you like to tell me about it?*
- *What catches your eye?*
- *What is important to you, at this moment?*
- *Did you gain any insights looking at your spider web results?*

5.4.4 Listening with intent

- Once a patient has filled out the spider web and you reflect together on aspects that may stand out and what is important to them, you have one very important task as general practitioner, namely to listen carefully to whatever comes up. Some people take their lowest score as a starting point, but equally often they will start talking about very different things. About what is on their mind, for example. This all provides you with context about them as a person. Things that you would otherwise not be aware of – despite the fact that you may already have been their physician for many years. Such background information may be the key to a solution. It is important that you emanate a sense of calm – practice *the art of slowing down* the conversation. Do not be afraid of silence, as these moments can provide the patient with the time needed to realise how they truly feel and, thus, find real answers to your questions. Much can be learned during the Positive Health training sessions; they will give you experience, as this type of conversation is practised extensively. Physicians often find it difficult to not break the silence – and, in this, they are not alone! It is tempting to fill a void by asking 'helpful questions'. After role-play training sessions, those in the role of 'patient' sometimes indicate that they were not at all bothered by the silence; they may even have found it rather pleasant. Some recounted how the so-called *helpful questions disturbed* them: 'I was just starting to realise how I felt, when your question interrupted my feelings and brought me straight back to rational thinking'.
- Furthermore, during an alternative dialogue, health care professionals really need to *set aside any preconceived notions* and preconceptions, *compliment* the patient when appropriate and to *trust* their wisdom. Patients are the expert with regard to their own lives and are very capable of describing what they need.
- To determine whether you are acting in the right way during the conversation, you may ask yourself: *who is working here – the patient or I?* It should be the former. You can relax and sit back, while listening attentively.

After patients have told you what they were feeling while filling out the spider web, and perhaps after a moment of silence adding another thing or two, the next phase of the conversation can begin. Are subsequent steps needed?

Here, the *metaphor of the taxi driver*, as mentioned in ▶ Chap. 1, is very helpful. Recount the fact that taxi drivers will never ask where you came from, but only *where you would like to go*. From there, the conversation may go in various directions – with the professional taking on *a coaching role*, rather than taking the lead. Help the patient find their own way by asking certain questions. There are various ways of doing so. Two are discussed below.

5.4.5 Two possible routes

— Ask solution-oriented questions
— Use the Action Wheel

5.4.6 Solution-oriented questions

Asking *solution-oriented questions* is at the heart of solution-oriented working methods. The aim of the questions is to help care providers make patients think differently and to create a context for change. Solution-oriented questions are about formulating a goal or dream (*'yearning for the vast and endless sea'*), about exceptions to the problem or medical complaints and about what patients are still able to do. Solution-oriented questions give hope as a positive perspective, which stimulates care providers and patients to continue. The two basic assumptions of solution-oriented work are (Bannink and Jansen 2017):
— When something works (or works better), do more of it
— When something does not work, stop and do something else

Asking solution-oriented questions is not about collecting information, it is about inviting patients to look for positive differences and making progress. Patients are considered to be experts when it comes to their own lives and finding solutions. Care providers need to listen for opportunities to talk about solutions, even when the conversation is filled with problems. Solutions will not surface automatically – if they were so obvious, the patient would have applied them already. Therefore, the solution-oriented care provider always needs to look out for the exceptions; interventions are intended to help patients shift their attention to the times when things are better or different, so that solutions appear as possibilities.

Many problems are perpetuated, simply because patients believe or say that they have 'always been there', but fail to notice the moments without those problems or the times when they are less obvious. Failing to notice those them means these times remain hidden. The attitude of solution-oriented care providers is therefore one of asking questions. A solution-oriented conversation can generally be held by asking four basic questions (Bannink 2019):
— *What do you hope for?*
— *What difference will that make?*
— *What will be effective?*
— *What will be the next sign of progress? Or: What will be your next step?*

Case no. 6: Four solution-oriented questions

Suffering a myocardial infarction is a terrifying experience, whereby the emphasis is on survival, during the acute phase. Its impact on the victim's life and that of their loved ones often becomes clear during the subsequent period of rehabilitation. Questions that can play a role in the process of rehabilitation may for example include: 'Why has this happened to me/what does this mean/what will be the impact on my life?'

A general practitioner visited a 58-year-old patient of his who had suffered a myocardial infarction three months prior. The man's two daughters and partner were also present during the home visit. The practitioner asked the man how his recovery was going. The man answered: 'The rehabilitation is disappointing; I don't seem to make any progress.'

The practitioner asked: 'What are you hoping for?'

To the practitioner's surprise, the man said: 'I wish I felt calmer.'

'What difference would that make?', he asked him.

The man swallowed and says: 'That I would have a better relationship with my children.'

The practitioner commented: 'I see that this question makes you emotional.'

The man burst out crying.

'Do you often see your father crying?', the practitioner asked the daughters.

'This is only the second time in our lives,' they said.

'And do you remember the first time?', he asked.

One of the daughters answered: 'It was three months ago. When you ran in with that machine (she meant the defibrillator (eds.)) and daddy was calling 'I'm dying!'

'Am I right to conclude', the practitioner asked, looking at the man, 'that the relationship with your children is as important as not wanting to die? And that realising this is making you emotional again?'

The man nodded in agreement. The daughters had meanwhile also started to cry.

The practitioner asked: 'Who could help you, in this respect?'

The daughters both put up their hand.

The man continued saying that he kept feeling so tired after the infarction. He appeared restless and agitated because his recovery was not going well and he was taking his frustrations out on his family. He realised that he was being short-tempered and unfriendly, and would like to change that.

The practitioner asked: 'What could be a first step in that direction?'

His wife said: 'How about you start by asking nicely when you want your children to tidy up, instead of ending with the comment that they never clean up after themselves?'

Everyone had to laugh at this heartfelt message. The man promised to do his best.

The general practitioner asked everyone to let this short talk sink in (it had lasted less than ten minutes) and if anyone wanted to talk about it some more, they would always be welcome to come see him. Two weeks later, the man showed up at the surgery hour. He said he wanted to find out what he could do to improve the atmosphere at home. Together, the practitioner and the man decided to make an appointment with the mental health practice nurse to find out why he was feeling so agitated and what he could do to improve the atmosphere at home.

In this case, the general practitioner was most impressed by the positive effect of using the four solution-oriented questions. These do make it easier to discuss certain subjects, and the answers illustrate what is really going on with the patient and what they need most. Moreover, the questions also put the patient in charge – what they would like to change and how they will go about doing so. All general practitioners need to do is follow their patient's lead. This does not cost them any energy and yields amazing results.

5.4.7 The Action Wheel

The *Action Wheel* is used in the Positive Health training. The process is represented in a cyclic depiction. See ◘ fig. 5.6.

The questions from the Action Wheel that you can discuss with your patients, possibly with the picture attached, are:

— *How are you doing now?* This question has been answered by filling out the spider web. Looking at the spider web, what do you notice? How do you feel you are doing?

— *What do you wish for?* What is important to you? As a result of filling out the spider web, would you like to pay more attention to a certain aspect or would you like to change something? And if so, what would that be? This could either be a small step in the direction of achieving your dream, or about something that bothers you and that you would really like to change. And then also consider whether this is really what you want to do?

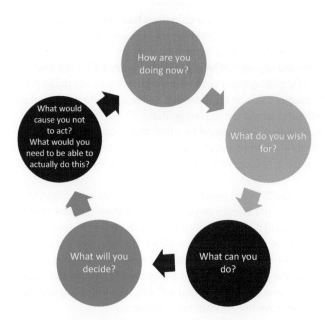

◘ **Figure 5.6** The Action Wheel describes the steps that can help you to make a feasible decision for taking action. (Source: inspired by P. Krijger, ▶ www.atma.nl)

- *What can you do?* This is the question about what would be feasible for you to do. Can you be honest with yourself about that?
- *What will you decide to do as a first step?* Be sure to make it small and doable. This will help you to stick with it, which in turn will strengthen your self-confidence so that you can take a next step.

And then comes the question related to *resistance*, a completely normal human characteristic, but it does help to be aware of it and to talk about it. This prevents disappointment afterwards.

- *What would be the reason for you not to act?* How does your resistance manifest itself? Are you too busy? Do you not feel like it, after all? Or is there something else going on?
- *What would you need to be able to actually do this?* People can only answer that question for themselves. It helps to provide them with insight into who or what they would need to support them in taking the first step towards their goal or desire to change.

This brings the discussion full circle and wraps up the conversation – for the time being. This cycle can always be repeated at a later point in time, possibly with a different theme.

Two tips:

- Letting patients formulate their answers to these questions is important. It is a known fact that the most effective advice is the one we give ourselves and *say out loud* (Lupyan & Swingley 2020) (► www.sciencedaily.com).
- With respect to someone's dream or what they would like to achieve, *an image* that represents it can be very helpful. Positive Health training sessions use a set of beautiful pictures as inspirational cards (► www.zorgvoorbeter.nl), but in practice you could also ask patients to bring their own photograph or image (e.g., from a magazine) that represents their dream or goal.

Please note:

Take the time to try out which questions suit you the best. Some professionals purposefully ask all the questions of the Action Wheel, but sometimes only a few questions are enough to provide insight and to take the next steps. Questions that already reveal a great deal about what someone would like to do and is able to do are simply these: *'What do you hope for? What do you find important? What could you do yourself?'* For you as a health care professional, the answers do not require you to take any action yourself; you do not have to solve the problems. In any case, the answers will show you the direction into which the patient wants to go. This puts the patient more in control and triggers less of a *'repair reflex'* in the care professional. Surprisingly, the direction of the solution often turns out to be different from what the professional had initially considered. As health care providers, we often think that reducing the pain or the complaint is what is expected of us, but sometimes patients need something very different.

After this first conversation, it may be useful to arrange for a follow-up appointment, if the patient so wishes. This is to see how the patient has been doing and what they have achieved, so far, with respect to achieving their goals. Sometimes, many things are revealed and a follow-up appointment could be used to focus some more on one of the dimensions of the spider web of Positive Health. A next conversation can also be planned with the physiotherapist, practice nurse, or mental health practice nurse, depending on what the patient wishes to work on or change. This will help patients to stay true to their intentions. Health care professionals should remain in their coaching role, also during a follow-up appointment, and allow patients to retain their personal responsibility. When people bring a photograph or image to the surgery, this helps to make the conversation even easier. Listen to what they can tell you about it and let them advise themselves!

Case no. 7: The Action Wheel

Sophie, a cheerful 8-year-old girl with Type 1 diabetes, came to the surgery with her mother, complaining of abdominal pain. Her mother was very worried about her daughter's pain and asked to be referred to an internist. The general practitioner talked to the mother about her concerns and asked if she had already discussed these symptoms with the paediatrician (whom the girl has been seeing for the last three years for her diabetes). The mother answered that the paediatrician had been unable to find anything unusual and had tried to reassure her – apparently rather unsuccessfully. Her mother worried about Sophie continuing to have such pain in her abdomen, so often. Further anamnesis and examination also did not provide any new leads. Functional abdominal pain was considered, but the mother insisted on further investigation. At the end of the consultation, the general practitioner proposed to take some more time to look at Sophie's abdominal pain symptoms and her general health and well-being. They agreed to make a new appointment to do so. In preparation, Sophie was asked to fill out the Children's tool on ▶ www.mypositivehealth.com. The practitioner told Sophie that she was very curious to see whether Sophie would be able to show her how she was doing, using all those funny emojis.

At the next appointment, they discussed what Sophie thought about filling out the spider web. Her mother had brought the printout. The practitioner asked Sophie how she was doing and what she felt was important to her. Sophie indicated that her friends at school were important (she scored rather low on 'Participation', but also on 'Your body', because she still had the abdominal pain). Then came the question: 'What could or would you like to do to feel better?' Sophie indicated that she would like to go and play at her friends' houses or stay the night. Because of her diabetes, her mother never allowed her to go anywhere, except to school (the school teacher was the only one, besides her parents, who knew what Sophie needed for her diabetes and when she would need to be injected). Her mother wanted to always keep a close eye on Sophie's insulin. The practitioner asked what could be a first step towards her being able to participate more. Sophie asked her mother if the mothers of her friends would also be allowed to monitor her diabetes. Her mother then told her that she had just received a new diabetes sensor, with a patch, which meant that she would not need to be injected every time. This would make things easier, although the mother admitted that she still found it difficult to let go of her daughter.

During the discussion, the mother did suggest that she would explain to the mothers of Sophie's friends about Sophie's condition, and to talk to her DM nurse about how she could involve her family more. The practitioner asked what could stand in the way of this terrific plan and, when she asked the mother what would cause her to not go ahead with this plan, the mother was close to tears, saying she still found it difficult to accept her daughter's diabetes. When asked what she would need to follow through, she stated that she would like some help with this. The practitioner advised her to talk to the mental health practice nurse. Sophie joyfully asked her mother when she would be able to have a sleepover at her best friend's house? Her mother took her hand and said: 'I promise you that I will make an appointment with your friend's mother very soon'.

This was quite a while ago, and the general practitioner has not seen Sophie or her mother since then, and certainly has not heard any more about her abdominal pain.

5.4.8 The alternative dialogue and time

An often-heard barrier to holding an alternative dialogue is the aspect of time – that it takes up more of a practitioner's time. Practitioners consider this a problem – and it is true: talking about the Positive Health spider web is difficult to do within the timeframe of a 10-minute consultation. But once you have some experience, and depending on the patient, the process of self-reflection can often be initiated during a double consultation. Which can then be continued in a new, follow-up appointment. There are general practices that have established a special Positive Health surgery, once a month for one hour per patient, for example in deprived neighbourhoods. Others have reserved a few half-hour slots in their agenda. This allows for having extensive conversations about the spider web, which patients often have already filled out beforehand. There are also practices, such as the practice of one the authors of this handbook (HPJ), which have come to an agreement with health insurance companies that they will no longer be paid per consultation but receive a fixed subscription rate per patient. Being able to take the time needed provides peace of mind.

However, there is also another aspect to consider, with respect to time – and that is quality. The ancient Greeks had two principles of time: Chronos and Kairos (Hermsen 2015; Slagt 2018). Chronos refers to duration, i.e., clock time: 10 minutes, or perhaps 15 or 20 minutes for a consultation. Kairos, on the other hand, stands for the qualitative aspect of time. Earlier, we mentioned the importance of *making real contact* and the power of *paying attention* to the other person during the conversation. When those qualities are present, patients will feel both seen and heard within a few minutes time, and feelings may surface that result in many other things being set in motion.

This type of attention and attitude during a consultation takes some practice. Once you have mastered this skill, you will run out of time much less often and the contact with patients will give you more satisfaction than before.

Incidentally, general practitioners are certainly not the only ones able to carry out alternative conversations. Others, including the practice nurse and mental health practice nurse, or those who have a feeling for it and have been trained, are able to achieve good results with the alternative dialogue.

5.4.9 When and with whom to hold an alternative dialogue?

There are a number of presentations and training courses for health care profession-als who are interested in working with Positive Health (see ▶ Chap. 8 and the related hyperlink QR code at the end of this chapter). A frequently recurring question is that of: 'In which cases could the concept of Positive Health be applied?' The answer is sim-ple: 'Generally speaking, the concept applies to all people – all of those registered at a general practice.' Patients who come to the practice with physical or mental-health-re-lated complaints can be provided with medical advice or treated with medications. Applying the concept of Positive Health means that a large number of contextual factors as well as background information on the complaints come into the picture, through which the source of complaints can be traced. As a general practitioner, Posi-tive Health makes it easier to talk about issues such as leading a meaningful life, mak-ing ends meet, belonging (loneliness), self-acceptance, gratitude and dealing with change.

In fact, one or more of these themes always play a role when patients consider coming to the practice. Whether these themes actually become a subject for dis-cussion depends on the situation. By filling out the questionnaire of the spider web of Positive Health, patients already obtain a certain insight into the background of and coherence between their complaints. The alternative dialogue allows patients to reflect on their health situation. There is no blueprint for the appropriate occasion. It is up to the health care professional in the general practice to assess this on the basis of the information provided by the patient, either verbally or non-verbally, in combi-nation with the professional's own experience and intuition. These conversations are satisfying for both patient and practitioner (see ◻ fig. 5.2) – or, as a practitioner once put it during a workshop: 'This is why I became a general practitioner!'

All conversations conducted on the basis of Positive Health are in line with the *core values* of primary care: *person-oriented, medical generalist, continuous and together*. These patient–physician conversations are particularly *person-oriented*, the patient is at the centre, and together you look for a suitable and befitting care solution. Examples of general medical consultations and Positive Health can be found in ▶ sect. 5.5, and the core value *'together'* is explained in ▶ sect. 7.5. Positive Health also has added value when offering patients *continuity*, which is at the core of pri-mary care.

In an implementation project on having an alternative dialogue (Voer Eens Het Andere Gesprek) in Leidsche Rijn, care providers were asked to determine the patient groups with which they would like to have the alternative dialogue. Both the Positive Health spider web, as well as another model (4-domains model) were applied. (Van den Brekel-Dijkstra et al. 2019). As ◻ fig. 5.7 shows, the alternative dialogue was used in one third of the cases for people with psychological complaints, in one third of the cases for recurrent somatic complaints, and the remainder for lifestyle questions, people with a chronic illness or intakes of new patients. The patients with recurring somatic complaints were those suffering from headaches, fatigue, back pain, dizzi-ness or insomnia.

Positive Health is especially suited to having an *alternative dialogue* with the fol-lowing types of patients:

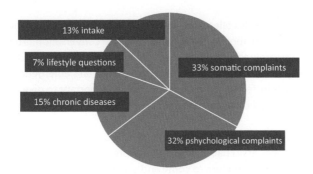

'The alternative dialogue' can be applied in various situations

- 13% intake
- 7% lifestyle questions
- 15% chronic diseases
- 33% somatic complaints
- 32% pshychological complaints

In total 167 conversations were registered in medical record.

◖ Figure 5.7 With whom to hold an *alternative dialogue*? (Source: ▶ www.lrjg.nl/andergesprek 2020)

- People with chronic diseases, to help them integrate the disease into their lives. To change from *being ill* to *living with a disease* and for them to experience that they are more than their disease. Often, these conversations also manage to motivate them to improve their lifestyle.
- People with mental health problems, such as anxiety, mood changes and burnout.
- People who have had COVID-19. Rehabilitation should not only be physically functional, but should also serve a higher purpose and an ideal.
- Elderly people with loneliness issues.
- People with all kinds of medically unexplained physical symptoms (MUPS).
- People who consume a lot of medical care, in the Positive Health concept also referred to as *'hotspotters'.*

In addition to general practitioners, practice nurses are also very much involved in the continuity of care, such as to support patients with chronic diseases and frail elderly people (practice nurse somatics/elderly). The mental health practice nurse plays a major role in cases of psychological problems. Many general practitioners and other general practice staff will not immediately start applying the concept on complex patients. This is understandable. However, in the authors' experience, in these patients with whom you hesitate about approaching them differently, the level of resistance can be surprisingly low and new courses of action may develop. In addition, there are patients with complex problems who visit the practice rather often. The 10 % of patients who come to the practice most often account for over 40 % of the total workload (Te Brake et al. 2006). There are many of these types of patients. A general practice in the Dutch town of Zoetermeer decided to actively approach their frequent patients (the so-called *'hotspotters'*) and invite them for a 'Positive Health conversation' (see case no. 8).

Case no. 8: Positive Health conversations with regular users at the General practice Zoetermeer

Together with three of his colleagues, Marco Ephraim, a general practitioner in Zoetermeer, invited 'hotspotters' for a Positive Health conversation. 'These are people with many problems, who often fall through the cracks in regular health care and go from pillar to post. They often go to a hospital's emergency room and are unnecessarily transferred to secondary care. It is important to give these people sufficient attention, to find out what could give them more meaning and control over their own lives.'

An example of such a case is that of a man with COPD, heart problems and bladder cancer. Ephraim recounts: 'I had a feeling that there could be a story behind the man's health problems and invited him to come and see me. As he was filling out the Positive Health spider web, I noticed him scoring very low on his personal perception in all areas. I started by asking him: 'What do you think is the most important problem?' His answer was rather surprising; he said that his neighbour —who was also his landlord – was his biggest problem. They had a conflict, there was a certain amount of nuisance, so he was sleeping poorly, which caused him to exercise less and he did not always take his medication on time. Because of this situation, his life was in a negative spiral, on all fronts.'

Ephraim's asked the following questions: 'What is standing in the way of solving those issues?' 'Who or what could help you?' and 'What could be a first step towards a solution?' It appeared that the man's son was good at dealing with situations of conflict and he stepped in to help his father. They started a lawsuit against the neighbour and this led to them reaching an agreement. The man has since moved house and rebuilt his life – he is doing better in many different ways.

What is the impact of holding an alternative dialogue with such 'hotspotters'? Ephraim: 'With this particular patient, we only had two conversations. Per patient, we have two to four of such appointments per year, each lasting between 30 and 45 minutes. I have found that I get to know patients whom I have known for years in a completely different way. My job satisfaction has also increased in dealing with these complex patients. And the same is true for my colleagues' (Medisch Ondernemen 2019).

Exploring a patient's daily life through these *alternative conversations* is very appropriate, both for frequent visitors to the practice and those with simple medical complaints; for example, by asking them: 'What are you hoping to achieve?' It can help to discover why the patient came to the surgery in the first place, and this often determines what the rest of the conversation should focus on.

Please note:

When holding an alternative dialogue, health care providers should not lose sight of the fact that people are all different, with differing views of their own health, who may look at it from a different perspective, depending on their character, age, gender, level of education, literacy and social status.

As early as in 1988, Calnan described two of such ways:

- Health as the absence of disease, where health care is primarily focused on treating disease.
- A more positive approach to health, where health care involves not only the treatment of disease but also considers the promotion of health an important factor (Calnan 1988).

A literature study (Jung 2003) shows that health care can be approached by patients either *actively* or *passively*.

■ **Active approach**

In the active approach, patients themselves actively seek information about their complaint or disease, they ask to be referred sooner, there is a preference for a certain type of treatment, they want to be involved in the decision-making process, and health checks receive a more positive rating. Patients who prefer this active approach are generally younger, better educated, have a higher income and are in better health than those who are less assertive.

■ **Passive approach or low health skills**

Patients with a preference for a more passive approach to health care, on the other hand, generally place more emphasis on the continuity of health care, see a greater role for the general practitioner in case of chronic diseases (are preferably seen by the same practitioner every time), are more likely to opt for a wait-and-see policy, are less interested in participating in decision-making on treatment, and require the general practitioner to take on a more dominant role. They attach less importance to preventing disease or simply lack the health skills needed to help prevent disease. On average, this group of patients is older, lower educated, with a lower income and poorer health than those in the first group.

The younger the patient, the more general practitioners are inclined to involve them in the decision-making process. With older and/or less healthy patients on a lower income, the medical-analytical model of thinking is applied more often.

This shows that patients have their own framework of thought that can be either more or less in line with the ideas of Positive Health. In particular, concepts such as self-management, self-reliance and resilience may be misunderstood by patients with a more passive approach to health care. A good example is that of a patient who came to the practice of one of the authors of this book, and said: 'My problem? I am not happy. Doctor, do something about it!' At times, it takes patience, empathy and explanation to ultimately arrive at the *alternative dialogue*. In this respect, it is also important to realise that patients have learned how to behave in health care. Illich (1974) speaks in this context of social iatrogenesis or the medicalisation of daily life and of cultural iatrogenesis or the loss of traditional ways in which people deal with suffering. If patients are accustomed to physicians approaching them and their needs in a medical-analytical way, then it will take some getting used to when their general practitioner asks: 'What do you think is important for your own health?' It is therefore important for physicians to realise who they are talking to; whether patients have insight into their disease, what level of health skills they have, and whether they are able to self-manage. This will determine which approach and support would be the most suitable.

Case no. 9: Simple tool in cooperation with guidance for people with an intellectual disability

A general practitioner was asked to make a house call to a 27-year-old man with a low IQ, autism, moderate obesity and recurrent luxating patella, who was staying in an assisted living environment. His personal counsellor asked if the practitioner could provide support because rehabilitation of the knee has been stagnating. The physiotherapist was at a loss as to what to do with the young man, who usually did not want to do anything. And when asked why he was not cooperating and if there was anything that he would want to do, he would invariably reply: 'I don't know'. Because of COVID-19 measures, the physiotherapist at that time was only allowed to make video calls. That did not work for this patient. The counsellor indicated he was worried about him; and the general practitioner was asked to speak firmly to this patient about him really needing to start exercising. In the hope that this would help.

The general practitioner made another suggestion, and asked the counsellors to fill out the Simple tool of Positive Health with the patient, so that the results could be discussed during the visit. The physiotherapists were unfamiliar with the concept, but were interested in trying it. The young man scored low on the subjects of physical complaints, participation and meaningfulness. Instead of focusing on what was wrong with his knee, the young man's dreams and wishes were discussed. It turned out that he would like to move to a different home; in his current residence, he felt that he had to do too many things himself, and he would also like to be surrounded by more people closer to his own age. A different type of home, in other words. This was no surprise to the counsellors; they were already aware of this wish, and the discussion was therefore yet another reason for trying to find a different living environment, with the help of his family. Furthermore, the young man indicated to be very fond of holidays and that he would very much like to travel by train again.

When asked what he would need to achieve this, he said that he would first have to learn to walk without a brace and do better with his exercise. In the past, often he had gone for walks with the counsellors, but over the past weeks he had not been outside. He talked with one of the counsellors about having their daily talk while walking, and he also practiced with the physiotherapist to walk the stairs using crutches, and slowly increase the distance. He felt that this would be a very good plan. In spite of the challenge of his intellectual disability, and with the help of the support staff, he managed to shift his focus from *having* to do something to *wanting* to do it.

Medical diagnostics remain important, although a good conversation is always appreciated (see case no. 10 'Patient suffering from gloominess and fatigue').

Case no. 10: Patient suffering from gloominess and fatigue

An 80-year-old woman came to the surgery because of worrying, gloominess and fatigue. She attributed her complaints to her having moved from a beautiful farm to a small house in the village, where she felt she had lost her freedom and she was unable to get used to the new situation. She was invited to fill out the spider web, where she scored low on meaningfulness. In the subsequent conversation she had with the general practitioner, she explained how, on the farm, she used to work in the vegetable garden every day and also tried to grow vegetables for her children and grandchildren. When that stopped, so did her daily physical activity. She believed that this was an explanation for her symptoms.

During the conversation, it was suggested that getting a dog as a pet could increase her physical activity level and give her cause to go outside more often. She decided to think about it and a follow-up appointment was made. A few weeks later, she asked the general practitioner to take a look at a spot on one of her breasts. On inspection, this turned out to be part of a large ulcerated process that, ultimately, proved to be breast cancer with metastases and anaemia. This could also be a good explanation for her fatigue. During a house call, after the diagnosis, the practitioner felt uncertain about how the patient had experienced the conversation about meaningfulness and the possibility of her getting a dog, while in fact something very different had been the matter with her. The woman, however, said that she had really enjoyed the conversation and looking at her health using the spider web, and that she really felt heard. She did not blame the practitioner for not having discussed the possibility of a medical problem at the time.

When you first start using the Positive Health concept, case no. 10 is probably the most worrisome. As a general practitioner, it always remains important to also use your *medical antenna*. The risk of *missing* a medical diagnosis can often be avoided by following a two-track method: be alert and listen to *your professional intuition* (the 'feeling in your bones') while also making a broad inventory of the context or background of a patient's complaint. Good follow-up and subsequent appointments are also important here.

5.5 Primary care core tasks and Positive Health

As described in ▶ Chap. 4, five core tasks have been formulated for primary care: *general medical care, emergency care, terminal palliative care, care coordination and preventive care*. First, some context is provided for the elaboration of each core task (Toekomsthuisartsenzorg 2020). Subsequently, various case studies are used to illustrate the added value of Positive Health.

5.5.1 Core task: *general medical care*

General medical care refers to general practitioners clarifying and assessing complaints, problems and queries in a variety of areas, from a medical perspective. For their diagnoses and working methods, the general practitioners also take into account their patient's history and personal circumstances, such as work and family life, their personal wishes and expectations, as well as their preferences.

An important task of general practitioners and their team is to determine the urgency of complaints. Which issues require immediate attention or within a few hours (emergency care) and which of them can be discussed later on during the regular hours of surgery. The practice is easily accessible to patients, so they can ask their general practitioner and practice staff all kinds of questions about health and disease. Determining the real nature of medical questions and problems forms the basis of primary care. It is part of the general practitioner's profession to make a proper assessment of where the observed problems originated from; whether there are somatic, psychological or social problems, or perhaps a combination of some or all of them.

After determining the nature of a patients request for help, the general practitioner or practice team member describes the problem or makes a diagnosis, either directly or after further investigation. Various treatment options are subsequently discussed. Depending on the problem or the diagnosis, the decision is made to, for example, wait while keeping a close eye on the situation, stimulate self-care, provide treatment or counselling within the general practice, or refer the patient to another care provider or institution. A relationship of trust is important when choosing the type of treatment. General practitioners take into account what their patients considers to be important. Practitioner and patient, together, determine what the patient would like to change and what would be needed to make this happen. General practitioners are able to deal with the majority of medical complaints themselves within the practice.

In cases when complaints cannot be solved by general practitioners or are not in line with the core tasks of primary care, the practitioners have an overview of the various domains within and outside the health care sector and function as a coach or guide for the patients concerned. This coaching function has an important social benefit, contributes to optimal and efficient care and is highly appreciated by patients (Nivel 2019). In cases where general practitioners feel other care providers would be more competent in a certain area, they will refer the patient to that specific field of care. This may, for example, be other care providers within primary care, secondary care, mental health care (GGZ) or social care providers in the community.

The medical-generalist character of primary care means that there are limits to the diagnostics and treatments that are provided by general practitioners themselves. Although questions of a non-medical nature are dealt with outside the general practice, the practitioners can advise patients on the type of other care they may need and refer them to the appropriate discipline. The alternative dialogue helps to determine the right type of care in the right place. The results from the spider web can be used to discover what patients would like to change. Practitioners and patients, together, can discuss whether further support by other care providers is needed (Mol 2002). Sometimes, general practitioners can decide to leave it up to patients themselves – for example, by informing them about certain self-care options (in the Netherlands, this can be an online health care website: ▶ GPinfo.nl) and letting them choose whatever suits them best. Case no. 11 describes a patient with a frequently heard complaint of fatigue and headaches.

Case no. 11: Patient with recurring somatic complaints, such as fatigue and headaches

A 42-year-old woman came to the surgery hour with complaints of fatigue. She described how she would wake up in the morning already feeling tired, which would get progressively worse over the course of the day, at which point she would also develop a headache. This had been going on for a few months. She really wanted to know what could be done about it. She indicated that she would prefer a hospital referral for further examination, as she was very worried. An aunt of hers also had headaches and this turned out to be a brain tumour. After an extensive anamnesis and general physical examination, the general practitioner explained to her that fatigue and headaches are symptoms that can have many causes, and that in such cases a twin-track approach is usually followed. This includes, excluding physical causes by means of blood tests on the one hand, and looking at broader to her health situation with the spiderweb of Positive Health, on the other. The patient agreed to this proposal and the practitioner asked her to make a new appointment and to complete the Positive Health online questionnaire in preparation for the next appointment. When she returned for her next consultation (a double appointment), the blood results appeared to be good. They then looked at the spider web she had filled out beforehand. At this point, some patients can see themselves what it is that makes them so tired, and that was also the case with this patient. Apart from the fact that she was happy to see that the results confirmed that she felt her life to be meaningful (she had a good job) and she also scored well on participation (a nice social network), she did notice that she had difficulty concentrating, did not feel fit, and that, often, she would stretch the limits of what she could endure. In order to keep all the plates spinning, both at home and at work, she felt that she was running behind, every day, all day. She indicated that she was not used to asking others for help – that she was actually just too busy and trying to cater to everyone's wishes while completely disregarding her own.

The general practitioner asked what her first steps towards changing this situation could be. She indicated that she first wanted to discuss the various tasks within the family with her husband, and how she would like to get more help with the children. She also decided, there on the spot, that she would like to work one day less a week and that she planned to discuss this with her employer. She said she had gained sufficient insight now, and that she had enjoyed achieving them through filling out the spider web. Sometimes you need a mirror before you know what to do, she said. She actually did not understand why she had not thought of the cause before then and how she was no longer worried about other physical causes. She indicated that, for the time being, she was able to move forward with her insights and steps to take, and that she would make a new appointment if she would need further support. To date, she has not been back to see the general practitioner.

Patients are able to prepare themselves well by filling out the questionnaire, which provides them with more insight into their own situation and makes them feel that there is attention for the whole person rather than just their medical complaint. With Positive Health, care givers work in a way that is different and feels less stressful. Patients provide insights themselves and, by asking questions, general practitioners can support their patients in taking the appropriate action. In a medical-analytical context, the initial request for help would lead to a referral to a specialist, whereas with Positive Health, the solution may be found closer to home. The following text box describes a case with a mental health assessment using the alternative dialogue method of Positive Health.

Case no. 12: Mental health problems

A 29-year-old secondary school teacher complained about having been extremely tired of late. He had difficulty concentrating and noticed that, come the middle of the week, he would have no energy left for the last two days of school. The practice assistant, on hearing these complaints, immediately booked him in for a double appointment and asked him to complete the online questionnaire at ▶ Mijnpositiev-egezondheid.nl, in preparation for the consultation. During the consultation, the patient talked about his complaints and took out his mobile phone from where he accessed his filled-out version of the questionnaire. He indicated that his mental and physical scores were lower and that he was not doing so well in other areas of his life, either. Lately, he was lacking energy for friends, felt he was withdrawing more and more. In addition, managing money and time has never been his strong suit, either. He particularly wanted to do something about his forgetfulness and concentration problems – issues that were also getting in the way of work. Furthermore, he was feeling less cheerful, had less energy and would like to improve his fitness level.

The general practitioner asked him what he would need to change these things and what the first small step could be, something that he could do himself. The man thought for a long time and did not know where to start. He had done an online test to check whether he had a burnout, and asked the practitioner if he perhaps had that. He also considered ADHD; as a child, he could be excessively active and during his studies he used to have trouble concentrating. He would like this to be examined further and possibly receive treatment. Together with the patient, the general practitioner decided to refer him to the GGZ (the Dutch Association of Mental Health and Addiction Care) for diagnostics and advice. The general practitioner informed him of a possibly long waiting period before he could be seen by the GGZ, and asked him what he thought he could do himself, in the meantime. To work on his level of fitness, the patient indicated that he would try to bicycle to work every day.

When asked by the general practitioner how he felt about this consultation, the man said that, with the help of the results from the spider web, he came to realise for the first time that he really wanted to take action to change certain things. He also realised that he himself had to take the first steps. Since that time, the patient has not been back to the practice, although he did wave at the general practitioner, one day, when they met while he was out on the bicycle.

5.5.2   Core task: *emergency care*

Emergency care is care that cannot wait until a regular appointment can be made with a health care provider. Emergency primary care is intended for health complaints that, from a medical standpoint, need to be looked at immediately (or within a few hours) and for which the general medical view of the practitioner is of added value. The medical-analytical perspective is needed to make a quick, likely diagnosis and rapidly get the patient to the right place for any follow-up treatment or examinations. Here, the general practitioner acts as a gatekeeper for follow-up care.

Determining the degree of urgency by the general practitioner as a medical generalist is of added value; for instance, in cases of assessing frail or elderly patients at home, terminally ill patients and children with fever or shortness of breath. Unnecessary referrals can be avoided by addressing the concerns and wishes of the patient and by agreeing on what should be done is cases of deviations from the expected course.

Emergency care starts with a request for care that the patient considers to be acute. Who would be the most appropriate care provider to provide such emergency care depends on the assessment of the seriousness of the symptoms and is related to the patient's medical history and context. In some instances, emergency care is not required although the patient does expect to receive it. Here, it is the task of the primary care provider to explain this to the patient; for instance, using the information on ▶ GPinfo.nl. Positive Health can also give the patient insight into the origins of complaints that may seem acute but are not. This is illustrated by case no. 13.

Case no. 13: Palpitations disappeared after paying attention to meaningfulness
An Eastern European woman who had moved to the Netherlands with her family because of her husband's work regularly visited the general practice's surgery hour. Each time, this woman in her thirties spoke of the same complaint, namely an indefinable feeling in her chest. It made her rather anxious. During and after her first visit, neither a blood test nor a blood pressure measurement or listening to the heart revealed any cardiac arrhythmia. At the next consultation, a cardiogram was made and a Holter was used – after which serious pathology was excluded.
Two cardiologists, who had the patient perform a bicycle test, confirmed that she would not have to worry about coronary artery disease. She had only had incidental, innocent premature ventricular contractions. However, the woman could not be reassured; she continued to visit the general practice with complaints of vague feelings in her chest and the anxiety this was causing her. She also regularly went to the hospital's emergency department or made use of out-of-hours services.
After yet another such visit, the general practitioner decided to telephone her and invite her to come to the surgery for an alternative dialogue. The general practitioner was not worried about her heart, but wondered whether other things might be going on. He said to her: 'I notice how you regularly visit my surgery with the same complaints, but that you have not yet been able to find a solution to those complaints. Shall we take a broader look at what may be the underlying cause of your complaints?' When she agreed to this, the general practitioner asked her to make a double appointment for this purpose.
In discussing her filled-out spider web, the patient herself concluded that she did not feel physically fit, and was not doing very well, mentally, either, and scored low in terms of meaningfulness. On the positive side, the results also confirmed what she knew what was going well with respect to her family and living conditions. The patient indicated that she would like to feel fitter, and be able to understand her symptoms and do the things that would give her more energy. Without explicitly mentioning it, the focus was shifted from fear of heart disease to areas that she would like to improve on, such as sense of purpose and physical fitness.
To help the patient understand her palpitations, which were still bothering her, the general practitioner advised her to go back to the cardiology clinic, this time to participate in a heart monitoring programme (Hartwacht 2019) whereby patients

are provided with a sensor so they can monitor their own heartbeat via an app. The general practitioner thought that if this patient would see what was going on when she felt uncomfortable, perhaps she would be able to let go of her anxiety more easily and realise she did not need to worry. In this way, the woman gained more insight into her complaints and became increasingly more confident about her health.

After this consultation, there were no more messages from the out-of-hours service, and, for a long time, the general practitioner did not see her again at the practice. The next time was when one of her children had to visit the surgery. When the general practitioner asked her how she was doing, she said she hardly had any heart complaints and felt much more energetic. The latter was partly due to a community project that the general practitioner had informed her about (Indekerngezond, ▶ www.indekerngezond. nl; see ▶ Chap. 7). This project intends to stimulate people to take control of their lives themselves and lead a healthy and meaningful life. In the meantime, she had been doing voluntary work and gained many social contacts. That she was doing all right was underlined by the fact that she had already returned the heart sensor from the heart monitoring programme – she no longer needed it (Van den Brekel 2019).

Emergency care means that the patient immediately receives the type of care that is needed. For people with an acute coronary syndrome, for example, the Positive Health approach is not the right one. However, such an acute incident, also often in the emergency department, can be a window of opportunity for having a conversation about behavioural change. For example, when someone comes to the hospital with yet another COPD exacerbation; if they continue their smoking habit, at some point, the only thing left is for them to have oxygen at home. Or following a heart attack in an obese patient, a conversation about lifestyle change may be in order. What can patients learn during their recovery from a heart attack about what and why this happened to them, for example? A person-oriented conversation, using the Positive Health approach, may help the patient gain insight into the things that they value, and perhaps in a roundabout way achieve a lifestyle change.

Of course, it is better for people to start adopting a healthy lifestyle before they develop a heart attack. The core task of *preventive care* describes the role of the general practitioner, in this respect. ▶ Chapter 7 further explains how this can be done in cooperation with the social domain, using the programmes of exercise and well-being offered within the community.

5.5.3 Core task: *terminal palliative care*

Positive Health is not the first thing that comes to mind in the last phase of life. Two cases (14 and 15 and the tip in ▶ sect. 5.4), illustrate the added value of having an alternative dialogue in the phase in which death is imminent.

Every general practitioner has general medical knowledge and expertise to provide terminal palliative care. In addition, general practitioners know the personal context and history of their patients and have insight into their living environment and social network. General practitioners have a special role in this final phase of their patients' lives, which is to be a steady and trusted point of contact in the entire care process.

In addition to the general practitioner, other care providers also play a significant role, such as informal caregivers, district and specialist nurses and pharmacists. The general practitioner has a coordinating role regarding the general medical care for the terminally ill patient in his or her home situation and, if necessary, makes use of the possibility of consultation (for example, from other physicians, medical specialists or specialised consultation teams). When general practitioners take over the coordination from secondary care, it is important that they are informed in due time about the disease process. The importance of personal continuity by general practitioners themselves increases as the end of a patient's life approaches. In this phase, the patient's condition deteriorates and symptoms often appear simultaneously, which may necessitate daily treatment adjustments. To connect with what is still of value to the patient, an alternative dialogue on the basis of the Positive Health approach may be worthwhile.

Case no. 14: Terminal palliative care and the spider web

In 2015, the Positive Health northern Meuse valley network developed a questionnaire to accompany the spider web. This was derived from the list of questions by the Institute for Positive Health (iPH) and the extended questionnaire on ▶ www.mypositivehealth. com. It was also the year in which the general practice in Afferden started to implement Positive Health to see if using the questionnaire would also be helpful with terminally ill patients. They found two such patients willing to fill out the spider web together. Both patients were in the last weeks of their lives, both were bedridden and cachectic, in pain and aware of their situation. The general practitioner expected to see low scores on several dimensions of their questionnaire, but to his surprise both patients were rather satisfied with all six dimensions of their Positive Health, despite the pain and other discomforts and despite being aware of their very limited life expectancy.

This was confusing to the general practitioner; perhaps the newly developed questionnaire was less suitable as a conversation tool to determine how these types of patients were doing? He discussed this with the two patients. Both indicated that they were resigned to what was coming and accepted their fate. Yes, they were in pain and bedridden, but they felt surrounded by the love of the people closest to them, which even gave them confidence about the future and allowed them to enjoy life in their own way and feel healthy, or whole, in a way. This was an important eye opener for the general practitioner. Without such a questionnaire, he might have been tempted to do something about the pain they were experiencing. In light of the overall picture, it became clear that both of them preferred to have a little more pain, in exchange for not being in a daze due to the painkillers. In this way, they were able to have full contact with their surroundings for longer. Also, without this questionnaire, general practitioners of course always talk with their terminally ill patients to see what would be the most sensible thing to do and they put the patient's needs and wishes first. Nevertheless, the general practitioner, in this case, was surprised by the results of using the spider web with terminally ill patients. It had been the basis for two extraordinary conversations.

The case in the text box on 'Terminal palliative care and the spider web' makes clear what is still of value to people in the last phase of their lives. The wishes of these patients are of course discussed with them by the general practitioner and also with the patient's immediate family. The use of Positive Health can be a good addition for obtaining more insight.

> **Case no. 15: Pain in relation to cancer and advanced care planning**
> It was unclear why a 50-year-old man with metastasised pancreatic cancer and many fluctuating pains, continued to have such erratic pain patterns. During a visit, his general practitioner asked how he was doing, using the various dimensions of Positive Health as a guide for the conversation. This showed that the patient attached great importance to his independence. He wanted to be able to drive his vintage car until the very end. Beautiful cars had always been his passion in life. He had great difficulty with the regime of painkillers, such as morphine, in the final phase, and always went his own way. Suddenly, his general practitioner realised why; the man took the morphine in the evenings because he thought he could then still drive during the day, which is also why he continued to refuse using the morphine patches. Unfortunately, his situation deteriorated rapidly over a number of months, and continuous pain medication was required.
> There was increasing unease, also amongst the teenage sons in the house, about how long their father would have to remain in bed. During the practitioner's next visit, he indicated that a conversation about the possibilities surrounding the end of life could create peace and clarity. The now familiar spider web was brought into play again. This time, the themes that were now considered to be of value had changed. Meaningfulness, gratitude, faith and the burden placed on his partner and children as to how and where he would die were the themes that determined his scores.
> The patient absolutely did not want euthanasia, and if his family could still cope, he preferred to stay at home with palliative sedation, until the very end. Two weeks later, he died at home.

5.5.4   Core task: *care coordination*

The project on future primary care (Toekomst Huisartsenzorg) describes the core task of *care coordination* as follows: 'The general practitioner maintains an overview of the patient's care pathway with regard to medical care. The general practitioner knows which care providers are involved and what their tasks and responsibilities are. The general practitioner coordinates the general medical care and has a signalling function. General practitioners are not responsible for the coordination of specialist (follow-up) care in secondary care, nor for the daily care or support of the patient. The general practitioner works within a broad network of care providers and caregivers and is often seen as the first point of contact in the coordination of care around the patient. The coordinating tasks of the general practitioner are related to the medical field. The general practitioner is not responsible for coordinating tasks regarding nursing care or those that concern the social domain.'

For the cooperation with other care providers, various guides have been drawn up. For examples of care coordination and Positive Health, see ▸ Chap. 7.

5.5.5 Core task: *preventive care*

With regard to prevention, general practitioners are mainly focusing on preventing disease, while the promotion of health is still of lesser importance, in most primary care practices. There is, however, much to be gained with respect to health if there would be a focus on optimising the health skills of patients. In the elaboration of the general practitioners' core task of preventive care they focus on the individual people with indicated and care-related prevention. The Dutch Public Health authorities are responsible for universal and selective prevention, with a focus on the general population. Indicated prevention is aimed at people who have not yet been diagnosed with a disease, but do have the risk factors or symptoms that precede a particular disease. Examples are cardiovascular risk management or the detection of lifestyle factors such as smoking or problematic alcohol consumption without a disease being present.

Care-related prevention focuses on people with a disease or condition and prevents an existing condition from leading to complications, limitations, a low quality of life, or death. Examples include the coaching and treatment of patients with chronic diseases, such as cardiovascular diseases, COPD, and diabetes mellitus 2 with healthy diet, lifestyle and/or medication. This concerns, for instance, the lifestyle and obesity modules of the standards of the Dutch College of General Practitioners (NHG) or other guidelines. This type of care is often offered by the practice nurse, in cooperation with other care providers. In preventive care, using the Positive Health approach, patients obtain insight into what is important to them and discover their intrinsic motivation, for example, with respect to making lifestyle changes (see ► sect. 5.7). In these cases, prevention is actually a response option with which care providers may give patients a push into the right direction.

Positive Health contributes to a meaningful life. The focus is therefore not necessarily on the prevention of diseases through lifestyle changes, but on appealing to the intrinsic motivation of patients to develop resilience and to make the necessary changes in their lives. Here, Positive Health functions as a mirror, through which patients see their own health reflected back at them. Positive Health poses a central question to patients about what they would like to change, and subsequently looks at how this could be done. Lifestyle adjustments can be part of that approach. Thus, first the intrinsic motivation must be encouraged, after which health progress can be achieved, possibly with lifestyle adjustments.

5.6 From spider web to action

The *alternative dialogue* stirs up the intrinsic motivation. After which it becomes important to discover what patients are able to do themselves. How they could take action, and what the appropriate *perspectives for action* could be. Physicians, sometimes, believe they should be able to provide expert advice on subjects in all dimensions. Whether that is such a good starting point is debatable. According to the *core values*, general practitioners are *general medical* experts and that clearly defines the scope of their work. This does not alter the fact that it is useful to be in contact with professionals who are skilled on subjects within the other dimensions of the spider web. However, before a patient is referred to someone else, for example, within the social domain, it is important to first ask the patient the following questions:

- *What are you thinking of?*
- *Which subsequent step could you make yourself?*
- *Who or what could help you with that?*

It is surprising how great the self-solving ability of people is towards taking a first step. Here too, as a rule, people are often their own best advisors! It is good to remember that many solutions are smaller in scope and closer to home than general practitioners tend to think. In practice, we hear of solutions patients have come up with themselves, such as going on walks with a neighbour, partner or friend, having a coffee with others or participating in a certain sport. Informal care can also often provide a solution. There are also cases where patients are at a loss about what to do. Therefore, below, a number of pathways are described that can be used as starting points:

5.6.1 Apps available online

If people need suggestions about which courses of action to take and they have good self-management and digital skills, there may be useful apps for them to download. In the Netherlands, there is the GGD AppStore, which is set up, filled and maintained by the Community Health Services (GGD). Their goal is to offer health apps that are in line with the six dimensions of Positive Health. Selection criteria for inclusion in the Appstore – out of the many health apps available today – are respect for privacy, comprehensibility and, where possible, effectiveness. The apps are ordered according to the dimensions of Positive Health and, for each app, an indication is given for which dimensions it can be of use (▶ www.ggdappstore.nl, ◨ fig. 5.8).

▶ Section 5.5 provides examples of how Positive Health can contribute to the core tasks of the general practitioner. This includes various response options on all six dimensions. The things on offer include, for example, voluntary social work and

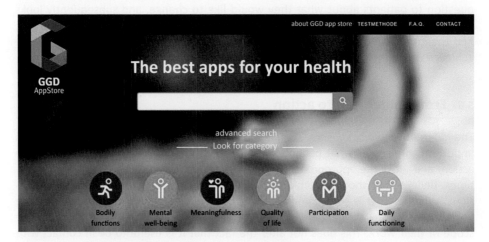

◨ **Figure 5.8** The homepage of the Dutch Community Health Services (GGD) AppStore, translated in English, with apps suiting the dimensions of Positive Health. (Source: ▶ www.ggdappstore.nl)

the programme on *Social Prescribing* (in Dutch: Welzijn op Recept), and are often all available locally, although sometimes they are difficult to find (see ► Chap. 7). An overview of useful links about what is on offer can be found at the end of the book.

5.6.2 Psychosocial complaints

In cases of psychosocial complaints, or if there is a need with respect to the social domain, there are many possibilities in the community, both related to informal and formal care (also see ► sect. 7.6), possibly in addition to the mental health practice nurse. The supply will vary per district, village or neighbourhood, and the social map is leading, here (► Chap. 7). If psychological problems are more serious, the general practitioner knows the way to mental health care for children and adolescents and to basic or specialist mental health care for adults. In the Netherlands, there are growing numbers of these GGZ mental health institutions that work with Positive Health. In this way, patients can already start by taking small steps themselves towards recovery while waiting for their treatment to begin. Patients appreciate it if the subsequent care providers all speak with one voice (see the case in ► sect. 7.5).

5.7 Positive Health and a healthy lifestyle

Lifestyle advice is an important part of primary care. For people with chronic diseases or at risk of these diseases (e.g., because of obesity or smoking), this falls under the core task of preventive care, as indicated and care-related prevention.

The general practitioner and the practice nurse play an active signalling and motivating role in this. Health care professionals often find it difficult to encourage lifestyle change and think it takes a lot of time. As a general practitioner, it is important to identify unhealthy lifestyles and to discuss it openly. If the patient is overweight or obese and is motivated, a lifestyle consultation can be arranged with the practice assistant (see ► sect. 5.7, lifestyle consultation). The general practitioner can invite a patient for a separate lifestyle consultation or pay attention to lifestyle counselling during a regular check-up. A combined lifestyle intervention (CLI) may also be appropriate (see ► Chap. 7).

More than 80% of patients say they appreciate the mention of obesity by the general practitioner. Less than 1% feels that this is not appropriate. Research (Aveyard 2016) shows that a 30-second advice by the general practitioner with a targeted referral to a group intervention yields significantly greater reduction in weight than merely the practitioner's advice to lose weight. If good lifestyle services are available in the local community, a brief indication and referral can therefore already be of added value (► Chap. 7). The effect of group interventions has been demonstrated before; whereby long-term interventions yield greater weight reduction than short-term interventions. This is why, in the Netherlands, basic health insurance was recently expanded to also include combined lifestyle interventions for people with obesity (► sect. 7.7).

The challenge is to start – getting someone to realise that they want to start working on a better lifestyle – and then to keep going. General practitioners have an important role in identifying and discussing lifestyle issues. The research mentioned above shows that this not necessarily takes a large amount of the general practitioner's time.

5.7.1   The lifestyle conversation

In cases where general practitioners or practice assistants want to encourage their patients to change their lifestyle, the alternative dialogue may be of help. Professionals are sometimes rather quick with giving advice, and whether this is always in line with the patient's wishes or desires is debatable. A person-oriented conversation can reveal what is important to patients themselves, with regard to their general health. Case no. 15 on lifestyle illustrates how Positive Health can be used to talk about someone's lifestyle.

Case no. 16: Lifestyle
A 23-year-old man visited the surgery with complaints about his musculoskeletal system. The general practitioner noticed that he was obese (BMI 32). Out of curiosity, she asked him if he wanted to talk about his obesity. The man indicated that he had already tried many things to lose weight, but that if there would be something new for him to try, he would be open to it. The general practitioner explained that she first wanted to take a broader look at how he thought about his health in general. For this purpose, she asked him to fill out an online questionnaire, at home, which would provide an indication of his degree of satisfaction about subjects on 6 dimensions of Positive Health. The general practitioner also asked him to have the assistant book a double appointment for next time, to discuss this (◘ fig. 5.9).
The following week, the general practitioner and the patient discussed the completed spider web. The patient appeared to lead a meaningful life and to be happy with his mental health. He also scored positively on the dimensions of participation and daily functioning. He said that this was the first time that he realised which things in his life were going well. The many years of being overweight had always put the emphasis on him being 'too fat' and on the things he was doing wrong, in that respect. This had made him eat more rather than less. He indicated that he was happy with his newly obtained insights; he would like to continue to function well in his work and daily life, in which there were many things he enjoyed, and he would like to continue being in these good spirits, with his friends and rich social life. However, he did have some physical complaints. There he scored much lower, and these things were not improving his quality of life.
His own conclusions and insights were that he really wanted to change his physical condition in order to continue living his life. 'I won't be able to do that for long, with this body', he admitted. The general practitioner asked what he would like. He said he did not like dieticians and well-meaning advice, but that he would need some support, because he could not manage to lose weight by himself. The general practitioner provided him with a number of possibilities in the local community and region, and they made a follow-up appointment.
Two weeks later, the man returned to the surgery and asked for a referral for a combined lifestyle intervention, saying that he really wanted to work on changing his lifestyle, under his own steam. The general practitioner asked him what he would still need from her in order to achieve his goal. He said: 'Nothing really, but I'll know where to find you if I do relapse'. Since then, the patient has not been back to the surgery.
A few months later, the general practitioner was talking to his mother and asked her

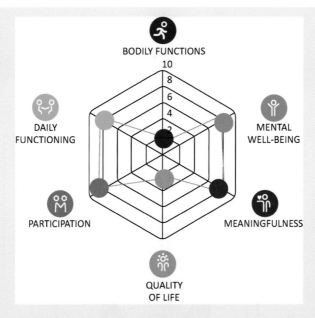

BODILY FUNCTIONS
10
8
6
4
2

DAILY
FUNCTIONING

MENTAL
WELL-BEING

PARTICIPATION

MEANINGFULNESS

QUALITY
OF LIFE

◘ **Figure 5.9**   Filled-out spider web of overweight patient

how her son was doing. 'He has already lost 10 kilos', she said, 'and really wants to make this change for himself'.

These three consultations with the patient, paying attention to the six dimensions of Positive Health, have possibly contributed to a saving of health care costs (related to obesity/chronic disease), and resulted in a satisfied patient and a satisfied physician. These are the types of consultations that make the general practitioner happy: 'I hardly had to do anything'. The patient became motivated and improved his lifestyle with his own insights and intrinsic motivation.

The Dutch physicians and lifestyle association (Vereniging Arts en Leefstijl) works to implement the use of lifestyle medical science in the consulting room and supports health care professionals in advising their patients. The association has developed the so-called Lifestyle Wheel (◘ fig. 5.10). The Lifestyle Wheel provides concrete examples of areas in which patients themselves can work on their lifestyle. The spider web and the Lifestyle Wheel complement each other rather well. In the first instance, Positive Health appeals to people's intrinsic motivation. The Lifestyle Wheel indicates practical small steps that the patient may choose from, in order to achieve concrete behavioural changes, step by step (▶ www.artsenleefstijl.nl).

How does the spider web relate to this Lifestyle Wheel? Both tools are about improving people's health. Both can be used separately or next to each other in the consulting room. They can also reinforce each other, as illustrated in ◘ fig. 5.11. If patients decide to change their lifestyle, the Lifestyle Wheel offers perspectives for taking action in this respect. Together, the spider web and the Lifestyle Wheel support the process of behavioural change towards living a healthier life (from insight to overview, to prospects and taking action). The spider web brings out people's intrinsic motivation which is needed

Personal information

Date: _____
Name: _____
Date of birth: _____

The lifestyle wheel

'The lifestyle wheel provides tools to set the right course for a healthy lifestyle.
You are in the driver's seat and can make adjustments yourself.
The lifestyle wheel is always in motion, it gives direction and makes connections.'

Arts en Leefstijl
For tomorrow's care
www.artsenleefstijl.nl

Nutrition
☐ Eat at least 250 grams of vegetables and 2 pieces of fruits per day
☐ Eat as little sugar as possible and other fast carbohydrates
☐ Eat fresh and unprocessed foods (not ready-sliced or -bagged)
☐ Eat three full meals per day, and as few snacks as possible
☐ Drink unsweetened drinks, preferably water and coffee or tea
☐ Eat unsaturated fats, such as extra virgin olive oil and nuts
☐ Eat more vegetable products and fewer animal products
☐ Do not smoke. Do not use drugs and drink as little alcohol as possible
☐ Stop counting calories

Social
☐ Spend time with friends and loved ones
☐ Invest in friendships and a social network
☐ Be kind and show an interest in others
☐ Make physical contact
☐ Surround yourself with people that give you energy

Relaxation
☐ Leave the house every day and go into the countryside
☐ Find a relaxing activity or hobby
☐ Turn off your smartphone more often
☐ Meditate or do absolutely nothing, from time to time
☐ Take short breaks during the day

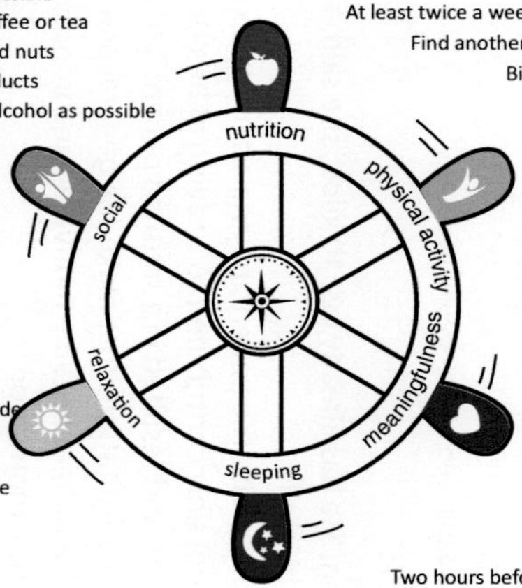

Psysical activity
☐ Every week, do at least 150 minutes of moderate to vigorous exercise
☐ Try to take 10,000 steps per day (using a pedometer or fitness app)
☐ At least twice a week, do muscle- and bone-strengthening excercies
☐ Find another person to join you in physical activities or sports
☐ Bicycle to work or go on walks in your lunch breaks
☐ Take the stairs instead of the elevator
☐ Avoid sitting still for too long

Meaningfulness
☐ Focus your attention on what makes you happy
☐ Set your personal goals and aim in life
☐ Replace negative thoughts with positive ones
☐ Be grateful for the positive things
☐ Continue your personal development and try out new things
☐ Develop mindfulness and compassion

Sleeping
☐ Make sure your bedroom is cool and well-ventilated
☐ Do not drink cafeine shortly before bedtime
☐ Ensure a regular sleeping pattern
☐ Sleep 7 to 8 hours per night
☐ Two hours before bedtime, turn off all electronic visual displays

And furthermore
☐ _____
☐ _____
☐ _____
☐ _____

(wheel labels: physical activity, meaningfulness, nutrition, sleeping, social, relaxation)

Figure 5.10   The Lifestyle Wheel of the physicians and lifestyle association. (Source: Arts en Leefstijl, ▶ www.artsenleefstijl.nl)

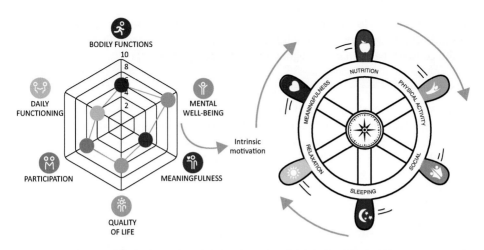

◻ Figure 5.11   The Lifestyle Wheel and spider web enhance each other. (Source: ▶ www.allesisgezond-heid.nl 2020)

to achieve behavioural change. More reading material on this subject can be found in the handbook for lifestyle medicine ('Handboek voor leefstijlgeneeskunde' (in Dutch), De Vries and De Weijer 2020). Both tools increase people's ability to self-manage. Moreover, it would be useful for care providers to experience both of these tools for themselves. This will have a significant and positive impact on using them in practice.

When patients become motivated to change their lifestyle and perhaps already want to take small steps towards their goal using the Lifestyle Wheel, there are many useful tips provided in the care modules on lifestyle by the Dutch College of General Practitioners (NHG). These provide guidance on subjects such as alcohol, exercise, smoking and nutrition, in daily practice (NHG 2015). General practitioners or practice assistants can provide information about lifestyle and the effects and risks of certain lifestyle choices on current and future health. The website ▶ GPonline.nl has information that supports this educational material, and there may also be information available online, in your country. In the Netherlands, there are many apps on lifestyle, such as from the GGD Appstore (▶ www.ggdappstore.nl, see ◻ fig. 5.8). Periodically, the general practitioner or practice nurse and patient, together, can assess whether the patient is succeeding in achieving his or her goal. This assessment can be made using an individual care plan, in which those involved (patient, care providers and caregivers) write down the objectives and targets, their agreements, actions and at which time the next assessment is to take place.

In general medical practice, various successful initiatives have been developed to support people in their desired lifestyle, such as counselling to stop smoking and the combined lifestyle interventions available under the Dutch Health Insurance Act. In some countries, health promotion is organised on a national level, by national public health services and/or locally organised in community prevention programmes. Many people find it difficult to make lifestyle changes on their own. The lifestyle conversation under the Positive Health concept supports patients in obtaining insight and taking action in accordance with their own needs and at their own pace. In this way, self-management is stimulated. If necessary, patients can subsequently be referred to locally available services. To ensure that patients continue with the lifestyle intervention methods in the right way, conducting an alternative dialogue according to the Positive Health concept, beforehand, is highly recommended (► Chap. 7).

Reflection

Do you have enough insights into how to start conducting the alternative dialogue in your practice? And what do you think about filling out the spider web yourself?
What is important to you? What would you like to change in your life?
What is your experience with taking concrete action?
Did you do it? Or, if not: What made you not do it? What would need to happen for you to do what you would like to do?
How could you apply your own experiences in practice?

This chapter is about the consulting room, the direct contact between people.

However, the consulting room is part of a greater whole. How to connect the general practice to this larger realm? This is discussed in ► Chap. 6.

5.8   Conclusions

This chapter focuses on the consulting room and discusses how to conduct the alternative dialogue. Positive Health first focuses on your personal experience, advising you to fill out the spider web for yourself. Once you have become an 'experience expert' and have achieved results with your own health, you will be more convincing in interactions with your patients. The chapter subsequently pays extensive attention to the person-oriented style of conversation, which follows on from the spider web, with examples of two possible ways of conducting the so-called alternative dialogue: asking solution-oriented questions and using the Action Wheel. The chapter looks at how to start and what questions to ask, in order to encourage patients to find solutions and take action themselves. Based on the core tasks in primary care, this chapter discusses the target groups with whom to have the *alternative dialogue* on the basis of the Positive Health concept. How to experience applying Positive Health in practice is described according to a number of examples, the four tools, materials, case studies, tips and pointers.

For more information, background or videos about this chapter scan the QR code.

SCAN ME

References

Allesisgezondheid (2020). Accessed in June 21 of ► https://www.allesisgezondheid.nl/evenementen/webinar-het-andere-gesprek-in-de-spreekkamer/.

Aveyard, P., Lewis, A., Tearne, S., et al. (2016). Screening and brief intervention for obesity in primary care: A parallel, two-arm, randomised trial. *Lancet, 388,* 2492–2500.

Bannink, F. (2019). *Handboek oplossingsgerichte gespreksvoering.* Amsterdam: Pearson.

Bannink, F., & Jansen, P. (2017). *Positieve gezondheidszorg. Oplossingsgericht werken in de huisartspraktijk.* Amsterdam: Pearson Benelux B.V.

Calnan, M. (1988). Towards a conceptual framework of lay evaluations of health care. *Social Science and Medicine, 27,* 927–933.

Campion, P., Foulkes, J., Neighbour, R., & Tate, P. (2002). Patient centredness in the MRCGP video examination: Analysis of large cohort. *BMJ, 325*(7366), 691–692. ► https://doi.org/10.1136/bmj.325.7366.691.

CRU+ (2019). *Praktisch lijn onderwijs communicatie en attitude (2019–2020).* Utrecht: UMC. Accessed in June 21 of ► https://students.uu.nl/gnk/geneeskunde-b/onderwijs/studieprogramma.

De Maeseneer, J. (2017). *Family medicine and primary care.* Lannoo Campus: At the crossroads of societal change.

De Saint Exupery, A. (2012). Citadelle, posthum, 1948. In Van der Kaap A. *Het eindeloze verlangen naar de zee.* Histoforum didactiek. Het online tijdschrift voor geschiedenisdidactiek. Accessed in August 2020 of ► http://histoforum.net/columns/column14.html.

De Vries, M., & De Weijer, T. (2020). *Handboek leefstijlgeneeskunde. De basis voor iedere praktijk.* Houten: Bohn Stafleu van Loghum.

Hartwacht (2019). Accessed in October 2020 of ► www.cardiologiecentra.nl/patienten/ons-zorgaanbod/hartwacht/.

Hermsen, J. (2015). *Kairos, een nieuwe bevlogenheid.* Amsterdam: De Arbeiderspers.

Huber, M., Van Vliet, M., Giezenberg, M., et al. (2016). Towards a 'patient-centred' operationalisation of the new dynamic concept of health: A mixed methods study. *BMJ Open, 2016*(5), e010091.

Illich, I. (1974). *Medical nemesis.* Londen: Calders en Boyars.

In de kerngezond, Leidsche Rijn. ► www.indekerngezond.nl.

Jung, H. P., Baerveldt, C., Olesen, F., Grol, R., & Wensing, M. (2003). Patient characteristics as predictors of primary health care preferences: A systematic literature analysis. *Health Expectations, 6,* 160–181.

Lupyan, G., & Swingley, D. (2020). *It doesn't mean you're crazy – talking to yourself has cognitive benefits, study finds. Science daily.* Accessed in June 2021 of ► https://www.sciencedaily.com/releases/2012/04/120417221613.htm.

LRJG (2020). *Rapportage Implementatie van het persoonsgerichte 'andere' gesprek in de huisartspraktijk.* Accessed in October 2020 of ► www.lrjg.nl/nieuws/ander-gesprek.

Mauksch, L. B. (2017). Questioning a taboo. Physicians' interruptions during interactions with patients. *JAMA, 317*(10), 1021–1022. ► https://doi.org/10.1001/jama.2016.16068.

Medisch Ondernemen (2019). *Ephraim M. Positieve Gezondheidsgesprekken geven huisartsenzorg een boost.* ► https://www.medischondernemen.nl/search/node?keys=positieve+gezondheidsgesprekken+geven+huisartsen+zorg+een+boost.

Mol, S. S., Dinant, G. J., Vilters-van Montfort, P. A., Metsemakers, J. F., Van den Akker, M., Arntz, A., Knottnerus, J. A. (2002). Traumatic events in a general practice population: the patient's perspective. *Family Practice, 19*(4), 390–396. ► https://doi.org/10.1093/fampra/19.4.390.

NHG (2015). *NHG Zorgmodules.* Accessed in September 2020 of ► https://www.nhg.org/sites/default/files/content/nhg_org/uploads/nhg-zorgmodules_leefstijl.pdf.

NIVEL (2019). *Burgers over kernwaarden en kerntaken,* Accessed in October 2020 of ► https://www.nivel.nl/nl/publicatie/burgers-over-kernwaarden-en-kerntaken-huisarts.

Ospina, N. S., Phillips, K. A., Rodriguez-Gutierrez, R., et al. (2019). Eliciting the patient's agenda- secondary analysis of recorded clinical encounters. *Journal of General Internal Medicine, 34,* 36–40. ► https://doi.org/10.1007/s11606-018-4540-5.

Oude Weernink (2020). *Een persoonsgericht gesprek in de Huisartspraktijk – Een Haalbaarheidsstudie.* Accessed in June 2021 of ► www.lrjg.nl/nieuws/ander-gesprek.

Slagt, E. (2018). *Chronos loopt, Kairos vliegt. Over tijdsperceptie en het juiste moment van handelen.* Amsterdam: Brave New Books.

Te Brake, H., Van Lieshout, J., & Verhey, R. (2006). Grootgebruikers in de huisartspraktijk, een last voor de huisarts? *Huisarts en Wetenschap, 12,* 597.

Toekomsthuisartsenzorg (2020). *Kerntaken in de praktijk.* Accessed in June 2021 of ► toekomsthuisartsenzorg.nl.

Van den Brekel-Dijkstra, K. (2019). Hoe Positieve Gezondheid bij kan dragen aan gezonde leefstijl. *Bijblijven, 35,* 70–79.

Van den Brekel-Dijkstra, K., Cornelissen, M., & Van der Jagt, L. (2020). De dokter gevloerd. Hoe voorkomen we burn-out bij huisartsen? *Huisarts en Wetenschap, 63*(7), 40–43. ► https://doi.org/10.1007/s12445-020-0765-8.

Chapter 6

Macro
Regional /
national

Meso
District / community

Micro
Practice / organisation

Nano
Patient / citizen

I will maintain an open and verifiable attitude,
and I am aware of my responsibility towards socity.
I will promote the availability and accessibility of
health care. I will not misuse my medical knowledge,
not even under pressure.

Thus, I will uphold the profession of physician.

This I promise

or
So help me God Almighty

Positive Health in practice

© Bohn Stafleu van Loghum is an imprint of Springer Media B.V., part of Springer Nature 2022
M. Huber et al., *Handbook Positive Health in Primary Care*,
https://doi.org/10.1007/978-90-368-2729-4_6

> **Main messages**
> — Without a yearning for the vast and endless sea, there can be no true inspiration, implementation and embedding of Positive Health in practice.
> — Positive Health is located mainly in the second quadrant of the time management matrix.
> — Which of the aspects of Positive Health are implemented first depends on the care provider's mission, vision and strategy and their position within the general practice.
> — Distinguish between introduction/inspiration, the implementation process and the embedding of Positive Health in the practice, and pay an equally large amount of attention to each of these three elements.

6.1 Yearning for the endless sea

As de Saint-Exupéry, in the motto at the beginning of this book (de Saint Exupéry, 2012), made his sailors yearn for the endless sea, so in primary care general practitioners must make their colleagues yearn for working with Positive Health. Not by imposing it on them, but by letting them experience the benefits. This is also in line with this chapter, which raises the question of how one could successfully implement Positive Health into a general practice organisation. The main message, here, is that it is not enough to see Positive Health as a clever trick; for example, by letting patients fill out the spider web – analogous with instructing the sailors to collect wood. Instead, everyone in the general practice will need to share the vision of Positive Health contributing to realising what the practice stands for (i.e., they must all yearn for the endless sea).

Only then will Positive Health be embedded in the organisation in a way that is needed to really change the way in which the general practice operates. But how to do that? Why change? How do general practitioners get others to share their enthusiasm? What difference would this change make? And how to ensure the new working method continues? How to keep the team involved? This is what this chapter is about. Drafting a vision and mission for the practice will reveal the elements that would need to change. The time management matrix proves to be very useful, in this respect. This chapter discusses how to become acquainted with Positive Health, how Positive Health can be implemented in practice and how the practice team will remain motivated to continue working with Positive Health.

6.1.1 Positive Health, yes, but...

When it comes to applying Positive Health in the primary care organisation, there are roughly two ways of doing so:
1. One way is to first reflect, together with all practice staff, on the mission and vision of the general medical practice, to determine the possible place of Positive Health within it. This can then be worked out in a concrete strategy for the organisation. Sections 6.2 and 6.3 are in line with this method.
2. The other method is to choose a topic that appeals and that seems promising for the particular general practice. That is when the work starts. For example, to first become acquainted with Positive Health to see if it is something that would

suit the care providers in the practice, or because the practice is already working on its official accreditation (i.e., primary care quality standards) and a concrete improvement project seems suitable (with the added question of how to introduce Positive Health when some practice staff members may never have heard of it). Subsequently, a new subject within the concept is chosen. This handbook and this chapter, in particular, may help general practitioners to determine which topics they find most appealing and most appropriate (see ▶ sect. 6.4–6.8).

Which of the two approaches is most appropriate depends on the situation, personal preferences and working style. For practice staff who are front runners with respect to wanting to work with Positive Health, discussing the new way of working and holding a fundamental discussion about the practice's mission and vision will only succeed if they are given sufficient opportunity to do so by the other staff members. There are countless arguments against starting to work with Positive Health (see ▣ fig. 6.1). Being general practitioners themselves, the authors understand only too well that it takes time and dedication to immerse yourself in something new. And this time is not always available. However, the perspective of the Positive Health concept is that, in practice, general practitioners and other practice staff will be better able to provide the right care in the right place. This will benefit the patients and give general practitioners themselves a large degree of job satisfaction.

Positive Health focuses on what is possible, rather than on what is not. General practitioners who have lived through certain events (diseases or loss) appear to develop a broader view of health, which makes it easier to start working with Positive Health (Huber 2014). Fortunately, this broader view is not a prerequisite.

A frequently heard remark amongst general practitioners and practice staff when they are first introduced to Positive Health is: 'But I am already doing this!' It may indeed be the case that they are already asking questions from a broader perspective, when patients visit them with a particular complaint. But it is debatable whether this is the same as working with Positive Health. These kinds of responses are sometimes an expression of resistance. This can only be determined by asking more questions. For practitioners who are unable to convince their colleagues, the advice is to focus on a small element of Positive Health and demonstrate how, in practice, this provides many benefits for both patients and physicians and try to build on that.

6.2 How to start?

┌─ Reflection ───

In preparation for this chapter, practitioners who would like to start working with Positive Health should give themselves some time to answer the following question: 'What would you like to do differently in your practice that, if you were to do this regularly, would have an enormous positive effect on your job satisfaction?' Please write down your answer, as we will come back to it.

└──

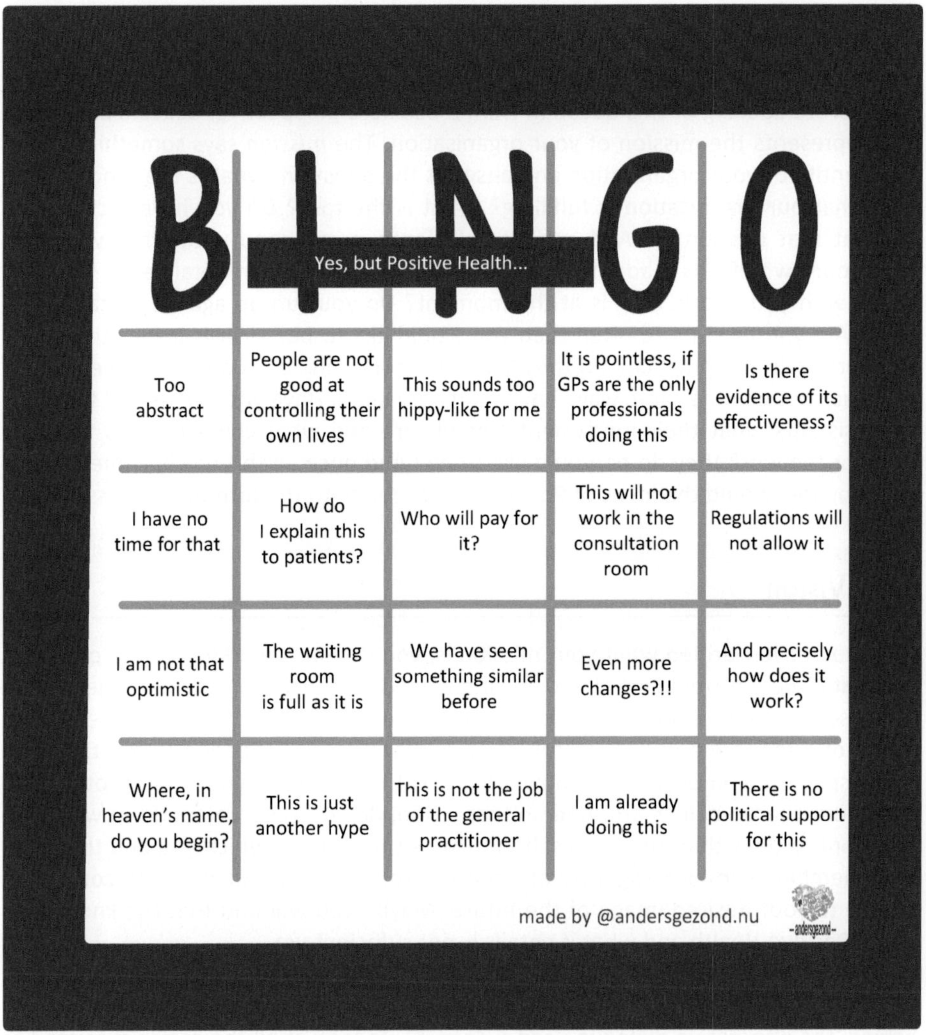

Figure 6.1 Positive Health, yes, but…. (Source: ▶ www.andersgezond.nu)

A good starting point to ponder the question of how to apply Positive Health, in practice, would be to reflect on what the proverbial 'yearning for the endless sea' actually means to you. How would you like to implement the concept? How would you like to enter into discussions with other practice staff members? And how do you ensure that the core values of the general medical profession (see ▶ Chap. 4) will be upheld? You can organise this yourself, but you may also enlist the support from organisations to assist you with training and implementation (see ▶ sect. 6.4).

6.2.1 Mission

The *yearning for the endless sea* could also be translated into the question: 'Why am I here?'. Looking at this question from a business perspective, delivers an answer that represents the mission of your organisation. The *mission* says something about the identity of your organisation and answers the question: what is the fundamental need that our organisation is fulfilling? What is the task? Do you have a clear idea of what that mission is? And does it sufficiently correspond with what you want from your own life? Is it adding something to your own fundamental needs? Are you happy with your work, as it is at the moment? Do you run up against certain problems? Are you tired more often than you would like to be? How is it for others who are working in the practice? Do they know what the mission is and does everyone in the practice think the same way? This is not very likely. Have you ever asked the nursing assistants what their fundamental needs are and what consequences this may have for the work they do or would like to do? And once all this has become clear as a group, how would the ideas of Positive Health relate to the formulated mission?

6.2.2 Vision

Once you have clarified what your mission is, you can start working on the question: 'In what direction would we like to go, and what do we want to achieve?' The answer to these questions represents the *vision* of the organisation. What is the shared image of a feasible and desired future and what would be needed to get there? In this respect, it is important to know what it is that connects you to each other and what your shared beliefs are. And, in that vision, do you see a relationship with who you want to be within the organisation? This is the point at which you and the other staff members can look together at what the concept of Positive Health could contribute to your desired image of the future. Maybe you will find that the knowledge about Positive Health and what it entails is not sufficient yet.

The iPH website contains some videos with background information (iPH 2019b). In addition, workshops can be organised to practice completing the spider web and having 'the alternative dialogue' (see ▶ Chap. 5). To look at all the material related to this chapter, please scan the QR code provided at the end of this chapter.

6.2.3 Strategy

If you feel that there is sufficient knowledge within your organisation about what Positive Health is, the subsequent step will be to determine what actions you will be taking next; what issues you will be addressing, and what will be the priorities. In business terms, this represents the *strategy*. It is essentially about making the right choices: about striving for results that are not only desired but also achievable by the organisation. This takes into account the goal, as well as the means available to achieve that goal. Once your practice has gone through all these steps, it will be clear how Positive Health relates to the mission of the practice, how Positive Health can contribute to the desired future of the practice and which concrete Positive Health activities you would like to implement. In management terms, you will have formulated a Positive Health strategy and business plan! It is essential that this is seen as a joint process, one to which everyone has contributed. Only in this way will you create support and a joint 'yearning for the sea'.

Mission and Vision pathway of the general medical practice Afferden

In 2016, the staff of general medical practice Afferden (workplace of author Hans Peter Jung) got together on four occasions, for half a day, to work on the mission and vision of the practice. In addition, a smaller group, consisting of one general practitioner and three practice assistants, met regularly in-between these meetings to prepare follow-up steps. They brainstormed to identify the topics that they thought were important to our mission and vision, and submitted these to the entire practice staff in the form of a questionnaire. Staff members could rate these questions in terms of importance and also add topics. This in turn served as input for the meetings in which they formulated the mission and vision together. Explicit part of the journey was to clearly discover what Positive Health could contribute to the mission and vision of the practice.

At the end, they wrote a mission and vision statement that reflected the process of how they arrived at their mission and vision, and that was also considered to conclude a period in which the practice was refocused on the challenges that lay ahead.

What was striking to see was that, during the process, the staff got to know each other in a different way and that this contributed to a feeling of solidarity and togetherness. A special moment was also when one of the nursing assistants taped a printout to the wall of the assistants' room which read: 'It's a beautiful thing, when a passion and a career come together'. The message reflected the insight that this process had given her. The mission and vision are on display in several places around the practice. At each of their monthly practice meetings, they repeat the mission and vision, and one of the participants keeps a record of the decisions taken during the meeting and to which of the elements of the mission and vision these decisions are contributing.

Mission of the general medical practice Afferden ('What is our purpose?'):
- To provide good primary care[1]
- To achieve a good relationship between care provider and patients/the community
- To provide a workplace where people enjoy working[2]
- To establish a good organisation in which the above-mentioned mission can be achieved

---

1   What do we consider good primary care? Evidence-based, but also pragmatic, involved, patient-oriented, accessible, based on trust, Positive Health as a starting point, if possible from disease and care to health and behaviour, cooperation, use of connecting (non-violent) communication, (sufficient) time.

2   What is enjoyment? Key words offered by practice staff include: balance of workload/carrying capacity, appropriate workload, meaningful work, team spirit, appreciation, attention, being yourself, safety, being heard, pleasant environment, relaxation and humour.

Vision of the general medical practice Afferden ('Where are we heading together?'):
- We want to work on the basis of Positive Health
- We want to have a good working atmosphere in our practice
- We want there to be a good balance between carrying capacity and workload amongst the practice staff
- We want to work according to the principles of the Triple Aim – improved population health, quality of care and cost-control.

Strategy of the general medical practice Afferden:
'From our mission and vision, there are three topics that are most crucial to work on, in our practice: (1) Construction of a new building; (2) Connecting, non-violent communication; and (3) Good organisation.'

6.3 The time management matrix

In order to properly determine which tasks should be given priority in the general medical practice, we looked at Eisenhower's time management matrix, which is also described by Stephen Covey (Covey 2004). Important here is the distinction made between tasks that are important/not important and urgent/not urgent. Important tasks are those that bring you closer to your goal ('the yearning for the endless sea')! It is essential that you know your mission and vision. A task that is truly important contributes to achieving your mission and fits in with the core values of the profession of general practitioner. An urgent task, on the other hand, is a task that has to be done quickly and cannot be postponed. It is important to realise that people tend to react to urgent matters, but addressing important issues that are not urgent requires a proactive attitude and making a conscious decision. It is good to realise that important tasks are not always also urgent and urgent tasks may be not important. ◲ Figure 6.2 shows this in a matrix that distinguishes between tasks that are urgent and important, urgent yet unimportant, not urgent but important and those that are neither urgent nor important.

The time management matrix can also be applied to classify the tasks encountered in a general medical practice. Does the practice decide for itself which tasks are put in which quadrant? All time in the practice is spent on one of these four classifications, urgent, important, not urgent and not important.

6.3.1 Time management matrix primary care

Consider the four quadrants of the time management matrix (◲ fig. 6.3). Quadrant I contains issues that are both important and urgent. These are important, and include things such as emergency care and terminal palliative care, which require immediate attention. Quadrant I attract people who are eager to tackle problems – preferably other people's (in which many general practitioners will recognise themselves, I am sure), but it also attracts the so-called procrastinators, people who first need to be faced with a deadline before they take action.

	Urgent	Not urgent
Important	I. Activities: - Crises - Pressing problems - Projects that are deadline-driven - Reactive	II. Activities: - Precautionary measures/quality - Working on relationships, cooperation - New possibilities - Recognition/Innovation - Proactive planning, relaxation - Schooling/training

Not important	III. Activities:
	
	- Interruptions:
	- Some phone calls, certain mail
	  pieces, some e-mail messages,
	  some WhatsApp and other text
	  messages, certain reports, some
	  meetings,
	- Niceties to others
	- Reactive
		IV. Activities:
		
		- Trivia
		- Certain mail pieces
		- Certain phone calls
		- Leisure
		- Social media
		- Pleasant activities

Figure 6.2   The four quadrants of the time management matrix. Source: adaptation of Covey (2004)

6.3.2   Quadrants I and IV

Quadrant I issues – important and urgent – are readily available and often also rather satisfying for general practitioners. Or, as described in Covey's book, they are the tasks that make you greatly appreciated by others! However, these are also the things in which you can become fully engrossed, making you run ever faster and forces you to constantly hurry from one urgent situation to the next.

You may lose your grip, fall victim to the issue of the day. People who allow themselves to become engrossed in urgent matters to escape from the pressure, find refuge in unimportant, non-urgent activities, such as those in quadrant IV. They tend to spend most of their time firefighting (quadrant I) and the rest almost entirely on matters in quadrant IV. They have no time for the other quadrants. Chances are that, over time, this leads to more stress, to being overextended and eventually to burnout. Focusing on the matters in quadrant I tends to make them bigger and bigger. In this context, ► Chap. 1 contains the interesting observation that the medical-analytical method is a suitable approach to address patients' questions in only a fraction of cases. In reality, however, current medical education teaches future physicians to apply the medical-analytical method to all questions. In applying this method, many urgent complaints are turned into important problems and thus into issues of the first quadrant. This underpins the notion that such issues tend to grow and enhance themselves!

	Urgent	Not urgent
Important	I. Activities: - Disease and health care in central position - Emergency care (focused on the individual) - Crisis management (reactive) - Focus on shortcomings and pathology - Caring for, rather than ensuring that - Problem-oriented work method - From the medical-analytical perspective	II. Activities: - Health and behaviour in central position - Prevention (people and society in central position) - Work plans (proactive), e.g., more time for patients, from the mission and vision - Focused on possibilities and strong points, lifestyle medicine - Ensuring that, rather than caring for - Solution-oriented work method - From personal resilience and strength, self-management, ability to adjust
Not important	III. Activities: -Responding to inappropriate requests for help (reactive) -Additional work due to insufficient triage -Insufficient time -Inappropriate referrals -Requests for help addressed at the wrong party -Medicalisation of life questions -Applying medical-analytical method, instead of 'not knowing' attitude, not being able to say 'no'	IV. Activities: - Bureaucracy/administration - Some physical examinations - Certain meetings - Visits from pharmacists - Check lists multi-disciplinary coordinated care - Protocols 'for the sake of it' - Parts of practice accreditation (quality standards) - Red tape

Figure 6.3   The four quadrants of the time management matrix for primary care

6.3.3 Quadrant III

Because of medical-analytical working methods, many issues that actually belong to the *third quadrant* (urgent – not important) are addressed as if they belong to the first (urgent – important). In reality, these issues are urgent because they are a priority for other people ('I want my headache solved now', 'I want to be referred to a specialist', I want an earlier appointment for that examination'), or because general practitioners no longer have any control over the work that comes their way (e.g. patients who unnecessarily end up in the consulting room because of inadequate triage, or patients for whom the general practitioner lacks sufficient time to explain that a brain scan will not solve their problem).

The overflow of Quadrant I issues can partly be explained by short-term thinking, lack of organisation of the practice (insufficient triage by the nursing assistant) and being overwhelmed by additional tasks, as outlined in ▶ Chap. 1. However, it also has to do with underestimating the importance of having a sound mission and vision (with a focus on the *'yearning for the endless sea'*) and the related plans. The resulting time pressure will lead to superficial or poor relationships with both patients and practice staff. It also makes general practitioners dependent on others (patients, health insurance companies, politicians, municipalities and specialists). In this context, the key message of the book 'The 7 Habits of Highly Effective People' by Stephen R. Covey is that effective people (and this includes general practitioners who have effectively implemented Positive Health in their organisation) are continually ensuring that they take on *as few issues* from the third and fourth quadrants *as possible*. Because, urgent or not, they are not important. In addition, they limit the amount of work under the first quadrant to the bare minimum, and operate mostly within the second quadrant.

6.3.4 Quadrant II

According to Covey, focusing attention on the *second quadrant* is at the core of effective personal management and leadership. This quadrant contains activities that, although not urgent, are important, such as maintaining good relationships, writing a personal mission statement, physical exercise, long-term planning, paying attention to prevention, and investing in quality and innovation. These are all things we know we should be doing, but somehow, we just cannot get around to doing them – after all, they are not urgent.

6.3.5 What would you like to do differently?

Now, look at the answer you wrote down in response to the question about *what you would like to do differently in your practice – the thing that, when done regularly, would enormously increase your job satisfaction?* In which quadrant would you place the thing you wrote down? Is it important? Is it urgent? It most likely belongs in the second quadrant, because it is important or even very important, but not urgent. And because it is not urgent, you have not been doing it.

6.3.6 The time management matrix and Positive Health

What does the time management matrix tell you about implementing Positive Health in your organisation? When looking at ◻ fig. 6.4, the primary care tasks in the second quadrant are precisely those that belong to the important themes of Positive Health.

	Urgent	Not urgent
Important	I. Activities: - Disease and health care in central position - Emergency care (focused on the individual) - Crisis management (reactive) - Focus on shortcomings and pathology - Caring for, rather than ensuring that - Problem-oriented work method - From the medical-analytical perspective	II. Activities: - Health and behaviour in central position - Prevention (people and society in central position) - Work plans (proactive), e.g., more time for patients, from the mission and vision - Focused on possibilities and strong points, lifestyle medicine - Ensuring that, rather than caring for - Solution-oriented work method - From personal resilience and strength, self-management, ability to adjust
Not important	III. Activities: - Responding to inappropriate requests for help (reactive) - Additional work due to insufficient triage - Insufficient time - Inappropriate referrals - Requests for help addressed at the wrong party - Medicalisation of life questions - Applying medical-analytical method, instead of 'not knowing' attitude, not being able to say 'no'	IV. Activities: - Bureaucracy/administration - Some physical examinations - Certain meetings - Visits from pharmacists - Check lists for multidisciplinary coordinated care - Protocols 'for the sake of it' - Parts of practice accreditation (quality standards) - Red tape

POSITIVE HEALTH IN CENTRAL POSITION

Figure 6.4 The position of Positive Health in the four quadrants of the time management matrix of primary care

This means that if you organise your work in such a way that you spend most of your time on things in the second quadrant, you are probably already working quite often on the Positive Health of yourself, your colleagues and your patients! If you would like to take this even further and spend more time on these matters, then it is important to limit especially those things that belong to the third and fourth quadrants. This will free up time to spend on Positive Health. The things in the first quadrant – important as well as urgent – are the icing on the cake of primary care and, often, are very satisfying to work on. However, it is important to maintain a good balance between the first and second quadrants and, where possible, ensure that crisis situations are either anticipated or prevented. Limiting the work in the third and fourth quadrants and preventing crises that require immediate attention in the first quadrant, is of course a second quadrant activity.

6.3.7 Time management matrix and core tasks of the project on future primary care

It is interesting to compare the time management matrix for primary care against the core tasks as described by the committee of the project on the future of primary care at the Woudschoten conference (Toekomsthuisartsenzorg.nl 2019) (see ▶ Chap. 4). To conduct this comparison, the matrix can be rotated clockwise (see ◘ fig. 6.5) until the second and first quadrants are in bottom left and bottom right position, respectively. Consultation is the central core task of primary care, where general medical care is provided. Quadrant I (important and urgent) contains mainly emergency care and terminal palliative care, while Quadrant II (important and non-urgent) contains preventive care and care coordination. The illustration shows that there is an overlap of emergency care with Quadrant III. This mainly concerns urgent questions and claims by patients, which are not presented as urgent or are not urgent from the general practitioner's perspective, which are also not important (insufficient or the wrong type of triage, patients who made use of the out-of-hours service but could also have waited and been seen during regular practice hours).

The figure also shows that part of the care coordination may end up in Quadrant IV. This happens in cases where the general practitioner coordinates matters that could better have been done by others or by patients themselves. The green circle of general medical care during consultations surrounds the consultation at the centre of the matrix, covering all four quadrants. Here, the general practitioner's expertise and consultation skills determine in which quadrant most of the energy will be spent. General practitioners are primarily trained in determining what type of care would be needed, from a medical-analytical perspective. Serious pathology should not be missed, which is why, here, the most suitable approach is that of using the diagnosis–prescription model (also see tab. 3.3) and the control model with static equilibrium (see ◘ fig. 2.5). This belongs in the first quadrant.

However, only part of the questions can be addressed in this way. In the second quadrant, Positive Health offers ways to consider other appropriate solutions for some of the physical, mental, emotional and social issues that patients present during consultations. These are more in line with the *resilience* model, the adaptive capacity and the dynamic equilibrium of the adaptation model (see ◘ fig. 2.5). To medicalise or normalise? ▶ Chapter 5 discusses in detail what consultation skills are required to answer this question.

Preventive care and lifestyle medical science can be applied in this quadrant, and the general practitioner, in his role of coach and liaison, can coordinate care and determine which solutions could be found within the social domain (▶ Chap. 7). Many of the requests for help cannot be addressed using the medical-analytical model. Attempting to force non-medical questions in a medical straitjacket during consulta-

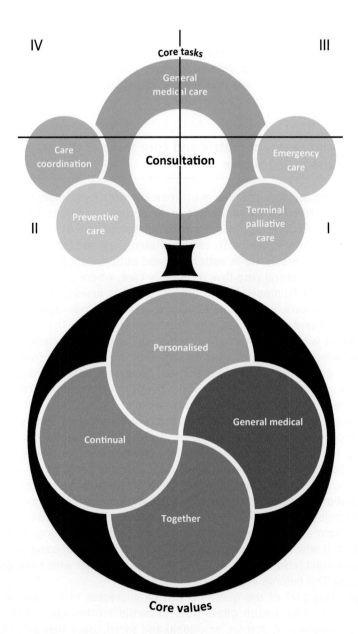

Figure 6.5   The four quadrants of the time management matrix projected on to the core tasks of primary care. (Source: ▶ www.toekomsthuisartsenzorg.nl)

tions, means working in the third and fourth quadrants, depending on whether the question is presented as urgent or not. Having sufficient time in the consulting room (meaningful conversations require slowing down) and the right conversational skills and attitude of the general practitioner are decisively important to enable working in the second quadrant, where possible, and therefore also working with Positive Health.

6.3.8 The importance of Quadrant II

When general practitioners try to find medical solutions or medical explanations for the many medically unexplained physical symptoms (MUPS), they will revert to further medical examinations or refer patients on to other medical specialists. The problem, however, is that there is no discernible physical cause for up to 40 % of physical complaints (e.g., headaches or abdominal pain) (Olde Hartman et al. 2013; Rosendal et al. 2016; Kroenke 2014). In certain specialisations of secondary care such as internal medicine and gynaecology, this percentage is even higher (60–70 %) (Nimnuan et al. 2001). Further medical examinations and referrals then turn into activities in the third and fourth quadrants. Lack of time can also be a reason for referring complicated patients on to others, often without much benefit to those patients. We are often aware of the fact that we are doing this, but feel powerless to do anything else. Sometimes we justify this by blaming the heavy workload. In these situations, ask yourself if that is really the reason. Could it be that you are trying to save time by limiting your work in the second quadrant instead of that in the third and fourth quadrants? Now you probably understand why, in the long run, this is a disastrous course of action.

So, make sure you have your mission, vision and strategy ready and have a good idea of your proverbial yearning for the endless sea, and which tasks should therefore be given priority. Make sure you know what matters, what is important. Is your daily schedule in line with your mission, vision, strategy and core values? Then ensure you make the right choices, from your own situation of Positive Health, and take the necessary steps to implement Positive Health in your practice.

6.3.9 What things to start with?

Your priorities or those of your practice with respect to the topics you would like to work on in relation to Positive Health will become clear from the process of formulating the mission and vision. It may be, however, that your practice is not yet ready for such a process. Or perhaps such an overall approach does not suit you personally, very well. Maybe Positive Health is also new to you, and you are curious, but first would like to gain some experience on a number of specific subjects, so that you will be better able to determine the value of working with Positive Health. Subsequently, choose the subject you wish to work on first. The authors of this book have given many workshops and training sessions on Positive Health, and their experience has taught them that, amongst care providers interested in working with Positive Health, there is a need for concrete advice with regard to three subjects:

1. *Inspiration:* how to get acquainted with Positive Health, and above all, do you feel the 'yearning for the endless sea'? What type of training is needed?
2. *Implementation:* how to organise this in your practice?
3. *Embedding:* How do you make sure that the changes you have made will take root and that your team stays motivated to work with Positive Health?

Concrete subjects to work on
Inspiration
- Inspiration/Learning/Training
- Inspiration lecture/workshop/training with primary care team or other community professionals

Implementation
- Which patients?
- How to organise having more time for patients?
- General practitioner (innovation theory by Rogers, see ▶ sect. 6.6)
- Practice nurse
- Mental health practice nurse
- Specific role of nursing assistants: triage/setting boundaries/Positive Health on the telephone
- The physical workplace

Embedding
- How to get and keep the team involved
- Positive meetings, reporting positive incidents (see ▶ sect. 6.8), discussing mission/vision at meetings
- Chain letter (see ▶ sect. 6.8)
- Small working groups (Positive Health team in the workplace)
- Connecting, non-violent communication

6.4 How to introduce Positive Health?

6.4.1 Inspiration

The website of the Institute for Positive Health (▶ www.iph.nl/en) provides a good impression of the various things going on in the field of Positive Health. If you would like to experience the Positive Health method for yourself, you can fill out the digital version of the spider web on the website and rate your own Positive Health on six dimensions (also see ▶ Chap. 5). It may also be interesting and instructive to have all the practice staff fill out a spider web questionnaire for themselves, and afterwards discuss the experience together. Both in the Netherlands and abroad, the iPH Academy also organises training sessions (lectures, workshops, the training working with Positive Health, webinars and master classes) (iPH 2019a). The inspirational page of the website provides many practical examples and developments. Over 100 certified trainers are affiliated with the Institute for Positive Health, who provide training sessions and workshops, and the Dutch association of nursing assistants (NVDA) also organises various training courses. Dutch inspirational stories can also be found at the websites of, for example, the Limburg Positive Health Movement, and the network for Positive Health of the northern Meuse valley. The website on solution-based working methods in health care (▶ https://www.positivehealthcare.eu/) also provides information, interviews and links to articles in English.

Other publications (in Dutch) that provide information and descriptions of Positive Health and may also serve to inspire include the Dutch magazine 'Bijblijven', which has dedicated a volume to the theme of Positive Health (Bijblijven 2019, no. 8 (in Dutch)) (Meyboom-de Jong 2019; Huber 2019; Bannink and Jansen 2019; Jung et al. 2019; Hesdahl et al. 2019; Kingsma 2019; Versteegde and Van Boven 2019; Walg 2019; Van den Brekel-Dijkstra 2019; Van Grinsven and Andries 2019).

Website of the Limburg Positive Health Movement

The Dutch Province of Limburg has its own Positive Health website (▶ https://limburgpositiefgezond.nl/ (in Dutch)). On the website are videos of 18 Positive Health inspirational sessions (one hour each), on various topics (primary care, mental health care, functional illiteracy, Positive Health in your organisation, healthy ageing, financial worries and health, nature and health, the Dutch Environment and Planning Act and Positive Health, sustainable employability of employees, Positive Health for vulnerable citizens and liveability and Positive Health in the community).

Network Positive Health northern Meuse valley

The website of the Positive Health network of the northern Meuse valley (Positive Health Noordelijke Maasvallei; Land van Cuijk and North Limburg) has published a number of videos about Positive Health (▶ www.netwerkpositievegezondheid.nl/videos (in Dutch)). It also contains an introductory game, the title of which translates to 'Positive Health, there is no escape' and a workshop about the leitmotiv of being in control and Positive Health as a starting point ('*Eigen regie de rode draad, Positieve Gezondheid als vertrekpunt*'). It is a type of 'escape room' game that introduces Positive Health in a fun and accessible way. At the end of the game, the players are introduced to a number of core concepts. In the conversation that follows, they find out what they could do differently, could stop doing, or continue to do, within their own profession. The game can be played in any room – from office, to garden pavilion or consulting room. It can be played 'as is', or be supplemented with lectures, workshops or be part of a symposium. The game can be bought or played under guidance of one of the directors of the Positive Health of the northern Meuse valley. A so-called 'leitmotiv' workshop deals with the turning point in health care that is necessary for working with Positive Health. The workshop is also available in a train-the-trainer programme. Besides the turning point, the workshop also clarifies the importance of personal control and cooperation.

6.5 How to organise Positive Health in the general medical practice

6.5.1 Implementation

Implementing Positive Health is a process that will cover multiple years. Several organisations in the Netherlands can help with this, such as regional care groups with which general practitioners are affiliated and the regional support structure (▶ www.ros-netwerk.nl). In addition, there are multiple organisations dedicated to the implementation of Positive Health (see text box).

> ### Positive Health implementation support
>
> There are a number of partners of the Institute for Positive Health (iPH) who can help care providers working with Positive Health. The Dutch website of *Anders Gezond* (andersgezond.nu) provides inspiration and transformational sessions on Positive Health and guidance for transforming health and welfare organisations to apply Positive Health in how they manage and organise their work processes (see ◘ fig. 6.1). The national Centre of Expertise for Long-term Care in the Netherlands, *Vilans,* supports long-term care organisations that want to start working with the Positive Health concept (▶ https://www.vilans.nl/about-us). The overall objective is for health care and the related support to match people needs, instead of the other way round. Dutch healthy lifestyle coaching institute *Visiom*'s mission is to bring health to health care (▶ www.visiom.nl); healthy employees, who are able to support patients with lifestyle coaching. Visiom is the main training partner of iPH, where interested parties can register to participate in the official training, the Training working with Positive Health.
>
> The *Positive Health network of the northern Meuse valley* has set up an implementation programme for Positive Health in general medical practice. This programme covers a period of two years (▶ https://www.netwerkpositievegezondheid.nl/files/media/a4-positieve-gezondheid_03.pdf-implementatieprogramma-hp.pdf).
>
> The *Bettery Institute* (▶ www.bettery.nl) coaches change processes in health care and welfare with the aim of making people feel responsible for their own health, to experience their health in a more positive way and to require less care by official care providers. Bettery works for municipalities and care organisations in the Netherlands that want to work with Positive Health by offering training and consultancy.

How to ensure you will have more time for your patients? What is the role of nursing assistants, practice nurses, mental health practice nurses and general practitioners themselves, and does working from the concept of Positive Health have consequences for the workplace and the layout of the building itself? This is discussed in more detail, in the following sections.

6.5.2 How to organise having more time for patients?

The most frequently mentioned precondition for implementing Positive Health is that of having more time for the patient. Since 2017, this has been one of the main focal points of the policy of the National Association of General Practitioners (LHV) (Lambregtse, 2017). LHV has created a separate page on its website for this very subject: Meertijdvoordepatient.lhv.nl ('more time for the patient', LHV.nl 2017). More time for patient in primary care can be achieved in a number of ways. LHV uses the following classifications: a smaller practice, deployment of staff, longer consultations, efficient practice management and limiting care.

Smaller practices

The aim of all projects in which the practice size was reduced (see Box) is to apply care effectively in order to reduce the increase in hospital care on the one hand (substitution) and to shift the focus from disease and treatments to health, behaviour and solutions in the local community and the social domain, on the other. Project evaluations show that the number of hospital referrals decreases as a result (sometimes, to a considerable degree, by more than 25 % in practices in the Dutch northern Meuse valley and Gorinchem). Job satisfaction increases, as does patient satisfaction. Fewer medications are prescribed and fewer diagnostic tests are conducted (Jung et al. 2018; Jung et al. 2019). Patients are given more time per consultation, while they also make fewer appointments at the general medical practice. A win–win situation.

An important point of attention here is the temporary nature of the experiments. There is currently no sustainable financial model, yet. This means that, for example, many general medical practices are forced to have a locum fill in the extra hours, possibly with less affinity with the Positive Health concept and therefore less understanding for the desire to reduce the size of the practice. A practice must also be able to accommodate an additional general practitioner, who also needs to be available when required. Nursing assistants, who invest more time in triage, also experience a heavier workload. In the Netherlands, perhaps the greatest objection, in this respect, is that it is not easy for general medical practices to come to financial agreements with health insurance companies. For example, in cases where general medical practices would like to reserve more time per consultation, from the desire to be engaged in Positive Health. This while, under the main agreement on primary care (Hoofdlijnenakkoord Huisartsenzorg 2019–2022), it has been agreed that more funding will be made available for initiatives related to more time for patients. In that context, the above-mentioned pilot projects are therefore partly intended to gather evidence to show the effectiveness of the intervention, which may bring structural solutions by government and health insurance companies closer. The best chance of success for realising smaller practices seems to be through regional talks with the preferred health insurance providers.

Dutch National Association of General Practitioners (LHV): More time for patients – smaller practices

At a number of locations in the Netherlands (northern Meuse valley (Boxmeer region) and Gorinchem), experiments are underway where practice sizes have been reduced to 1800 patients per full-time general practitioner (1 FTE). The northern Meuse valley was the first region in the Netherlands to start doing this. Nine general medical practices are now participating. The Gorinchem region first had 12 practices that worked this way, but in 2020, the entire region joined in. In Hoorn, too, four practices have reduced their practice size. Dutch health insurance companies Zilveren Kruis and CZ are supporting a number of general medical practices in the major cities of Amsterdam, The Hague, Rotterdam and Utrecht through so-called strong basic care (Krachtige Basiszorg). In these cases, additional FTEs in general practitioners are also being deployed, causing practice sizes to decrease below *1800 patients per full-time general practitioner* (1 FTE).

In the Deventer area, ENO health insurance company has provided the opportunity for creating smaller practices or hiring additional staff, in a three-year project, in which 20 practices are participating. In Twello, the Schilder-Spijkerman general medical practice is participating in this project; it has an additional locum for one day per week, more time per consultation, with a greater focus on solutions and less on diagnosis-oriented working methods. What are the experiences so far? According to the general practitioner: 'It provides peace of mind and better conversations with patients. Now, I have the time to really talk to a patient, ask more questions, explain choices. I can suggest to patients that they find out certain things for themselves, without them feeling that I am not taking them seriously or am rushing them out the door.'

Finally, in Munstergeleen, the general medical practice 'Hartje Dorp' has entered into an agreement with health insurance company CZ; they will reduce the size of the practice, based on the ideas of Positive Health, by deploying an additional locum and a practice nurse. The general practitioner wants to have more time to talk to patients about lifestyle and nutrition and to strengthen the network within the community, to work together with local citizens and the social domain (see ▶ Chap. 7). It is therefore not only about a structural change to create more time, but also about a change in culture, with a different mission, vision and way of working.

6.5.3 Staffing

Employing more staff can be a challenge, as it leads to a more complex organisation. Good reporting and communication become crucial elements; each team member must be kept well-informed. This requires an open culture and delegation based on trust. Using the Positive Health concept is an added value, in these respects, with everyone in the practice looking at the health and needs of patients from a broad perspective, with attention for the six dimensions of health. Practices that use more staff are indicating that the additional costs involved are not always reimbursed but the benefits of increased job satisfaction and reduced workload far outweigh those costs.

Dutch National Association of General Practitioners (LHV): More time for patients – more staff

The website of the National Association of General Practitioners (LHV) provides a number of possibilities for general medical practices to create more time for patients. These possibilities include employing additional staff members, such as general physicians, physician assistants (with a higher vocational education, e.g., with an occupational therapy or physiotherapy background), practice managers, nursing assistants with additional training to become general practitioner's assistants or who are trained in implementing 'lean thinking' in primary care, clinical nurse specialists (often with a district nursing background), practice nurses and mental health practice nurses. In practice, this almost always leads to general practitioners extending the length of their own consultations from 10 to 15 minutes per patient. Job satisfaction also increases and the perceived workload decreases. In certain practices, the extended consultation time has led to fewer disgruntled patients. By delegating certain tasks, general practitioners are able to invest more time in the more complex care issues of patients. As can be expected, this also leads to more teamwork and cooperation. A better atmosphere in the workplace was also reported, making it easier for some practices to find new general practitioner colleagues. In the city of Hengelo, a general medical practice used the additional time specifically to apply the Positive Health concept.

Longer consultations and more efficient practice management

Longer consultations

The conversion to smaller practices and additional staff, in most cases, leads to extended consultation times. This, in turn, has shown that patients are making use of the longer consultation time but also that they visit the practice less often. All the examples given in the text box on smaller practices and additional staff were taken from the LHV website. There has been a shift in the traditional way of dividing tasks between simple problems (with which the nursing assistant is able to help) and the more complex problems for which the general practitioner then needs more time. The COVID-19 era has shown that many simple problems can also be discussed digitally, leaving more time for other things. Practices and patients have gained experience with this online method because of the COVID-19 situation, and it is expected that these online possibilities will also continue to be used in the future.

Efficient practice management

Efficient practice management saves time. The LHV organises courses about how to manage general medical practices (▶ www.lhv.nl/academie) with the aim of showing general practitioners how to maintain control over their practice (LHV 2020). The courses provide advice on organising the practice, time management, such as how to deal with e-mails most effectively, time for administration and the distribution of activities that are indirectly related to care. They also discuss which consultation structures would be most suitable and how to organise them smartly. For example, by experimenting with implementing or abolishing a walk-in surgery hour. A specific approach that can help make the practice more efficient is the so-called 'lean thinking' method.

This method provides a new way of thinking about how to organise the practice while eliminating and preventing waste of both time and materials. It starts by looking at the organisation of materials and the set-up of the practice, followed by the processes. Are there things that involve wasting time that could be solved by organising them more efficiently? General medical practices that apply 'lean thinking' indicate that it saves time and provides peace of mind, because there is less going back and forth, no need to search for stuff or doing unnecessary things. Thus, there is more time for you as the general practitioner to hold an alternative dialogue with your patients.

6.5.4 Setting boundaries

Setting boundaries is essential for the general practitioner's own health. The high incidence of burnout amongst general practitioners is an indication of how difficult it is to monitor and limit the personal workload (Van den Brekel-Dijkstra et al. 2020). Deciding where to draw the line is very personal and differs from person to person. Some general practitioners focus on the medical domain and the related core tasks, from the notion that it is impossible to be responsible for the acute medical care of patients AND have time for their social problems. Adding the word 'medical' to the 'generalist' core value – as was the result of the Woudschoten conference (see ▶ Chap. 4) – also reflects this view. However, if limiting the type of care means that the tasks belonging to the second quadrant of the time management matrix (i.e., important, but not urgent) are no longer being carried out, this will have a negative effect on the physician's well-being, in the long term. In addition, general practitioners need to realise that patients often see health from a much broader perspective (see ▶ Chap. 2). Lifestyle medical science shows that, for many health-related problems, there is an overlap between the medical and the social domain. General practitioners are often asked in which domain a certain request for help could be solved. Many general practitioners enjoy the task of unravelling the social context of such requests, and some of them cooperate with social teams, where they submit cases that should be addressed by, or in cooperation with, the social domain (also see ▶ Chap. 7).

Setting boundaries. Number of patient contacts at the general medical practice Afferden 1998–2020

At the general medical practice in Afferden, the number of patient contacts tripled over the 1998–2008 period, from 5,000 to 15,000. During the same period, the number of registered patients barely increased (+ 10 %), which therefore cannot explain the increase in the number of contacts. A factsheet from the Dutch National Association of General Practitioners (LHV) shows that this increase is, in fact, a national trend (LHV 2019). In order to cope with his increased workload, Hans Peter Jung (one of the authors of this book and general practitioner at the general medical practice Afferden) decided to hire an additional practitioner (Hylke de Waart). However, this did not lead to a reduction in workload. Quite the opposite occurred; the first year of there being two physicians (2010), the number of contacts increased by 25 % – the largest increase ever: from 15,000 to 20,000 contacts in a single year. It appeared that the creation of additional capacity (i.e., the new colleague) led to an increase in the demand for care. In the years that followed, the number of contacts remained stable. In 2015, both colleagues came to the conclusion that things really had to change for them to be able to keep going. This led to an experiment with Dutch health insurer VGZ, in which the practice would no longer bill the insurance company for each medical service they were performing, but rather received a fixed amount per patient per year (i.e., a subscription fee instead of a service fee). In addition, the insurance company also paid for the recruitment of a third general practitioner (Saskia Benthem). The general practitioners decided to start working with the Positive Health concept with its six dimensions and alternative dialogue method. Interesting aspect here is that, when the second general practitioner joined the team without changing the work and financing methods, there was a strong increase in the number of contacts. However, after the arrival of the third general practitioner and with changes in how the work was organised and financed, the number of contacts declined sharply. The consultation times did increase, on average. From 2017 onwards, the number of contacts seems to be stabilising at the 2008 level. For the practice in Afferden, the conclusion is clear: maintaining the traditional organisation and methods will lead to a rapid increase in the number of contacts due to the additional capacity and a strong volume-based incentive, namely a fee-for-service system. Merely setting boundaries with respect to care and with an additional colleague does not appear to lead to a reduced workload if not also *a different way of working and/or financing* is implemented. That the Positive Health concept makes a big difference in the perceived workload as well as in job satisfaction goes without saying. In 2020, the number of contacts decreased further, as a result of the COVID-19 outbreak and subsequent lock-down. Patients became hesitant about making an appointment, mainly because they did not want to burden the practice with questions unrelated to COVID-19, but also out of fear of becoming infected by the virus themselves (◼ fig. 6.6).

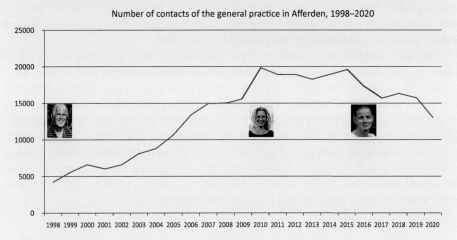

Number of contacts of the general practice in Afferden, 1998–2020

◼ **Figure 6.6**   Number of patient contacts at the general medical practice Afferden 1998–2020. Source: Jung (2019)

The solutions for freeing up more time for patients, as also mentioned on the LHV website, are described from the perspective of the general practitioner. From a patient's perspective, more time may mean that they have more room or possibilities for thinking of solutions themselves, which incidentally often lie outside the medical domain. Although, initially, spending more time per patient may seem like an investment, it can ultimately lead to those patients returning less often to the surgery. The other care professionals in the practice team can, from the vision of Positive Health, also help to increase the patients self-managing ability. Team members of the general medical practice may each fulfil a different role in this process and enhance each other's achievements. The following section describes, in more detail, the roles of the various team members in applying Positive Health.

6.6   General practice staff

Prioritising the work is an important step towards the implementation of Positive Health in primary care. The people working in the practice themselves are ultimately the ones who determine the extent to which Positive Health can be successfully adopted by the organisation. And the team members all have their own roles to play.

6.6.1   The general practitioner

General practitioners have the *final responsibility* for the care that is provided by their general medical practice and they are the *key figure* who decides whether innovative ideas are implemented in the workplace or everything stays the same. They are the ones to get others in the practice involved and acquainted with the concept of Positive Health. They themselves also need to be convinced that the changes in the organisation of the practice in relation to Positive Health are desirable and, subsequently, they have the responsibility to implement such changes and to ensure that the practice's team remains motivated to abide by them. These are all core tasks. Certain practices will be front runners in implementing the Positive Health-related changes, whereas others are more comfortable to wait and see, for a while.

The same applies to the staff members working in these practices. Some will be eager to get started on new things, while others cherish existing and familiar structures. The theory on the *diffusion of innovations* by Rogers (Rogers 2003) is enlightening in this respect. It is a theory about innovation life cycles. Rogers distinguishes five stages in which five different groups adopt an innovation or new idea. When applied to general medical practice, this means that the first general practitioners to work with a new idea serve as an example for the subsequent group. If the idea does not catch on with the first group, successful dissemination to subsequent groups of practitioners will be almost impossible. Rogers distinguishes five categories (see ◘ fig. 6.7): innovators, early adopters, early majority, late majority and laggards.

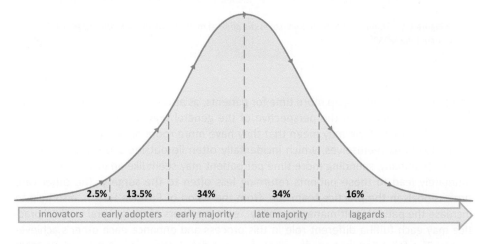

◘ Figure 6.7   Embracing a new idea according to the *diffusion of innovations* theory by Rogers. Source: Rogers (2003)

The first 2.5 % of users of a new idea are the *innovators*. They are the first to experiment with the idea. The innovators are followed by the group of early adopters, according to Rogers' theory, who embrace the idea. This group consists of another 13.5 % of users. A new idea can only be defined as successful if the early adopters are enthusiastic about the idea and are applying it, in practice. They are the most important group because they are the 'influencers' and therefore function as role models for the subsequent group of people interested in the idea. Once early adopters start applying an idea, others are likely to follow. The next group to also embrace the idea is called the early majority, which makes up 34 % of the total. This group consists of the people who like the idea, but are more cautious about trying it out and prefer to wait until they are persuaded by the enthusiasm of the early adopters. The next group is the late majority, which also comprises 34 % of the total and, in primary care, mainly concerns practices or practice staff members who are only prepared to apply a new idea if the early majority has already tried it out successfully, or if they can no longer avoid applying it. The last group in Rogers' theory is made up of laggards, who are the remaining 16 % of the total. Laggards value tradition and resent change. Laggards also tend to have little scope or energy to try out new ideas.

When looking at your own position within your medical practice and considering the adoption process according to Rogers, would you say you are an early adopter and in a position where you are able to promote a new idea such as working with Positive Health? And if so, who would be the first likely followers? Would that be a sufficient basis to start with Positive Health? Are you aware of who, if anyone, would rather 'wait and see'? Who would come up with arguments *against* working with Positive Health? These are the 'Yes, but...' people (see ◘ fig. 6.1); would they perhaps belong to the 'late majority' or the 'laggards'?

6.6.2 Practice nurse

Practice nurses supports the general practitioner in the treatment of patients with a chronic disease or physical condition. In most cases, this refers to diabetes, asthma, chronic obstructive pulmonary disease or bronchitis and pulmonary emphysema (COPD) and cardiovascular disease. The position of practice nurses was first created at the beginning of this century to support the general practitioner. For these chronic diseases, they successfully support the general practitioner by means of programmatic care (or multi-disciplinary coordinated care). In the Netherlands, as many as 85 % of patients with type 2 diabetes, for example, currently receive care that complies with the guidelines and standards. At first, this used to be around 66 % (Den Outer 2019; Klomp et al. 2020). At the same time, practice nurses face a number of fundamental problems when it comes to the interpretation of their work:

- Programmatic care is by definition *disease-oriented* and standardised in protocols and guidelines, but patients with a chronic disease are more than just their illness.
- In addition, there are increasing numbers of vulnerable older people with multiple chronic diseases for whom disease-oriented programmatic care is not the right solution.
- Furthermore, the administrative tasks involved in registering coordinated care are increasingly felt to be a burden.

— Programmatic care is often considered a straitjacket that leaves little room for a person-oriented approach or for patients deciding together with their physician what is important to them.

There is a clear need for providing a type of care that is based more on the wishes and preferences of individual patients. A more generic approach to patients with chronic diseases, integrating the various care programmes, seems desirable. This may also create opportunities for practice nurses supporting patients with other chronic conditions (heart failure, gout, hypothyroidism, chronic kidney damage, atrial fibrillation and osteoporosis). The most important development here for the practice nurse seems to be the change from protocol-based standard care to more personalised care.

The concept of Positive Health is ideally suited to bring the needs, wishes and ideas of patients with one or more chronic diseases to the surface, during the *alternative dialogue* between patient and practitioner. These needs and wishes can then be entered into an individual care plan. Lifestyle is an important theme in the various care programmes currently applied. However, the approach to lifestyle is often generic and differs hardly or not at all per particular chronic condition. The integration of care programmes offers opportunities for the more efficient organisation of lifestyle advice and support. A Positive Health approach can be used to determine what type of lifestyle advice would best suit the individual patient's needs.

If practice nurses move away from standardised programmatic care, they will be able to do more for very vulnerable elderly patients. This concerns a small share of the elderly who, due to an accumulation of chronic diseases in combination with mental conditions and social circumstances, are at risk of losing personal control. These very frail elderly people require a special form of integrated care and support that is person-oriented, proactive and coherent with ample attention for informal care. A publication by Wind and Ten Velde on vulnerable elderly who still live independently forms a guide to integrated care and community, and contains an overview of the roles and tasks that can be used in organising the support and care for this group of people (Wind and Ten Velde 2019) (also see ► Chap. 7). The publication explicitly mentions the importance of proactive care (early identification of problems to prevent later escalation) by practice nurses, amongst others, and the importance of looking at all life domains from a Positive Health perspective.

> **Practice nurses and Positive Health**
>
> Simone Dekker has been working at the Afferden practice since 2005. First as a nursing assistant, and later, because she wanted more fulfilment in her work, she chose to become a practice nurse. What she encountered was that the coordinated care (i.e., chain care) involved ticking off items on checklists more than anything else. For example, for the practice to be eligible to receive the maximum financing for chain care patients, 90 % of the required indicators must be detected in patients in this target group. At the same time, these strict guidelines also provided structure. When the practice started to focus more on vulnerable elderly people and Positive Health, those were uncertain times, at first. It took Simone a while to figure out how to apply the concept most effectively. This became better over time; with the pillars of the spider web of Positive Health providing a new type of structure.

It has become second nature to Simone to ask her patients about sleeping and eating patterns, whether they are happy with their living environment, and she enquires about her patients daily functioning, how they experience meaning in life, participation in society and their quality of life. She enjoys puzzling over complex patient problems. At the beginning of her career as a practice nurse, her work mainly covered the medical field. These days, it is also on a broader, more human level. She has noticed how satisfying it is to be an attentive listener, for herself as well as her patients. She recounts: 'How genuinely happy people can be when I visit them. To be able to see the person behind the disease, again. What is more beautiful and more enjoyable than that; that small things can make such a difference to another person. Just that little bit of personal attention.' When asked if she could name a specific patient as an example, she immediately thought of an elderly widow, well into her 80s, who was in the coordinated care system for diabetes and had her blood tests every three months according to that care system's protocol. The patient called the practice almost daily with numerous physical complaints. A little pain here, a little pain there, with much anxiety and a great need to be reassured about there not being anything seriously wrong with her. This was putting a lot of strain on the workload of the practice assistants and the general practitioners. Then it was decided that Simone would pay a home visit to the lady, every six weeks. Simone: 'Just to have a chat. How are the children doing? Are you worried about anything in particular?' It turned out that the patient was really looking for answers to certain questions, such as how to stay in control of her life – with her memory failing, here and there, and deciding what it was that she wanted. She agreed to the use of residential care when Simone convinced her that this could be important if she wanted to continue living at home for as long as possible. It became clear that the lady's greatest fear had been having to move house. Over the course of time, she then stopped calling the practice every day and was far less concerned about her physical complaints. The practice stopped the three-monthly checks of her blood glucose levels, as they had remained stable all these years, without any medication, and thus represented no added value for the patient. Her time was far better spent on really paying attention to what she herself was doing. For Simone, this was a good example of how working with Positive Health had changed her work as a practice assistant.

Group meetings on diabetes

Based on the concept of Positive Health, the practice nurse at the Spectrum Medical Centre in Meppel is holding group meetings with 10 to 12 diabetics. Over the course of six to eight meetings, diabetics learn how to do their own check-ups and they also learn from each other's experiences in how to stay fit. Either a dietician or physiotherapist are present at every other meeting to contribute to the participants' knowledge about the impact of their diet and lifestyle on diabetes. All the things related to diabetics, including medical issues, are discussed at these meetings. The participants include both new diabetics and people who have suffered the disease for many years. At the end of each cycle of meetings, the participants have acquired the skills to manage their own health, they have built a network of fellow patients, with whom they can keep in touch via a forum. In addition, by using the Positive Health *spider web*, they are coached to consider what they would like to change in their lives and what they could do to take the initial steps towards such a goal.

> The practice nurses at the Spectrum Medical Centre are very enthusiastic about these group meetings, and feel incentivised by this way of working to increase the self-reliance of diabetic patients in an interactive way, rather than doing the traditional check-ups and ticking boxes on lists.

6.6.3 Mental health practice nurse

In the Netherlands, the position of *mental health practice nurses* (who provide mental health care) was created in 2007. It filled the need for meeting the increasing demand for professional help with psychological and psychosocial problems and to reduce the rising costs of the relatively more expensive secondary care. In 2007, the Dutch Ministry of Health, Welfare and Sport commissioned the association of primary care organisations (LVG, currently *InEen*) to provide a description of the *mental health practice nurse* function, which resulted in a report on practice assistance in primary mental health care (*'Praktijkondersteuning GGZ in de eerste lijn'*) (LVG 2007). Since 2007, increasing numbers of mental health practice nurses have been active in the Netherlands. Their position has a special place in health care and therefore requires specific professional skills. Knowledge and experience with respect to a wide variety of psychological complaints and psychiatric disorders is vitally important. Mental health practice nurses work in shared responsibility with the general practitioner and independently supervise patients, at the general medical practice (Landelijke Vereniging POH GGZ 2020).

In principle, mental health practice nurses see patients whom are *not suspected* of having a psychiatric disorder (a disorder classified under the Diagnostic and Statistical Manual of Mental Disorders (DSM)), but only those with psychological complaints. In cases where a DSM disorder is suspected, mental health practice nurses will only see those patients with a low functional limitation, a limited impact of the symptoms and a low risk of serious neglect, violence, suicide or self-mutilation. In addition, patients with stable chronic problems, who require long-term monitoring rather than treatment, and who have a support system, can also be seen by mental health practice nurses.

Because of the nature of the complaints that are presented to mental health practice nurses, their approach will be more solution-oriented than disease-oriented. That is why the concept of Positive Health is so appropriate for the care offered by these care professionals. They are in the ideal position to look, together with the patient, for non-medical solutions for the presented complaints by focusing on mental well-being, meaningfulness, participation in society, quality of life and daily functioning. Once they have a good idea of the possibilities that are available within the community, they will be able to help patients increase their level of self-reliance, sometimes with help from their local community (i.e., *community reliance*). In addition, they have a good idea of the possibilities available within the social domain (well-being, social workers, community team) and will be able to make targeted use of those possibilities.

Group meeting led by mental health practice nurse

For some years now, Lili Jung, mental health practice nurse at general practice 'De Wit Huisartsen' in the Dutch city of Heerlen, has been organising group meetings for her patients. Originally, she provided mindfulness training courses, but gradually developed a Positive Health intake and Positive Health group meetings. Since then, she has coached more than 200 patients in these groups. Why did she start these group sessions and what has been the result? What does she advise other mental health practice nurses who would be interested in doing this, as well?

Lili: 'Working with patients using the Positive Health concept creates optimism and hope. This made me wonder what it would be like to work with this concept in a group. Would patients be able to motivate each other and thus give each other this good feeling? Could they do so in a more accessible way rather than through more traditional psychological treatments? I started with three such consecutive meetings, but soon there was a demand for more. Now, there are five group meetings, each time, with the emphasis on one of the six pillars of the spider web.'

One patient (28 years old) about her experience with such group meetings:

'I have been to group meetings before. They are a little scary, but this doesn't deter me and it's worth it to me. I know I am not the only one with these thoughts and feelings. The advantage of a group is that there is always so much recognition and acknowledgement when people share things that have also happened to me or match my experience. This is for me just that little bit of extra confirmation that, yes, I'm not crazy, I'm really not the only one. Some of the spider web topics in the group meetings have helped me a lot, such as 'mental well-being' and 'meaningfulness and resilience'. They taught me that, although I *have* thoughts, I am not my thoughts. By giving the worrying voice in my head a name, I managed to distance myself from my negative thoughts. This helped me to focus on more beneficial thoughts, such as What do I want? What do I believe? What would be effective? What has worked in the past? By allowing my feeling of insecurity about not being good enough, those feelings actually got less of a hold on me, giving me more room to try out new things despite my fear'.

Tips for mental health practice nurses who are interested in starting group meetings

Mental health practice nurses who want to start with Positive Health in group meetings are advised to do so by starting with the 'quality of life' spider web theme. With this starting point, the focus will automatically be on a patient's strength rather than their symptoms. In practice, this topic can be addressed in the first, initial conversation by starting with the particular complaint, but focused on identifying what the patient does *not* want. The next step is to clearly establish the opposite: what the patient *does* want or would rather want, instead. It will take only half an hour and 3 intake questions to clarify what 'quality of life' means to the patient concerned:

1. What do you wish for or dream of, with respect to topics such as your relationships, residential housing, employment, how you spend your days, finances, what you enjoy doing, what makes you happy, what you would like to develop over the next five years?

2. The miracle question: Imagine going to sleep tonight and waking up to a miracle having happened: your wishes/dreams have come true. At first, of course, you would not know that this has happened, so which things would immediately tell you that your dream came true? What would be different for how things are today? At what point, during that first day, would you notice something had changed? Help the patient imagine and visualise this in detail.

3. Which of those differences could you make happen yourself, in practice, in the short term – let's say within 24 hours – even if this is only a minor thing?

A 29-year-old patient recounts her experience at her intake for the group meetings: 'I thought the intake was very pleasant, because it was different. Looking towards the future gave me more clarity about where I want to go. It was also a very nice way of becoming acquainted; it showed me that going to a psychologist can also be fun. It lowered the threshold for me, and despite the fact that I was dreading it, it wasn't that bad. These things made an impression on me and were also good to talk about when I was back home again. After the first session I already left feeling more positive.'
The answers to the questions are always enlightening and goal-oriented, so that sometimes one meeting is already enough.
The benefits:

- Sharing information within a group is inspiring. Often, the participants also are each other's mirror and sounding board. Following the intake, it becomes easier to get people together.
- The themes of Positive Health appeal to everyone.
- As a mental health practice nurse, before conducting group meetings, you should consider which interventions you often use in individual consultations and apply them to the group, since such interventions become amplified in a group situation.
- The group dynamics are something very special, the same results can often not be achieved in one-on-one conversations.

6.6.4   Nursing assistants

Nursing assistants have a crucial role in the organisation of a general medical practice. This is also true when working with the concept of Positive Health. They particularly and to a large degree plan the surgery hour through *triage*, i.e., the dynamic process of determining the patients' level of urgency and follow-up actions. The patient and his/her request for care are central in this process (Dutch Triage Standard 2014). Most questions reach the practice by telephone. The assistant must process the questions as well as possible, often under serious time constrains. With the exception of *repeat prescriptions*, most *requests for help* are passed on to the general practitioner. The *degree of urgency* of these requests for help varies. Some patients require an emergency visit, but a number of them do not need to see a physician on that same day.

Some of the care needs may be addressed by other care providers, such as practice nurses or physiotherapists. Adequate triage differentiates between *care needs* on the basis of the type of care that is needed, its urgency, the type of care provider, and time required. The nursing assistant handles some of the care requests by telephone, giving self-care advice and referring patients on to the related website GPinfo.nl, and planning simple procedures for a *nursing assistant's surgery hour* (procedures include checking blood pressure, unblocking ears, measuring glucose levels and giving vaccinations or other injections). The remaining requests for medical assistance can be forwarded to the general practitioner or other care providers.

The *triage system*, thus, distinguishes between '*filtering*' and '*delegation*'. A useful tool for nursing assistants in the Netherlands is, for example, is NHG's Triage Guide – a structured method that can help assess the nature of the care that is needed (NHG, 2020). Research shows that correctly applied triage by the nursing assistant can lead to a *10 % reduction* in the number of visits to the surgery hour (i.e., 'filtering'). Referring to the website ▶ https://gpinfo.nl may facilitate this (Reitz et al. 2007; Spoelman 2016). In addition, the nursing assistant determines the required follow-up action (i.e., 'delegation'). If nursing assistants know about the concept of Positive Health, they can also apply this in a targeted way in triage. In particular, the solution-oriented questions of 'What are you hoping to achieve?' and 'What difference would solving your complaint make for you?' can help to gain insight into the patient's real needs. This can lead to a different follow-up action than if these questions are not asked.

On the one hand, it may help to offer solutions over the phone to questions that clearly can be solved by patients themselves, with some helpful advice, or for questions that do not even belong in the medical domain. On the other hand, when it becomes clear that questions about the meaningfulness or more complex problems are involved, nursing assistants can plan more time for such appointments at the practitioner's surgery hour. In this way, they play an important role in creating more time for patients. If they are able to reduce the number of consultations by 10 %, there will be *more time for the consultations* that require it. This does call for a different approach to some requests for help (see text box) and cause added pressure for the nursing assistants who are working with the concept of Positive Health.

Dutch association of nursing assistants (NVDA)

The Dutch association of nursing assistants is organising additional training courses on Positive Health and specific *courses on triage in combination with Positive Health*, especially for nursing assistants (for both members and non-members) (▶ www.nvda.nl/scholing/positieve-gezondheid/).

To ensure that general practitioners, practice nurses and nursing assistants have more time for their patients, it becomes even more important to prevent patients from coming to the surgery with questions that are not related to primary care. Some general practices that work with Positive Health, therefore, have consciously chosen to *increase* the availability of their assistants *on the telephone*, giving them thus more time for the patients that need it.

Common cold symptoms and triage by nursing assistants (towards self-determination and self-care)

When patients call for an appointment to have their lungs examined because they have a cold, it is debatable whether this is absolutely necessary. Nursing assistants can explain this and refer to the ▶ https://gpinfo.nl website, which contains a video explaining how a cold will generally go away by itself. It also provides information about when the general practitioner should be contacted. Because explaining this takes time, time that is sometimes not available, this is rather demanding on the nursing assistants. Patients may also become disappointed if their request for an appointment with the doctor is rejected. Because nursing assistants are basically trained to be helpful towards patients and work in a patient-oriented way, it is sometimes difficult for them to respond negatively to such appointment requests. Saying 'no' is always more difficult than saying yes. Especially when nursing assistants can see that there is still some time available at the next surgery hour.

If the general practitioner has no objections either (listening to the lungs does not take much time; it would be a quick and easy consultation and can be invoiced), an appointment is quickly made. The patient will be pleasantly surprised, it makes the nursing assistant feel good and it is not a burden for the practitioner. The only problem is that, if a practice has been dealing in this way with these kinds of requests for 25 years, patients will have learned that it is obviously useful to have one's lungs examined for a cold. In other words, this is medicalisation. The number of appointment requests will increase, as a result, and rejecting such requests when there is no time available within the surgery hour will become more difficult. 'Yes, but last time I was able to make an appointment for this symptom, too!'

Starting to do things differently in practice is not only rather demanding on the nursing assistants, but also on general practitioners themselves and certainly also on patients. It requires spending ample time on the telephone explaining and learning to deal with patients' resistance when their appointment requests are not answered in the usual way. In order to stimulate self-determination and resilience, it is appropriate to appeal to the patient's own responsibility. This requires an understanding attitude when a patient nevertheless wants an appointment to see the practitioner. Here, it is important for general practitioners to communicate the same message as their nursing assistants, with respect to the new way the surgery hour is being organised. Stay consistent. Even if it is very busy and it would actually be much faster to just have a quick listen to those lungs than to explain why you will not do so. Looking at the time management matrix in ◻ fig. 6.3, the willingness of the nursing assistant and the general practitioner to invest in certain matters is again evident. Matters such as classifying activities (e.g., important but not urgent), proper planning, with the emphasis on encouraging patients' own resilience, self-management and solving things for themselves. There will be fewer matters in the third quadrant (urgent but not important), such as appointment requests for non-medical problems, insufficient triage, not being able to say 'no', and requests for help addressed in the wrong place.

In practice, it is often difficult for nursing assistants to remain actively involved in working with Positive Health. This is due to the overly busy days and the many practical tasks of the nursing assistants. What may help in these cases, as well, is for the nursing assistants to gain more insight into the Positive Health concept by filling out the spider web for themselves and discussing the results amongst colleagues. In some general practices, nursing assistants already proactively fill out the *spider web* together with newly registered patients, in preparation for their intake interview with the general practitioner. Or, in cases where patients complain about fatigue and other burn-out-related symptoms, they will first fill out the spider web together with the patient concerned. Informing patients by communicating in various ways about the new way of working may also be effective. For example, publish this new Positive Health method on the home page of the practice's website, explaining what this may mean for patients. Send out newsletters or tell something about Positive Health in the local paper or in a leaflet or brochure about the practice. Nursing assistants can help to outline the most appropriate communication tools for this purpose and help to spread the message amongst the community.

6.7 The physical workplace

The easiest Positive Health-related adjustment to the physical workplace is that of placing brochures and flyers about the spider web in the waiting room, inviting people to fill out a spider web and then discuss this with the general practitioner. One of the authors once saw a patient who had made an appointment for back pain but who came into the consulting room in tears, leaflet in hand, saying: 'Oh, how wonderful that finally someone is asking me how I am doing!' In addition, posters can be hung up in the waiting room, see ◻ fig. 6.8, and an information stand can be placed in the waiting room containing booklets, brochures and leaflets. A video about Positive Health with patient information can also be played in the waiting room via a digital information system (▶ iPH.nl).

The most radical way to adapt the physical workplace is to design the entire practice according to the concept of Positive Health, in which the colours of its six dimensions are visible in the form of colour-coded navigation lines inside the practice (iPH 2019c). A good example of this is the Spectrum Medical Centre in Meppel (see text box). It is a nice way of drawing people's attention to the fact that the health care professionals in this health centre are looking at the whole person rather than only at people's symptoms and complaints. In a general practice in Arnhem, for example, all disease-oriented leaflets have been placed inside a cupboard, out of sight, in order to keep a positive focus on what people would like to achieve. Therefore, no posters showing the things that could be wrong or are bad for them, but rather those with images of what could happen in a positive sense, with a view towards a better future. In yet another practice, every two months, they show another theme of Positive Health in the waiting room.

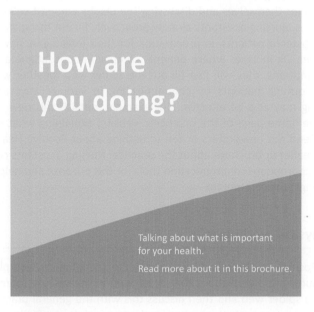

Figure 6.8   Poster inviting people to fill out the Positive Health spider web questionnaire. (Source: www.iph.nl)

Spectrum Medical Centre in Meppel ▶ www.spectrummedischcentrum.nl

In the Dutch city of Meppel, a number of general practitioners and therapists have joined forces to form a new health centre together. With the help of a number of experts, they have formulated a joint mission and vision in which Positive Health became an important cornerstone. Inspired by Machteld Huber's ideas, they looked for partners in the primary care sector who wanted to join them. A local entrepreneur supported their plans by providing a building that had previously housed a do-it-yourself building supplier. Together with the participating parties and with input from the patients' council, all disciplines were distributed across the available space, with separate spaces for meetings and mutual cooperation as the centre's leitmotiv. The various disciplines are housed around a spacious, central waiting room, with the general medical practice in central position.

From there, six wings were formed, corresponding with the six domains of Positive Health, containing the consulting rooms of the cooperating disciplines of the respective domains. Some of the staff of the general medical practice are therefore located in another wing; for example, the practice nurses have their consulting rooms close to the dietician, physiotherapists and podiatrist. The architecture of the health centre reflects the vision that the centre aims to promote. In total, the centre houses about *30 different disciplines*. The smaller first floor contains a meeting place for all of the centre's employees, where they can have their coffee or lunch breaks and talk about developing new cooperation initiatives, under the motto 'Better together!'

6.8 How to keep my team motivated?

As shown earlier on in this chapter, changing working methods in practice is a complex undertaking. The changes, subsequently, also need to be firmly embedded in the organisation – something that is often underestimated or forgotten about. It must be realised that this is a process of many years, during which time there will be periods with a lot of energy and enthusiasm and periods when the attention for Positive Health fades into the background. According to a publication by Wye and McClenahan, 'Progress is not linear, but three steps forward and two steps back' (Wye and McClenahan 2000). InEen, the Dutch association of primary care organisations visualised the sustainable implementation of the *alternative dialogue*, in everyday practice (◘ fig. 6.9). The figure shows what is involved in embedding this new working method. InEen supports the advocates of person-oriented care. What makes general practitioners and other care providers want to apply the alternative dialogue? What do they need to apply this approach, and what does their practice need in order to continue doing so (*reminders*)?

Studies of effective changes in patient care that look at factors explaining the successful and sustainable implementation of those changes always conclude the important role of mutual cooperation and leadership (Wensing et al. 2020). It is therefore not surprising that more projects were found to have been successfully implemented in cases where physicians themselves took the lead in improvement processes in health

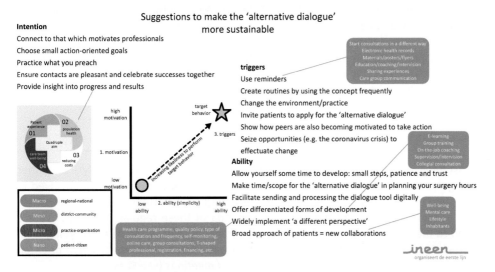

◘ **Figure 6.9**   *Embedding the* alternative dialogue

care rather than when external project leaders were involved (Weiner 1997). The organisational culture also plays a crucial role in the implementation and sustainability of changes. Achieving an organisation in which Positive Health has become part of the culture takes time (i.e., years), energy and money! The literature on the preconditions for an *organisational context* in which new working methods are successfully implemented shows the following matters to be important (Wensing et al. 2020):

— Effective leadership needs to have a consistent vision of improving care, setting concrete, ambitious goals and working according to strict deadlines. It also plays an exemplary role; enthusiastic management that delegates the actual implementation of changes to others does not seem to work.

— An open, change-oriented culture can be achieved by involving everyone in the organisation, continuously providing training courses for employees and establishing effective mutual communication.

— Effective management of change processes involves choosing people within the organisation who are committed to working on those changes. A project team should be formed in which they all participate, and successes should be communicated as soon as they are achieved (to promote the feeling that something worthwhile is being achieved for both patients and care providers alike). In addition, also allow sufficient time for the change to take root, and make sure that sufficient budget is available. ▶ Chapter 8 provides options for additional funding.

— Experience gained from numerous implementation projects also shows the great importance of embedding the implementation plan into existing organisational structures – use what is already there (Wye and McClenahan 2000). One such structure – already present in most practices – is that of regular staff meetings. Think of ways to use these meetings to keep a focus on Positive Health.

— Unambiguous documentation and registration of the *alternative conversations* may also contribute to a sustainable implementation. On this point, no agreement has been reached on how this should be done on a national level, as yet. In the Utrecht district of Leidsche Rijn, the ICPC P49 classification code is used (i.e., preventive treatment) to enter 'PH conversation' on the problem list (PH, in this case, stands for both person-oriented and Positive Health). A link to the filled-out spider web can be included here, as well, so that it is easy to retrieve from the patient's medical file. There are increasing technical options for including the spider web in someone's medical file. Then there are also the general practices that consider Positive Health as a physician-patient communication method that does not need to be specifically registered under an ICPC code.

6.8.1 General practice meetings

Most general practices hold regular meetings – daily, weekly or monthly – for either the general practitioners, the whole practice team or with other parties involved in care (e.g., residential care, welfare, physiotherapists, pharmacists). Positive Health can become a permanent fixture on the agenda of these regular meetings. We are used to meetings being about what needs to change, things that are not going well. In their book on Positive Health Care, Bannink and Jansen call them *problem-oriented meetings* and set them against *solution-oriented meetings* (see ◻ tab. 6.1).

Table 6.1 Differences between problem-oriented and solution-oriented meetings

problem-oriented meetings	solution-oriented meetings
focus on problems: on undesirable situations in either the past or the present	focus on a shared objective: on the desirable future situation
focus on what people or organisations do not want	focus on what people or organisations want
focus on what no longer works	focus on what works
focus on problems	focus on exceptions to problems
analysis of problems and bottlenecks, weaknesses of individual people and teams; forming hypotheses	analysis of positive characteristics, strengths and resources of individual people and teams; forming hypotheses
history of problems: looking for causes and/or indications of guilt	history of previous successes of individual people and teams: what worked before and how did that come to be?
suggestions by individual people and teams are not or insufficiently appreciated or used	suggestions by individual people and teams are appreciated and used
prediction, no action is taken	considering the next steps and taking action

From: Bannink and Jansen. Positive health care. Solution-oriented methods in primary care (2017, p. 192). (Included with permission of the publisher).

Meetings may take a different course if they have a positive start. The Afferden general practice has a monthly staff meeting for all staff members, and each meeting always starts by one of the employees mentioning some positive things about all of the people present. Subsequently, if they like, others can also add any positive events to those already mentioned. At the end of each meeting, members are asked who would like to volunteer to do this at the next meeting. Thus, this person will have a month to prepare and observe his or her colleagues. The practice in Afferden has been starting its meetings in this positive way for years and this method is highly appreciated by everyone. Furthermore, the positive atmosphere that it creates noticeably remains for the rest of the meeting.

Another example is a general practice in the Dutch city of Hengelo that uses a chalkboard on which successes are written each day and are subsequently discussed in staff meetings. It is good to experience each month how solution-oriented meetings and describing the things that are going well have a positive impact on the participants in the meeting. It is a regular reminder of how this approach could also have a positive impact on patients and this encourages applying the positive approach also during surgery hours.

A second regular feature of the monthly staff meetings in Afferden is that of one (alternating) team member during the meeting observing to what extent the things that are discussed and decided contribute to the practice's mission and vision and, thus, also contributes to working with the Positive Health concept. It ensures that the practice is reminded every month of its mission and vision and the related role of Positive Health, and it stimulates everyone present at the meeting to make a contribution towards realising this mission and vision.

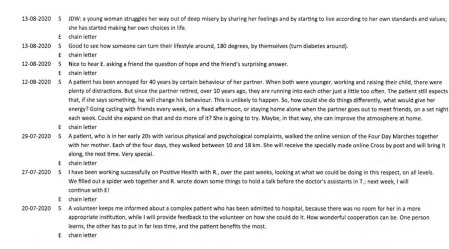

13-08-2020	S	JDW: a young woman struggles her way out of deep misery by sharing her feelings and by starting to live according to her own standards and values; she has started making her own choices in life.
	E	chain letter
13-08-2020	S	Good to see how someone can turn their lifestyle around, 180 degrees, by themselves (turn diabetes around).
	E	chain letter
12-08-2020	S	Nice to hear E. asking a friend the question of hope and the friend's surprising answer.
	E	chain letter
12-08-2020	S	A patient has been annoyed for 40 years by certain behaviour of her partner. When both were younger, working and raising their child, there were plenty of distractions. But since the partner retired, over 10 years ago, they are running into each other just a little too often. The patient still expects that, if she says something, he will change his behaviour. This is unlikely to happen. So, how could she do things differently, what would give her energy? Going cycling with friends every week, on a fixed afternoon, or staying home alone when the partner goes out to meet friends, on a set night each week. Could she expand on that and do more of it? She is going to try. Maybe, in that way, she can improve the atmosphere at home.
	E	chain letter
29-07-2020	S	A patient, who is in her early 20s with various physical and psychological complaints, walked the online version of the Four Day Marches together with her mother. Each of the four days, they walked between 10 and 18 km. She will receive the specially made online Cross by post and will bring it along, the next time. Very special.
	E	chain letter
27-07-2020	S	I have been working successfully on Positive Health with R., over the past weeks, looking at what we could be doing in this respect, on all levels. We filled out a spider web together and R. wrote down some things to hold a talk before the doctor's assistants in T.; next week, I will continue with E!
	E	chain letter
20-07-2020	S	A volunteer keeps me informed about a complex patient who has been admitted to hospital, because there was no room for her in a more appropriate institution, while I will provide feedback to the volunteer on how she could do it. How wonderful cooperation can be. One person learns, the other has to put in far less time, and the patient benefits the most.
	E	chain letter

Figure 6.10 Chain letter Positive Health from the Afferden practice's electronic information system; the 'S-line' always starts with the initials of the team member who has written the particular entry in the patient file

The three general practitioners of the Afferden practice hold weekly meetings. A fixed item on their agenda is a discussion of all referrals from the week preceding the meeting. Referrals are all sent and registered via *ZorgDomein,* a digital platform used by general practitioners to organise referrals to specialist care. This system is used by most general practitioners in the Netherlands. The application also generates weekly lists that can be printed out. The purpose of discussing the referrals during the meetings is to learn from each other about which considerations were involved in the decision to refer a certain patient and whether there could be alternatives for such referrals; for instance, by looking for a solution in the social domain or by paying more attention to one of the other dimensions of Positive Health. Applying this method in Afferden has played an important role in decreasing the number of referrals to secondary care (Jung 2018).

6.8.2   The chain letter

A way of sharing your daily experiences with using the Positive Health concept (looking at what went effortlessly as well as at things that took rather more effort) is to create a 'fake' patient in your practice's electronic information system and to have each team member write things down in this patient file about what they have experienced that day in their work with Positive Health. In Afferden, this method has been applied for a number of years now, where they have created a patient file under the name *Mr P. Health* (see ▢ fig. 6.9). The subject line of the fake patient file was given the title *'chain letter'*. The patient file is regularly read by all team members, which ensures that Positive Health stays on everyone's mind. Some staff members are more fanatical about filling the file with examples, others less so. Sometimes a wake-up call is needed to increase the level of discipline (▢ fig. 6.10).

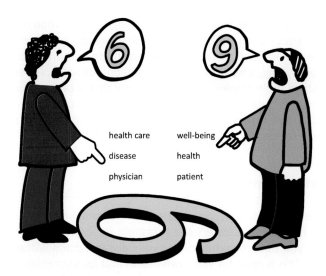

health care   well-being

disease   health

physician   patient

◻ Figure 6.11   Effective communication?

6.8.3   Working groups on Positive Health

Another possibility is to set up small working groups of practice team members, for example consisting of a nursing assistant, a practice nurse and a general practitioner, and have meetings every six weeks around a Positive Health theme. This could be a chapter from this handbook on Positive Health, or giving each other an assignment to practice with solution-oriented questions, to practice with the spider web or to think of appropriately wording some information about Positive Health on the practice's website.

6.8.4   Effective communication

An open culture that is focused on change, to be achieved by involving everyone, continuously training employees and achieving effective mutual communication, seems to be an important condition for introducing and securing new working methods (Wensing et al. 2020). This also applies to introducing and embedding the Positive Health concept. It can therefore be good to take a critical look at how team members communicate with each other, as well as which elements of this communication contribute to an open, change-oriented culture and which do not. Communication is often used to judge each other's behaviour. By doing so, we create distance rather than make a connection (see ◻ fig. 6.11), resulting in expressions such as: 'You're not listening', 'This is not what we agreed', 'You know I don't like doing small procedures halfway through my surgery hour', and 'Has that full container of needles still not been replaced? Is that what you call working according to lean principles? (for information on lean thinking, see this chapter's text box on efficiency).

This type of communication deprives people of the possibility of really connecting with each other. Speaking in this way, we think and communicate from what we think is wrong with the behaviour of others. We apply the same to ourselves. It focuses our attention on determining how wrong something is rather than on our needs and those of others. Focused on problems rather than solutions. Not on what is going well or what we would hope to achieve. This has to do with irritations about things we encounter every day, where we point to someone or to ourselves as the person responsible, instead of first looking at our own need that is causing the irritation. This causes us to become stuck in feelings of frustration, anger or sadness when interacting with others. It also makes it very difficult to communicate those needs, which is why they become repressed.

6.8.5 Connective communication

One form of effective communication is *connective communication*. Connective communication is a method that lowers the threshold for expressing what is bothering you by teaching you how to communicate your dissatisfaction without pointing the finger at anyone. This is good for your own health and for your relationship with others. Connective communication was developed by Marshall Rosenberg who called it non-violent communication (Rosenberg 2003). In his publications, Marshall Rosenberg explains in simple terms how to distinguish the content of the message from the way it is delivered and, subsequently, how to communicate without harming oneself or others. It teaches you how to say what you want and to hear what the other person is saying. It is a language of compassion that transcends power struggles and moves towards cooperation and trust. In this way, communication is disarming, more effective and leads to connection.

Connective communication provides structure to a conversation, ensuring the focus remains on the goal, even when emotions are involved. It also gives peace of mind, because it enables combining people's own needs with those of others and enables holding each other accountable for certain moral values. It also shows where responsibility begins and ends; people are responsible for their own interpretations, feelings, needs and behaviour. In communication, one can take control while allowing others to do the same. In this way, irritation, anger or other emotions can be channelled in a way that does not break up the conversation, but keeps it going. Rosenberg chose two animals to convey his ideas in a powerful and clear way: the jackal and the giraffe. They symbolise two qualities in humans. The jackal focuses on the problem and blames emotions such as sadness or anger either on himself (I am wrong) or on others (you are wrong).

The giraffe aims to find a solution within himself (making people aware of their own feelings and needs) or in others (making them aware of the feelings and needs of the other). It can be very useful to train in connective communication as a team. By practising with each other, team members get to know each other better and it becomes easier to speak a common language. The jackal and the giraffe can become concepts and part of this common language. This makes it easier for team members to help each other stay connected with themselves and others, in difficult situations. In the Netherlands, numerous courses in this type of communication can be followed that have been certified by the centre for nonviolent communication (CNVC 2020).

Recognising emotions through connective communication

Imagine you are a nursing assistant. The time is five to five in the afternoon; the answering machine is about ready to be switched on. It has been a busy, hectic day. And you know that the general practitioner who is working today has to pick up her young children from the day care centre before half past five. So, you were on a tight schedule that day. In fact, you had been feeling that pressure all day long. Nothing was allowed to go wrong. And you felt responsible for that. Then the phone rings. This cannot be, but it is: Mr B. always calls at the end of the day and, yes, he's asking for a house call from the general practitioner.

These are the situations where you run the risk of making wrong decisions, based on emotions. Mr B. always calls for unimportant things, you think, and there is really no time for another appointment today, anyway. You brace yourself on the phone. Mr B. notices your resistance and reacts by becoming very angry and more demanding about an immediate house call. You are unsure about what to do next and, in the end, you put him through to the general practitioner – feeling guilty. A few moments later, the general practitioner walks past the counter, holding her doctor's bag, without saying a word, but the look in her eyes says it all: this is a terrible day.

Connective communication teaches you to recognise your emotions as soon as they occur. If you are able to do so, you will be more able to respond to another person's request (in this case, Mr B. and his house call request) and put yourself in the other person's shoes. Even when the clock says five to five. It provides the opportunity to listen to the other person, who then does not have to brace himself against any negativity from your end, and makes him feel heard – even when you are not honouring his request.

You need to be aware of where your responsibility begins and ends. You cannot help the fact that children need to be picked up at the day-care centre before a certain time, and neither can Mr B. You put the decision about whether or not a home visit is necessary in the hands of the general practitioner herself. Putting her on the phone to Mr B. means she will be able to decide whether an appointment is urgent or can wait until another day. She will be able to discuss this with Mr B. and organise the time for the appointment.

In this other situation, a few moments later, the general practitioner could walk past your counter without her bag, wave at you with a smile and say: 'I'm off, you have a good evening!'

General medical practices are embedded in the local community. How does a practice relate to this community? That is the subject of ▶ Chap. 7.

6.9 Conclusions

This chapter is about the organisation of the general medical practice and the role of the various team members. How to successfully incorporate Positive Health in your organisation? The key message is that it is not enough to see Positive Health as a clever trick to apply; for example, by instructing your team members to fill out the spider web questionnaire. Everyone in the practice needs to be convinced of Positive Health contributing to the realisation of the core values of their practice. Only in this way can Positive Health be part of the organisation, which is needed for working methods to really change. But how to do that?

Changes in working methods are considered by drawing up a vision and mission for the general medical practice. The time management matrix appears to be very useful, for this purpose. This chapter discusses how to introduce Positive Health, how Positive Health could be implemented in practice and how to ensure the team remains motivated to work with Positive Health.

For more information, background or videos about this chapter scan the QR code.

SCAN ME

References

Afferden-Limburg.nl (2019). *Analyse dorpsdagboeken Afferden*. Accessed in August 2020 of ► https:// afferden-limburg.nl/tag/dorpsdagboeken/.

Bannink, F., & Jansen, P. (2017). *Positieve gezondheidszorg. Oplossingsgericht werken in de huisartspraktijk.* Amsterdam: Pearson Benelux.

Bannink, F., & Jansen, P. (2019). Samenwerken aan een beter leven. *Bijblijven, 35,* 18–25.

Bannink, F., & Jansen, P. (2020). *Positieve Gezondheidszorg.* Accessed in August 2020 of ► https://www. positievegezondheidszorg.nl/#home.

Bijblijven. (2019). *Themanummer Positieve Gezondheid*. Volume 8, jaargang 35. Bohn Stafleu van Loghum, Houten.

Covey, S. R. (2004). *The 7 Habits of Highly Effective People: Powerful Lessons in Personal Change.* Free Press, New York.

Den Outer, B. (2019). Ketenzorg vraagt om een persoonsgerichte, geïntegreerde benadering. *De eerste lijns platform voor strategie en innovatie.* Accessed in September 2020 of ► https://www.de-eerstelijns. nl/2019/10/ketenzorg-vraagt-om-een-persoonsgerichte-geintegreerde-benadering/.

De Saint Exupery, A. (2012). Citadelle, posthum 1948. In: Van der Kaap A. (Red.), *Het verlangen naar de eindeloze zee. Histoforum didactiek. Het online tijdschrift voor geschiedenisdidactiek.* Accessed in June 2021 of ► http://histoforum.net/columns/column14.html.

Hesdahl, B., Houben, C., & Smeijsters, R. (2019). Positieve gezondheid helpt de huisarts naar mens én omgeving te kijken. *Bijblijven, 35,* 39–48.

Huber, H. (2019). Positieve gezondheid – de status anno 2019. *Bijblijven, 35,* 7–17.

Huber, M. (2014). *Towards a new, dynamic concept of Health. Its operationalisation and use in public health and healthcare, and in evaluating the health effects of food.* Maastricht: Maastricht University. ISBN 978-94-6259-471-5.

iPH Institute for Positive Health (2019a). *De iPH academie.* Accessed in June 2021 of ► https://iph.nl/academie/.

iPH Institute for Positive Health (2019b). *Samen werken aan positieve gezondheid.* Accessed in August 2020 of ► https://iph.nl/.

iPH Institute for Positive Health (2019c). *Positieve gezondheid op de tekentafel van architecten.* Accessed in June 2021 of ► https://iph.nl/positieve-gezondheid-op-de-tekentafel-van-architecten/.

Jung, H. P., Jung, T., Liebrand, S., Huber, M., Stupar-Rutenfrans, S., & Wensing, M. (2018). Meer tijd voor patiënten, minder verwijzingen? *Huisarts en Wetenschap, 61*(3), 39–41. ► https://doi.org/10.1007/s12445-018-0062-y.

Jung, H. P., Liebrand, S., & Van Asten, C. (2019). Uitkomsten van het hanteren van positieve gezondheid in de praktijk. *Bijblijven, 35,* 26–35.

Kingma, E. (2019). Kritische vragen bij Positieve Gezondheid. *Bijblijven, 35,* 49–54.

Klomp, M., Mutsaerts, J. F., Rempe, J., Neumann, R., & Vogelzang, F. (2020). *Denkraam integratie zorgprogramma's voor chronische aandoeningen.* Utrecht: InEen.

Kroenke, K. (2014). A practical and evidence-based approach to common symptoms: A narrative review. *Annals of Internal Medicine, 161*(8), 579–586.

Lambregtse, C. (2017). Meer tijd voor de patiënt. *LHV de Dokter, 8*(4), 8–11.

Landelijke Huisartsen Vereniging (2017). *Meer tijd, welke oplossing past bij uw praktijk?* Accessed in June 2021 of ► https://meertijdvoordepatient.lhv.nl/.

Landelijke Huisartsen Vereniging (2020). *LHV academie.* Accessed in June 2021 of ► https://www.lhv.nl/lhv-academie.

Landelijke Vereniging Georganiseerde eerste lijn (2007). *Praktijkondersteuning GGZ in de eerste lijn. Een eerste beschrijving van de functie praktijkondersteuning GGZ in de eerste lijn.* LVG, Utrecht. Accessed in June 2021 of ► https://www.praktijksteun.nl/huisartsenpraktijk/zorgverlening-poh-ggz.

Landelijke Vereniging POH-GGZ (2020). *Functieprofiel.* Accessed in August 2020 of ► https://www.poh-ggz.nl/poh-ggz/functieprofiel/.

LHV.nl Landelijke Huisartsen Vereniging (2019) *Factsheet.* Accessed in August 2020 of ► https://www.lhv.nl/actueel/dossiers/meer-tijd-voor-de-patient.

Meyboom-de Jong, B. (2019). Redactioneel ten geleide. *Bijblijven, 35,* 4–6.

Nederlands Huisartsen Genootschap (NHG) (2020). *NHG Triagewijzer 2020.* Accessed in August 2020 of ► https://www.nhg.org/triagewijzer.

Nederlandse Triage Standaard (2014). *Nederlandse Triage Standaard, ketenstandaard voor triage in de acute zorg.* Accessed in August 2020 of ► https://de-nts.nl/.

Nimnuan, C., Hotopf, M., & Wessely, S. (2001). Medically unexplained symptoms: An epidemiological study in seven specialities. *Journal of Psychosomatic Research, 51,* 361–367. ► https://doi.org/10.1016/S0022-3999(01)00223-9.

Olde Hartman, T. C., Blankenstein, A. H., Molenaar, A. O., Bentz van den Berg, D., Van der Horst, H. E., Arnold, I. A., et al. (2013). NHG-standaard somatisch onvoldoende verklaarde lichamelijke klachten (SOLK). *Huisarts en Wetenschap, 56*(5), 222–230.

Reitz, G. F., Stalenhoef, P., Heg, R., & Beusmans, G. (2007). Triage in de huisartspraktijk. *Huisarts en Wetenschap, 13,* 656–659.

Rogers, E. (2003). *Diffusion of innovations.* New York: Free Press.

Rosenberg, M. B. (2003). *Non-Violent Communication, A Language of Life.* Encinitas, CA: PuddleDancer.

Rosendal, M., Carlsen, A. H., & Rask, M. T. (2016). Symptoms as the main problem: A cross- sectional study of patient experience in primary care. *BMC Family Practice, 17*(1), 29.

Spoelman, W. A., Bonten, T. N., De Waal, M. W., Drenthen, T., Smeele, I. J., Nielen, M. M., Chavannes, N. H. (2016). Effect of an evidence-based website on healthcare usage: an interrupted time-series study. BMJ Open 2016;6:e013166.

The Center for Nonviolent Communication. Accessed in August 2020 of ► https://www.cnvc.org/.

Toekomsthuisartsenzorg.nl (2019). Accessed in Juni 2021 of ► https://toekomsthuisartsenzorg.nl/.

Van den Brekel-Dijkstra, K. (2019). Hoe Positieve Gezondheid bij kan dragen aan gezonde leefstijl. *Bijblijven, 35,* 70–79.

Van den Brekel-Dijkstra, K., Cornelissen, M., & Van der Jagt, L. (2020). De dokter gevloerd. Hoe voorkomen we burn-out bij huisartsen? *Huisarts en Wetenschap, 63*(7), 40–43. ► https://doi.org/10.1007/s12445-020-0765-8.

Van Grinsven, S., & Andries, M. (2019). Culturele interventies dragen bij aan positieve gezondheid ouderen. *Bijblijven, 35,* 80–90.

Versteegde, T., & Van Boven, K. (2019). Positieve gezondheid een onsamenhangend concept. *Bijblijven, 35,* 55–58.

Walg, C. (2019). Vertrekken vanuit Positieve Gezondheid vraagt om core, naast cure en care. *Bijblijven, 35,* 59–69.

Weiner, B., Shortell, S., & Alexander, J. (1997). Promoting clinical involvement in hospital quality improvement efforts: The effects of top management, board and pysician leadership. *Health Services Research,* 32(4), 491–510.

Wensing, M., et al. (2020). *Improving Patient Care: The Implementation of Change in Health Care*, John Wiley & Sons Ltd, ▶ https://doi.org/10.1002/9781119488620.fmatter.

Wind, A., & Ten Velde, B. (2019). *Kwetsbare ouderen thuis*. Handreiking voor integrale zorg en ondersteuning in de wijk. Accessed in August 2020 of ▶ https://www.beteroud.nl/beteroud/media/documents/han-dreiking-kwetsbare-ouderen-thuis-mei-2019_2.pdf.

Wye, L., & McClenahan, J. (2000). *Getting better with evidence*. London: King's Fund.

Chapter 7

Macro
Regional /
national

Meso
District / community

Micro
Practice / organisation

Nano
Patient / citizen

I will maintain an open and verifiable attitude,
and I am aware of my responsibility towards society.
I will promote the availability and accessibility of
health care. I will not misuse my medical knowledge,
not even under pressure.

Thus, I will uphold the profession of physician.

This I promise

or
So help me God Almighty

Positive Health in the community

© Bohn Stafleu van Loghum is an imprint of Springer Media B.V., part of Springer Nature 2022
M. Huber et al., *Handbook Positive Health in Primary Care*,
https://doi.org/10.1007/978-90-368-2729-4_7

❯ **Main messages**
  - The Hippocratic Oath says that physicians know their responsibility towards society.
  - General practitioners cooperate with other stakeholders in the community, in this respect.
  - Obtaining insight into what people want and are able to do is essential.
  - Citizen initiatives, informal care and other community initiatives can be more important for general practitioners to use or know about than is currently recognised.
  - Positive Health can be a catalyst for starting to work with all dimensions of the spider web within the community.

┌─ **Definitions** ──────────────────────────────────
For explanations and definitions of frequently used terms, such as self-care, citizens' initiatives, community strength, well-being, informal care, municipality, Community Health Services (GGD), district nursing, social domain and medical domain, see the appendix at the end of this chapter and book.
└───

The Hippocratic Oath states that physicians have *a responsibility to society*. What does this responsibility entail? Is it shared with others? How can human health take shape, both in society and in people's local living environment? What does this mean, in concrete terms, at the level of local communities or municipalities? When general practitioners are faced with questions or requests for help from their patients to which there is no suitable *general medical* answer, there is often still a certain blind spot for the possibilities offered by social and lifestyle services within the community. To be able to meet people's own needs and abilities, what they could and would like to do themselves, it is useful for general practitioners to know the options and possibilities outside the medical realm. ▶ Chapter 5 describes how Positive Health provides patients with insight into their own health situation, and how this may stimulate self-determination. Enhancement of this self-determination also occurs increasingly often in local communities where residents organise themselves to lead healthier lifestyles.

The ideal is for patient care *to be designed jointly* with other stakeholders from within the community. On an individual level this may mean, for example, more coordination with and around patients. On community level, this may involve designing integrated healthy community networks. Cooperation takes place not only between general practitioners and specialists, but also with many others in the community.

┌─ **Reflection** ──────────────────────────────────
Consider the following questions.
Write down the answers; we will come back to this.
  - *What group of patients are visiting the surgery hour rather often?*
  - *What could these patients do themselves to benefit their health?*
  - *Does the practice include other care professionals who could support these patients?*
  - *What could be the benefits of cooperating with other professionals around these patients?*
└───

7.1   Blind Spot

Health care still seems focused on diagnosing and treating diseases and applying care, with too little focus on health, behaviour, people and society (Polder 2011). Health is the starting point with people positioned at the centre, in an ever-more complex society. In the Netherlands, many domains are involved in achieving a healthier country. Could the existing possibilities within the community be less well-known to general practitioners?

The crises in primary care in the Netherlands could be prevented or alleviated if the workload of general practitioners could be reduced. General practitioners are easily accessible for people with health questions. However, many people present complaints that have other underlying causes, such as mental, social or lifestyle problems. Is the right care provided in the right place? How could health care be organised more proactively, rather than waiting for the time when diseases present themselves? This calls for more attention being paid to prevention and greater involvement of the people themselves. Person-oriented care creates a better picture of what people need to be in good health within their own environment.

As ◘ fig. 7.1 illustrates, we are facing a turning point, from a mainly disease-oriented approach (blue part of the pyramid) to a broader basis for prevention and self-management. The pink part of the pyramid can be filled with self-care, technological support with e-health, informal care, community strength, and social and lifestyle services. Here, a greater role is reserved for people themselves as well as for public health.

With a better notion of what people need in order to be in good health within in their own environment, care can be organised proactively instead of waiting for a disease to manifest itself. If diseases do occur, the emphasis will be on learning how to cope with them. For example, by focusing on what a patient is still able to do. There will be greater emphasis on a meaningful life. Integrated primary care remains very important, but also requires a change in mentality of the professionals. In addition, people's expectations of health care also need to change; from looking for medical

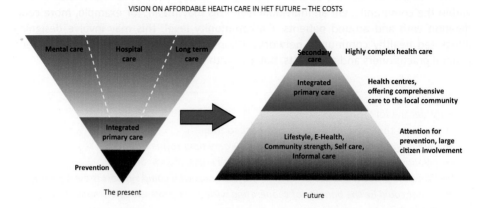

◘ **Figure 7.1**   Vision of the turning point in health care – from disease-oriented management to health care management. Source: B. Leerink, (formerly of Menzis)

Trial successful

Contact with fellow patients beneficial

SITTARD-GELEEN/HEERLEN

By Hennie Jeuken

A successful trial in South Limburg with contact between fellow patients and people with common interests should be repeated throughout the Netherlands People feel good about it and it offers an opportunity to save costs.

In Belgium, experience experts are used three times more often than in the Netherlands. In Germany up to five times as often, which saves the Krankenkasse (health insurance) alone half a billion euros, annually, explains Wim Venhuis of Burgerkracht Limburg.

His organisation works to achieve 'a society in which everyone participates'. The knowledge and experience of citizens who have lived through something, is currently utilised far too little. Venhuis: 'There is room for improvement. Not only does it save society a lot of money, it also makes people feel better.'

In Sittard-Geleen and Heerlen, Burgerkracht Limburg successfully set up a project called 'Zelfregietool.nl', which is unique in the Netherlands. A single digital platform where people have access to the knowledge and experience of others — quickly, easily and close at hand. This does not have to be limited to the subject of disease, but could also include issues such as debt and divorce. A total of 170 groups of people have joined the project.

Through Zelfregietool.nl, a network of corona experience experts is also being created for health care professionals, patients and former patients.

Health insurance companies, municipalities, the province and general practitioners in South Limburg are supporting the project.

'After volunteer work and family care, contact between people with similar experiences should become the third pillar of informal care'.

REGIO // **6-7**

◼ **Figure 7.2** Contact with fellow patients beneficial. Source Newspaper "The Limburger": Hennie Jeuken (2020)

solutions from health care professionals to seeking self-care. By promoting this type of self-management, the possibilities for implementing Positive Health on a community level will grow.

7.2 Why apply Positive Health in the community?

Positive Health is a leitmotiv in the Dutch National Policy Document on Public Health 2020–2024 ('Gezondheid Breed Op De Agenda', Rijksoverheid.nl 2020a) (see ▶ sect. 8.3). Health problems, generally, are not isolated issues, but are connected with challenging situations in various domains. Thus, an approach outside the health domain can also lead to health gains. Health in people's physical and social environment is one of the focal points of the policy document. Other health-related issues are the reduction in health inequities, the pressures of daily life on young people and adults, and healthy ageing. Positive Health can be applied to view these health-related issues from a broad perspective; it is a connecting theme for public health policy. The arena in which this transformation is taking place is shifting increasingly towards networks, local districts and regions (◼ fig. 7.3 and 7.4).

A healthy community approach adds value to the cooperation around relevant local health topics within the community. Agreements can be made with local community actors. Positive Health can be a catalyst for cooperation within communities or networks, on all aspects of the spider web. Positive Health appears to be a connecting and recognisable language for all stakeholders involved. The broad perspective on health places individual people in their residential environment in central position.

Health care can be seen to be moving from disease-oriented care to prevention, in the communities where health is organised in an integrated way. For example, data may provide insight into health topics that feature frequently in a community, village or municipality. With an integrated joint approach, health issues can be addressed with a greater focus on prevention and attention for cooperation between the medical and

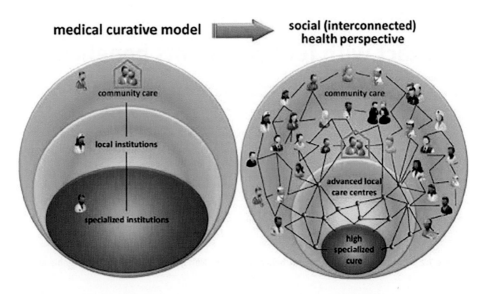

Figure 7.3   From a medical curative model to a network-oriented model (Guldemond 2015)

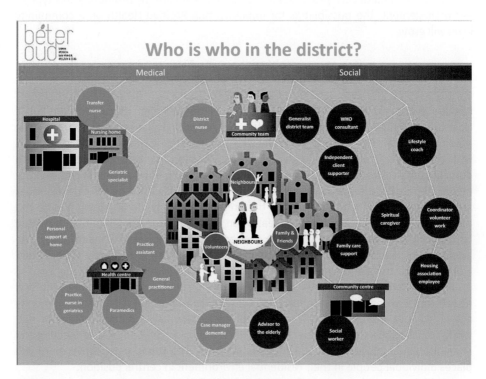

Figure 7.4   Who is who in the local community? (Beter oud 2019)

the social domain. For general practitioners, this could mean a lighter workload, as the many non-medical issues would not end up only in their consulting room. Social prescribing, as also mentioned in ▶ sect. 5.6, is a programme that is perfectly in line with this perspective. It supports general practitioners to lead social issues into the direction of the appropriate care service, when the outcome of an *alternative dialogue* calls for it. The new core value of *together* and core task of *care coordination* are very important, in this respect.

Has this sparked your curiosity about how Positive Health leads to more self-determination in patients? The pink base of the pyramid of ◼ fig. 7.1 will need to become much broader in the future. This chapter first describes what people themselves can do for their health It starts with self-care (sect.7.3.1), then the contact between fellow patients (▶ sect. 7.3.2), then informal care (▶ sect. 7.3.3), followed by how they could organise themselves with community strength (▶ sect. 7.3.4) and citizens' initiatives (▶ sect. 7.4) and what the basic steps would be in organising a healthy local community. These steps are important, in order to increase access to the available health care and where to find it, and to forge a good connection between the social and the medical domain. Positive Health in the local community is an added value for an integrated primary care – where primary care and the community, with a focus on people's personal environment, *work together on meaningful health care*.

7.3 The person in central position, the role of citizens

Putting people in central position requires knowing what is important to them. The research on which Positive Health was based shows that people have a broad view of health (▶ sect. 2.4). Positive Health follows their view, with the broad perspective on health including all six dimensions of the spider web. As general practitioners, we are accustomed to clarifying the issues presented to us by patients. In the first place, general practitioners deal with *general medical* complaints. However, these complaints often have other, underlying issues, such as psychosocial problems or lifestyle challenges.

An active role for patients has long been absent from the realm of health care, which is geared towards disease. This seems to have been changing, over recent years, with more attention for empowering patients by stimulating self-care and with a greater focus on prevention and health – not only in the Netherlands but also around the world.

It is important that patient themselves give the appropriate input, and that they understand what is going on, what they can expect with regard to what will happen next and what they could do themselves. In this respect, the person-oriented conversation of the Positive Health concept (▶ Chap. 5) can be very helpful. When discussing any goals patients may have, there are many possibilities for support available within the community, both in social and psychological areas as well as on lifestyle and meaningfulness. In order to determine where the best support could be found for a particular patient, it is important that general practitioners and their professional colleagues in primary care know the services available within their community and what they have to offer.

As care professionals, before we immediately go into solution mode, it is important to first wait and see what patients themselves are thinking. When discussing the spider web, the self-resolving ability of people may surprise us. People come up with various and often simple ideas. A patient who wanted to feel fitter said: 'From now on, I will take my bicycle to work, every day'. And someone who was trying to relax more said: 'I want to get back to doing yoga again'. Another patient with increased muscle tension in neck and shoulders that appeared to be related to stress at work, considered the first step to be: 'I'm going to talk to my employer about cutting down my hours', or someone who was overweight said: 'I'm going to stop drinking eight cappuccinos a day'. Although these may all seem like small steps at first, it is good to realise that many of our patients' questions do not always require a medical answer. And the best advice is usually that which people give themselves. It is good to be aware of this as a care professional, so that you can encourage patients to find their own solutions.

From the point of view of health care providers, it can be refreshing to look at patients from a different, broader perspective. In the medical world, we use the term *patients*. By doing so, we implicitly take the disease-oriented approach. Rather than looking at people as patients, should we not talk about people, citizens, residents and inhabitants? This would also give people a larger share in solving whatever ails them. The perspective then subtly shifts from *caring for* a patient to ensuring *that the person gains more insight* into what their possible complaint entails, how they could best deal with it, and what they could do themselves or where they could find the appropriate support. As described earlier in the text, the authors chose to use the term *patient*, from the perspective of the health care provider. To remind everyone that this is a nuanced term in the way it is used in this handbook, we explicitly emphasise this here, once again.

The section below discusses the various opportunities for people to help each other, within the community. Often, this is summarised under the umbrella term of *informal care* (▶ sect. 7.3.3). We first start with what you can do to take good care of your self.

7.3.1 Self-care

Self-care is a broad concept. Terms such as self-help, self-determination, self-care and self-management are often used interchangeably. The term self-management is often used in the context of chronic diseases. Nine out of ten chronically ill people consider themselves primarily responsible for the day-to-day management of their disease. They choose to be in charge of their own care and life, preferably with informal help from family and friends (Heijmans M. et al., 2014). A Dutch support organisation for self-care – called 'ZelfzorgOndersteund' ((▶ www.zelfzorgondersteund.nl), which has meanwhile ceased its operations and transferred its tasks to the insurance companies) – was helping care providers to support people with a chronic condition. They supported care organisations and projects with practical resources and funding – amongst other things, for care providers to use Positive Health in having *alternative conversations* in the consulting room.

Self-care is about what people can do for themselves around health and disease. A good example of how self-care can be stimulated, in practice, is the website of ▶ https://GPinfo.nl/ (the English version of an independent Dutch website for health information, developed and maintained by the Dutch College of General Practitioners and contains a selection of topics). This not only encourages self-care, but also leads to a decrease in the number of consultations. GPinfo.nl is a reliable website, with general medical information and advisory tools. It is useful for both practitioners and patients, and can be referred to for self-help. The website can also be used as an additional tool during a consultation. In the Netherlands, the use of ▶ www.thuisarts.nl (i.e., the Dutch version of GPinfo.nl) has increased enormously in recent years, and the content is regularly updated to include the latest developments in health care and society.

The website also features a decision tool to help people gain insight into certain decisions about their health. Research shows that after the launch of the website, the frequency of visits to general medical practices decreased by 12 %. On a national level, this means a monthly decrease of 675,000 in visits to general medical practices in the Netherlands. The results were published in the British Medical Journal (BMJ) and in a Dutch journal on primary care and science (*Huisarts & Wetenschap*) which is published by the Dutch College of General Practitioners (Spoelman et al., 2017). It is a good example of how the use of digital support can stimulate self-care, which also reduces the general practitioner's workload. During the COVID-19 crisis, when a large part of primary care could not always be provided in the consulting rooms of general medical practices, the Dutch version of GPinfo.nl was also widely used.

Self-care

GPinfo.nl: Reliable information about disease and health

GPinfo.nl is the Engels version of the Dutch website (▶ www.thuisarts.nl) that is intended for everyone who is looking for more information on health and disease:

- If you want to stay healthy
- If you want to know what you can do yourself about your medical complaints
- If you want to know how to deal with your medical complaints
- If you want to know who could help you, in this respect
- If you want to know whether you should go and see a physician
- If you want to prepare for your doctor's appointment
- If you want to take another look at the explanation and advice provided by your physician

Each text starts with a number of important aspects:

- What are my symptoms?
- What is causing those symptoms?
- What could I do myself about those symptoms?
- What treatments are available? Can I choose one myself? What are the advantages and disadvantages?
- When should I contact the general practitioner or specialist?

When, during an *alternative dialogue*, people discover what they need for their health, there are many digital referral possibilities to begin with. People look up information about their health, for example by using certain apps, wearables or other digital or technological support or gadgets. The younger generations are growing up with these possibilities and are autodidactic when it comes to gathering health-related digital information. GPinfo.nl has already been mentioned as a good example of an e-health application in general practice. This handbook does not elaborate in detail on the important theme of e-health. The text box provides some information about applications in primary care that stimulate and support self-care amongst citizens.

E-health

In primary care, e-health is becoming more and more popular and needed. Dutch medical professional organisations wholeheartedly support e-health (Van Tuyl et al., 2020). On the subject of e-health, the Dutch College of General Practitioners (NHG) states: NHG prioritises applications that help general practitioners in caring for their patients. This primarily concerns educational information and contact possibilities between general practitioners and patients.

Here, we focus on the following three themes (NHG, 2020):

- Online primary care services:e-consultations, online appointments and online prescription requests
- Support for self-management by patients, including the use of an individual care plan
- Supporting patients by supplying them with individual digital data from their electronic health record (EHR), for example to be used in a Personal Health Record (PHR)'

The NHG sees it as its task to critically monitor e-health applications, to develop guidelines and practical resources, where necessary, and to share knowledge. E-health can make a significant contribution to the increasing need for health care and the prevention of diseases. This does mean that everyone must be able to use the many e-health applications – which is currently far from being the case. These e-health applications are unclear or too complicated for many people, such as people with limited health skills, those who have difficulty reading and writing, and for many elderly people and people with an immigrant background.

They are currently making little use of e-health applications and it is precisely these people who could benefit greatly from the possibilities that e-health offers. Pharos, the Dutch centre of expertise concerned with health inequalities, is promoting the use of e-health applications through their eHealth4All programme (Pharos, 2020). As ▶ sect. 5.2 describes, a simple tool (▶ www.iph.nl/tools/eenvoudige-tool) has been developed in cooperation with Pharos to make Positive Health available to everyone. A programme has been set up to promote the digital availability of medical records (OPEN, ▶ www.open-eerstelijn.nl). The three Dutch national general practitioner organisations (InEen, LHV and NHG) support general practitioners in the secure online exchange of medical data with their patients. The OPEN programme offers practical support, such as training courses for professionals and educational material for patients. There is a great need for digitisation of information and more self-management by patients. In the Netherlands, one in seven people are currently working in the health care sector. As the demand for care increases over the coming 15 years, this number will rise to one in four. In the Netherlands, this will call for a regional and national joining of forces, also financially – which can be done, with sufficient support (InEen 2020)'. Much progress still needs to be made with respect to digitisation (NHG). The COVID-19 pandemic has taught us how to accelerate innovations, and the use of e-health has increased since the outbreak (Van Tuyl et al. 2020).

Particularly during the COVID-19 period, the delivery of primary care services changed due to circumstances. Simple medical-analytical procedures (rules-based precision medicine, value adding processes (see ▶ sect. 8.1.1)) were increasingly standardised and could be addressed via e-health (e.g., sending photographs) or by telephone. Videophones were used regularly for continuous, person-oriented care; for instance, for patients with chronic diseases or those with more complex mental or recurring physical symptoms. The Positive Health approach is particularly suitable for this last group of patients. Positive Health offers the individual digital tool for filling out the online spider web (e.g., in preparation for a consultation), to enhance self-reflection. Various courses of action can be followed, with many local possibilities that can be found online as well, such as local social maps and referral to online apps (GGD AppStore; ◨ fig. 5.8).

7.3.2 Contact between fellow patients

In addition to self-care and consulting the website GPinfo.nl or other digital support, the contact between fellow patients may also help people to increase their self-managing abilities. There are both digital and in-person options to achieve such contact between people in the same situation with respect to their health or with experience experts. In some areas (e.g., the Dutch Province of Limburg), contact between fellow patients is organised for people with certain syndromes or who are in similar situations. A newspaper article about the organisation 'Burgerkracht' describes the benefits of the contact between people with a certain disease or in a similar situation (◨ fig. 7.2). Burgerkracht Limburg facilitates easy access to self-help. Initiator Venhuis himself experienced the benefits of contact between fellow sufferers and, subsequently, set up the network. Venhuis: 'It is important that people know about self-help, and the various options that are on offer in their community. This citizen movement is growing around the country and it would be good if it also became more widely known amongst primary care providers.'

On an international level, there is already a great deal of experience with contact between fellow sufferers, such as the large worldwide platform of *PatientsLikeMe* (▶ www.patientslikeme.com). In Germany, a national organisation of self-help groups, Nakos, has been operational for the past 30 years (▶ www.nakos.de). Germany has over a 100,000 self-help groups on a wide variety of subjects. Local self-help groups are easy to find in regional networks (*Kontaktstellen*) around central municipalities. In these regional networks, the community supports these groups by providing them with accommodations, management, common support, PR and some degree of coordination. The groups themselves are autonomous, often linked to a patient association, which also supplies the related information. Research in Germany shows that not only is there an added value in terms of the provision of information, but there are also benefits in financial terms. The Social Return on Investment (SROI) tool calculates the added value to society for measures that have been or will be implemented. In Germany, every euro that is invested has been found to yield a social benefit of five euros, although the country does not want to talk about economic interests – the emphasis is on what people can do for each other, which is why structural embedding has been organised (zelfregietool.nl 2020).

7.3.3 Informal care

Informal care refers to various types of care that are not provided by professional care providers (Struijs 2006). In the Netherlands, this includes caregivers and volunteers. In a broader sense, this also includes the *self-care* and *contact between fellow sufferers*, as described above (Burgerkracht Limburg 2020). There are many local organisations in the Netherlands that support informal care. Unfortunately, not all informal care is well-known amongst care professionals such as general practitioners, practice assistants and consultants in social community care.

> **Pillars of informal care**
>
> **Fellow patients and experience experts**
> Experience experts have much to gain from each other; people suffering from the same disease or who are in a similar situation recognise each other's stories. Looking for and finding solutions together is a very powerful thing. It helps in emotional processing and it supports people to help themselves. More and more initiatives like the buddy system and the use of experience experts are being created (e.g., ▶ www.vved.org).
>
> **Family care**
> Family care is the care for and support of patients by family members or close friends from the community. It is provided in cases where patients require care-intensive assistance or in the palliative phase (▶ www.mantelzorg.nl).
>
> **Voluntary caregivers**
> This type of care is provided by volunteers in an organised setting. The Dutch website ▶ www.vrijwilligerswerk.nl and many others like it are examples of local and informal care networks in the Netherlands (e.g., ▶ www.nizu.nl (Utrecht region) and the Dutch national website: ▶ https://volunteering.nl/)

What can people, themselves, do to live their lives as healthy as possible, for as long as possible? How do they create an inclusive community that is focused on people who are in need of support, working together with actively involved local residents, informal caregivers and caring residents? Self-management with self-determination and organisation are key, in this respect. In civil society, people are already taking care of each other and the elderly, increasingly often. And people's own social networks are called on more and more frequently, with family members, neighbours and friends looking at where they could offer care and support. In this respect, volunteer support as a pillar of informal care is important. On both national and local levels, large amounts of support are on offer. Of the more than four million caregivers in the Netherlands, around 750,000 provide intensive and long-term informal care. A caring society is needed, particularly around the elderly, with social cohesion in local communities and villages, and where neighbours help and support each other. However, it is important that these informal caregivers remain fit and resilient. Positive Health can also be applied to support this group. It is therefore important that, throughout society, self-determination and self-management (the broad pink base of the pyramid in ◼ fig. 7.1) are increased.

7.3.4 Community strength

The COVID-19 crisis has caused social, economic and health damage. However, there were also positive developments within communities. During the *lockdown*, it was hardly possible to make use of physical health care services. People developed great self-resolving abilities when it came to medical complaints. They also started to take better care of each other. In the media, but also locally, many citizens' initiatives and help from the community could be seen and heard: from shopping services to helping neighbours. Informal care networks also became much more visible during this time. Citizens' initiatives are initiatives that are started without any obligation and are to the benefit of others or society as a whole. The concept of Positive Health shows that citizens see health in a much broader sense than mere physical and mental problems (the six dimensions). People are called on to show strength and resilience, both individually and as a community. It transcends the health care domain and, thus, gives general practitioners the opportunity to allow their patients to think of solutions themselves, those that are not strictly medical but are in the social domain (also see ▶ sect. 7.4 and 7.5). Community strength is the positive energy that is released when people help each other and increasingly achieve their goals by sharing their resources. Many citizens' initiatives use the building blocks of a basic social infrastructure for vital and social communities (Van der Aa and De Jager 2020).

In Germany, self-help groups are already commonplace, but in the Netherlands, citizens' initiatives are less well supported. For this reason, a network was set up of care initiatives in people's own local districts and villages, called *Nederland Zorgt Voor Elkaar* (NZVE) (▶ www.nlzorgtvoorelkaar.nl). Residents are helping each other by sharing knowledge, experience, problems and research. NZVE represents the interests of the initiatives by encouraging those involved in the health care system to work together with these citizens' initiatives.

Citizens' initiatives are encountering certain bottlenecks, which increase with the number of citizens actively engaged in offering services that were traditionally offered by professional organisations. For example, with respect to legislation and regulations, finances, municipal cooperation, care organisations and health insurance companies. Citizens who are organising health care themselves, within their own community, want the health care system to regard them as full partners in their own right (Bruijn 2016).

Cormac Russell, Managing Director of Nurture Development, the leading Asset-Based Community Development (ABCD) organisation in Europe, asks: 'What have we learned from COVID-19, in which a lot has happened within neighbourhoods and local communities?' The pandemic revealed which essential functions where present within these communities. 'People were home-schooling their children, they took care of people who wanted to die at home. If we don't help each other, nobody will,' says Russell. Many professionals encourage those communities and support them. This is about setting up citizens' initiatives from the notion that communities can do a lot for themselves (Russell 2020). The LSA (Dutch national cooperative of actively involved citizens) is a cooperative of people who are committed to their local communities and who, for example, work with the ABCD method in various places in the Netherlands (▶ www.lsabewoners.nl). The LSA encourages and connects residents and helps them to share knowledge and expertise with each other and with others. Community resilience is entirely in line with the Positive Health concept. It places citizens at the wheel, with health care professionals in a supporting role. Communities organise themselves as citizen cooperatives.

7.4   Citizens' initiatives in the community

Local citizens' initiatives are mushrooming: care cooperatives, care collectives and urban villages are taking matters into their own hands and are organising health care and support for the elderly and other vulnerable people within their communities. They give local residents the opportunity to be of service to others. The importance of these types of initiatives is also recognised on a national level – amongst others by the Dutch Ministry of Health, Welfare and Sport. In addition to, for example, the essential contribution of these initiatives to provide sustainable care for the elderly, they are also already providing quality welfare, housing and care facilities, lower health care costs and a new form of democracy (Van der Aa and Smelik 2018). Citizens' initiatives can also be supported, digitally. Online community platforms enable people to organise things together via the Internet, for the daily functioning of their own living environment. Often, many of the things that are very effective for local communities are invisible. With the help of local community platforms, meetings are organised for local residents.

Two community initiatives that work completely according to the Positive Health concept are elaborated below. Citizens describe what they consider to be important with regard to their own health and well-being and towards participating in the community.

7.4.1   'Indekerngezond', health for and by the community

In 2018, in the suburb of Leidsche Rijn (in the Province of Utrecht), the first community project based entirely on the Positive Health concept was launched. It challenges local residents to live healthier lives and to take the initiative for this themselves. Janine van der Duin (project leader of *Indekerngezond*) has experienced the power of Positive Health for herself and how much wisdom it can bring. The municipality of Utrecht has set up a community location in the suburb of Leidsche Rijn.

The community project is mainly organized for and by the local community. It is a meeting place where people can go to set up their own Positive Health projects, or to find something that will help them in their personal situation. All initiatives that arise there have one thing in common: they stimulate local residents to determine the course of their own meaningful and healthy life. They start from what people CAN do – instead of focusing on what they cannot. Indekerngezond's mission is for local residents to take control of their own lives in a meaningful and healthy way. *Indekerngezond* is a lively place, a meeting place, where everyone is able to contribute to the development of a healthy community.

Meaningfulness and participation

Local residents say that sense of purpose, participation and development are the most important reasons for them to contact *Indekerngezond*. Many go there to meet with others and play a meaningful role in some way. *Indekerngezond* does not give advice, but allows people to try and find their own direction, what works for them and what the areas are for them to take steps forward. Because people themselves set to work on the basis of their own intrinsic motivation, the chances of them succeeding are much greater. *Indekerngezond* also combats loneliness by stimulating participation. Amongst other things, local residents are able to initiate or participate in all kinds of workshops, all linked to the philosophy of Positive Health. For example, about nutrition, stress prevention, physical exercise and Positive Health, neighbourhood meals, helping children to handle emotions and much more. There is also a general workshop on Positive Health, in which people can get acquainted with the concept; and there are local residents who have followed the training 'working with Positive Health' and are conducting Positive Health-style conversations with other residents of the community. In addition, student internships are provided, for example, to enter into Positive Health conversations with people who are new to the neighbourhood. *Indekerngezond* is part of a healthy community cooperative network Leidsche Rijn–Vleuten-De Meern (see ▶ sect. 7.6.1).

What are the benefits?

For local residents: 'At *Indekerngezond*, there are opportunities for people to develop their own initiatives. Here, I can make a contribution by passing on Positive Health to the neighbourhood. People can meet each other here and learn new things.'

For care professionals: People often visit the general medical practice with questions related to the dimensions of physical and mental well-being. After completing the spider web, however, the goals they wish to pursue often are in very different domains. *Indekerngezond* is primarily a place where people can go with questions about participation and sense of purpose. Volunteers at *Indekerngezond* can also hold Positive Health conversations with local residents. This can relieve the workload of the professional care providers.

Here are some tips for those who want to set up a similar community project:
- Let citizens themselves come up with such initiatives.
- Initiatives should be managed by project leaders who have sufficient amounts of both time and knowledge. These are not activities that can be done 'on the side'.
- Ensure a good combination of offline and online services. Thus, not only provide a digital platform, but also a cosy, recognisable meeting place in the community, where people can physically meet.
- Connect with various partners in the community and with the municipality. There will be a lot of common ground when working according to the Positive Health concept.
- Professionals tend to quickly jump on an initiative and bend it to their will. And, soon, such citizens' projects will turn professional again. This should be avoided.

7.4.2 'Texel Samen Beter' (*Texel better together*)

Local residents of Texel, one of the Dutch Wadden Sea islands, were concerned about the future availability of care facilities in their community. They saw opportunities to do something about that situation, and, in 2014, they joined forces and set up the care cooperative *Texel Samen Beter* (TSB). TSB made sure that good health care and support for all islanders ended up on the agendas of official health care and welfare providers and the municipality. In 2016, a cooperative was formed by working according to the Positive Health concept. The programme for a healthy island of Texel (*Gezond Texel 2030*) was developed to realise the joint ambition to strengthen, broaden and accelerate the movement towards greater health, to maintain quality of life on the island of Texel and to reduce and redirect the pressure on care facilities. The goal is for health care to remain available, also in the future, for those who really need it. The programme works along three interdependent courses of action, to improve the health of all people living on the island of Texel:

1. Strengthening the resilience of inhabitants and communities
2. Dealing with physical, mental and socially challenges in a healthy way
3. Texel-wide cooperation based on a shared vision

(On the website of *Texel Gezond 2030* you will find more information about the second and third points; for website links to the examples, see the QR code at the end of this chapter.)

Examples of the first point of action that particularly affect the inhabitants include:

- Community building: stimulate, make visible, smart connections, and scale up inhabitants' initiatives;
- The 'Tuunen': inhabitants make arrangements together about life in their community, using the environmental model for Positive Health and the local living environment (▶ www.buurtskapdetuunen.nl).
- Hooray, it is today! Elementary school pupils are gaining experience with Positive Health; Iceland model: the municipality of Texel works with the Icelandic preventive approach to health for young people to reduce the use of alcohol and stimulate sports and exercise. After working with the Icelandic model for three years in 6 Dutch municipalities, the next step in Texel will be to start with a combination of the Icelandic Model and Positive Health. This is an interesting group to start with, since this age group is difficult to reach via other care professionals (Smeets et al. 2019).

As a local residents' cooperative, TSB was a co-initiator of the coalition on Positive Health in Texel (CoalitiePositieveGezondheid Texel) and the driving force behind the movement towards greater health on the island. It is a good example of cooperation within a Positive Health Network (see ▶ sect. 8.3.1), on citizen, local community and regional levels. ▶ Section 7.6. explains the connection between the medical and social domains and the integrated cooperation.

As general practitioners working with the Positive Health concept, the authors of this handbook are experiencing the more active role of patients, on a daily basis, as well as the added value of citizen initiatives. We also see the added value of a broader basis (◻ fig. 7.1) for more self-care, community strength, prevention (also see ▶ chapt. 5) and e-health. What does this movement *from aftercare to preventive care* mean for care professionals? Integrated primary care continues to play an important role, with more emphasis on care coordination. How to optimally cooperate around patients? Positive Health as a single language for a common broad perspective on health may help. In the examples of Utrecht and Texel, and many others in the Netherlands, the initial approach was on a small scale, so that Positive Health could really become firmly implemented in practice. This is an organic process that starts small and gradually gains wider support. The spread of Positive Health will have a ripple effect, as more and more local residents and organisations start to speak the same language.

7.5 Elaboration of core value 'together' and core task 'care coordination'

Now that the various opportunities for and by the community are becoming more widely known, the question is what influence this has on *the role and tasks of general practitioners*. People are used to going to their general practitioners with health questions. In recent years, these questions have become increasingly complex. It is therefore not without reason that the 'generalist' core value for general practitioners was redefined to '*medical generalist*'. In a *person-oriented* conversation (i.e., the *alternative dialogue*), an overall inventory can be made of what patients want and are able to do for themselves.

7.5.1 Taking on a different role: from gatekeeper to coach or liaison

Physicians and future physicians, first and foremost, learn about diseases and how to diagnose and treat them. The change in mentality from a disease-oriented perspective to one that is more broadly health-oriented, also changes the role of general practitioners. In the Netherlands, this is still mainly the role of gatekeeper – i.e., every hospital referral goes via the general practitioner. Part of the role of gatekeeper was also to prevent medicalisation and keep health care costs under control. However, instead of resulting in the envisaged cost reductions, it greatly increased the administrative workload. In countries where there is no such gatekeeper role for general practitioners such as Belgium, Germany and Switzerland, patients appear to turn to their general practitioners with more focused questions and positive expectations (Terluin 2013). Whether the Dutch role of gatekeeper towards secondary care still suffices, these days, is debatable. One could argue that general practitioners no longer are gatekeepers, but have taken on the role of coach or liaison.

The committee of the project on future primary care in the Netherlands (*commissieToekomst Huisartsenzorg,* see ▶ Chap. 3), has published the following about the core value of '*together*', on their website (▶ www.toekomsthuisartsenzorg.nl): 'General practitioners, together with their patients, determine which type of care would be appropriate. They provide this general medical care together with other care providers'. On the core task of 'care coordination', the committee says: 'General practitioners operate within a broad network of care providers and are often regarded the first point of contact in the *coordination of care* around a patient. They are not only ultimately responsible for the care provided by their own team, but are often also the connecting factor in the care chain and the first point of contact for other care providers who have medical questions about those patients'. General practitioners ensure that the care of their patients who have complex medical problems is properly coordinated.

The coordinating tasks of general practitioners are in the medical field. General practitioners are not responsible for coordinating nursing care or care in the social domain. Together with their team, they help patients with social problems to find the right kind of help. It is therefore important that, in order to make the appropriate referrals, they know what is available. Equally essential, from this perspective, is the written or oral information provided to general practitioners about the policies of other care providers.

Cooperation around patients is becoming more network-oriented (see ◘ fig. 7.3 and 7.4). Patients have more control over their own lives, and are given access to their medical records. Also, more and more care networks are emerging. The *Parkinson network*(▶ www.parkinsonnet.nl) is a good example of such an organisation in the Netherlands, for people suffering from Parkinson's disease. In addition to cooperation related to a specific disease, there are also organisations for broader stakeholder groups, such as vulnerable elderly people. The coordination and cooperation of general practitioners with other professionals and local residents, informal caregivers and volunteers is also crossing over into other domains. This is happening both physically, in people's own local environment and digitally in Personal Health Environments (PGOs). Here, too, Positive Health often proves to be a connecting language. It can be applied effectively, in the light of its core value 'together', focused on the cooperation around patients in their community.

7.5.2 Cooperation around patients in the community

The growing numbers of initiatives and movements around and with citizens or patients require good connections between medical and social domains. ◘ Figure 7.3 shows how patients themselves are in a more central position, with the care network surrounding them.

The movement from the linear and medical curative model to a more health-oriented network organisation represents a paradigm shift in health care (see ◘ fig. 7.3). As the tilting pyramids of ◘ fig. 7.1 show, the system is moving towards smaller institutions for highly complex care, broad health centres close to citizens and a high degree of citizen involvement. In ◘ fig. 7.4, citizens are primarily surrounded by family, neighbours and volunteers, who, in turn, are surrounded by various formal and informal services in the social domain. In the medical domain, from the perspective of care networks, general medical practices are increasingly incorporated in local community centres and health squares (see ▶ sect. 6.7 on the Spectrum medical centre in Meppel). Cooperation around patients or local residents can then be designed more efficiently in an ever-more complex society.

What do these changes mean for the role of general practitioner? To organise the coordination of general medical care in alignment with other professionals in the network around a patient, the role of the general practitioner becomes more that of *coach, organiser, team member or liaison*. This is why the core value of 'together' had to be added to the other core values of primary care. *Care coordination* and alignment are applied in practice, at the following levels:

— The consulting room. Here, at the level of personal interaction, the appropriate type of care is chosen, as well as which things the patients are able to do for themselves (see ▶ Chap. 5 on person-oriented care using the *alternative dialogue* and joint decision-making; ▶ sect. 4.5).

— The medical practice. At this organisational level, the general practitioner, together with the other practice staff, provides patients with sensible care (see ▶ Chap. 6 on the change in task).

- The community. At this level, general practitioners and the members of their practice team with general medical expertise work together with other caregivers and care providers in the community to provide the right type of care in the right place (see elsewhere in this chapter).
- On a regional and national level, general practitioners, together with other members of the medical profession, work to promote the quality of primary care (► Chap. 6).

In the second picture of ◻ fig. 7.3 and in ◻ fig. 7.4 it is shown how many people and organisations can be involved around the health and disease of individual people. The 'Better old' programme concerns the care of vulnerable older people (Wind and Velde 2019). In addition to specific indications, having a good conversation with elderly people is important here. This can then be used, for example, in a multidisciplinary meeting to discuss the required follow-up care and any other wishes of the patient. A preparatory *alternative dialogue* can be very helpful in clarifying what is important for the particular patient. Various care professionals work together on caring for the elderly in the local community, such as community teams, welfare, informal care, district nurses and primary care (general practitioners, paramedics and pharmacists). A mobile geriatric team and geriatric specialists can also work together on behalf of the elderly. General practitioners, district nurses and paramedics have long been partners in the coordination around people with chronic diseases and the elderly in their community.

Case no. 17

Positive Health for vulnerable elderly people

A 74-year-old woman with mental health problems and Parkinson's disease was making a heavy demand on the general medical practice during the day, with complaints of chest pains. These were repeatedly diagnosed as hyperventilation and, during one of her visits to the surgery, she was given an oxazepam which calmed her down. In spite of this diagnosis, she also very often called the out-of-hours service with this same complaint and, at several occasions, an ambulance was rushed to her location. Each time, after having arrived at the hospital's emergency department, no cardiac abnormalities would be found and she would end up being taken home again. Despite the fact that her medical file stated that her complaints were related to her personality and that several analyses by cardiologists had not revealed any heart issues, when once again she would call the general medical practice or out-of-hours service, the triage staff on duty would not dare to take any risks and would send an ambulance to her address anyway. This may be related to the time pressure at the particular service not allowing for lengthy telephone calls with patients (such as those in which the other dimensions of Positive Health could be discussed). As the pressure on the day surgery also increased due to the woman's many phone calls, the general practitioner decided to hold an *alternative dialogue* with her, based on the Positive Health concept. This revealed that loneliness was an important factor. The general practitioner was able to connect her with a volunteer from the community, who proved to be very capable of dealing with her personality problems. The out-of-hours service was also no longer approached, and slowly the woman began to discover that her loneliness played a role in the manifestation of her physical complaints. This helped her to decide not to continue living by herself at all costs, but to opt for a nursing home. From there, she also continued to be in contact with the volunteer from the community.

Positive Health is very applicable to the elderly. In case no. 17, the *alternative dialogue* was conducted by the general practitioner. Other professionals involved in the care of the elderly can also conduct a Positive Health conversation. For example, a practice nurse (geriatrics), physiotherapist, remedial therapist or district nurses. District nurses are close to patients, and observe and hear a lot. A Positive Health conversation can give direction, and a nurse can also refer a patient on to other care providers in the social domain. Instead of focusing on disease and limitations, they look at what the elderly person still can and will do for themselves. In keeping with what they still value in their lives. Elderly people, in particular, often are very resilient. Being aware of this fact and using this resilience is much more important than 'fixing' whatever physical aspect is not working properly. Although what also matters, in this respect, is the patient's expectations and fear of physical illnesses. Elderly people are sometimes better off if they are helped with what they need in order to have a good life and living it in a healthy way.

The guidelines for applying Positive Health in elderly care ('*Handreikingen bij de toepassing van Mijn Positieve Gezondheid bij ouderen*' (in Dutch)) discusses the ways of using Positive Health in elderly care. There are different conversation methods for awareness, self-reflection, having an *alternative dialogue*, and how to guide people into action (iPH 2019f). There is also a video (in Dutch) on the practical application of Positive Health for professionals. In it, practitioner for the elderly, Brenda Ott, tells how she gets to know her patients even better through the use of Positive Health, and how she arrived at surprising new insights for an older patient whom she had already known for a long time.

When many care providers are involved around a vulnerable elderly person, Positive Health may be useful as a connecting language. For example, the *alternative dialogue* can also be applied to discover how people think about the end of life (i.e., advanced care planning). This is particularly appropriate for addressing issues of meaningfulness. Some believe it is not appropriate to present the spider web questionnaire to people in the last phase of their life. In this phase, however, it is important to talk about what is meaningful and what may be helpful when looking back at one's life. (iPH 2019f). In ▶ Chap. 5, there is also an example of the spider web having been used with a patient in the terminal phase (i.e., case no. 14).

7.5.3 Positive Health as a common language

As already mentioned, the common language of Positive Health may support the communication between care providers, both in the medical domain and when crossing into other domains. ▶ Chapter 6 describes how the cooperation and care around individual people is organised within the team of the general practice. Positive Health can be used in the local community by other professionals, such as those in the social domain, welfare, sports, youth care, district nursing (e.g., in geriatric care) and many other disciplines. There are also more and more paramedics working with the Positive Health concept. It does not matter who holds the *alternative dialogue* with a patient, what matters is that someone does. It is of course necessary that certain agreements are made in this respect, about the transfer of such patients between cooperating partners. In addition, there is also a growing number of specialists and nurses in hospitals who are aware of the Positive Health philosophy and are embracing the concept. It is not without reason that Positive Health is included in the vision document for medical specialists, 'Medisch Specialist 2025', by the Dutch federation of medical specialists (Federatie Medisch Specialisten, 2015). The Jeroen Bosch Hospital has embraced the concept of Positive Health and speaks mainly of promoting health-related well-being (▶ https://tinyurl.com/hier-staan-wij-voor). The experiences at the Jeroen Bosch Hospital in the Dutch city of 's-Hertogenbosch show that the hospital's nursing staff also have an important role to play. For example, in cooperation around cancer patients (Van den Brekel-Dijkstra and Van Rixtel, 2020). Working according to the Positive Health concept helps in the cooperation around patients, so that care providers are all talking about the same thing, the broad view of health, with a more health-oriented mindset. It creates clarity amongst professionals about the impact of listening with intent and stimulating self-management. Speaking this common language has been found to be very valuable, with everyone moving into the same direction (also see ◻ fig. 6.11).

7.5.4 Cooperation between social and medical domains

Positive Health as an elaboration of: *Health as the ability to adapt and self-manage in the face of social, physical and emotional challenges*, as applied in the spider web (see Chapters 2 and 5) is also suitable as a joint vision on a level of local communities or the

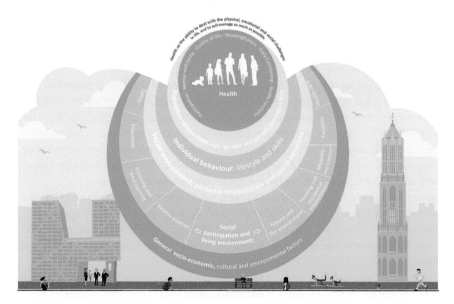

◻ **Figure 7.5** Positive Health in the policy document on public health of the municipality of Utrecht, 'gezondheid voor iedereen' (*health for everyone*). Source: Municipality of Utrecht (2019)

municipality. For health care providers, policymakers and citizens, Positive Health is a joint 'umbrella', a foundation for the broad perspective on health. Thus, a reference to Positive Health can also be found in many policy documents of Dutch municipalities, as well as, since 2020, in the Dutch Government's National Policy Document on Public Health (see ▶ Chap. 8, iPH 2019e).

How this is done in practice differs per municipality. In some regions or provinces, the ideas of the broad view of health are described in the policy document, but lacks concrete applications in practice. In other regions, the connection between the medical and the social domain is stimulated from a common vision of Positive Health. The health of the local residents is in central position, as it is in the policy document on public health ('Health for all') of the municipality of Utrecht (see ◘ fig. 7.5).

Part of the broad approach to health is the cooperation with others. Municipalities provide support and make connections. For the organisation of care that also involves other domains, it is important to have clear roles and tasks of the various parties involved and to know everyone's formal and legal responsibilities. The emphasis is on care that can be provided within a patient's community and the promotion of personal responsibility and self-reliance. Many questions now end up unnecessarily in the health care system, whereas they have their origins in totally different areas, such as the problems related to *parenting, work, school, housing, or relationships*. The patient in ◘ fig. 7.4 is surrounded by the medical domain in blue and the social domain in pink. Ideally, the care for people's health should be a joint effort. General practitioners who know the possibilities offered by the municipality can more easily refer patients with social problems to the right places. With vulnerable elderly people who remain living at home for longer, good cooperation is essential. This handbook uses case studies to show how Positive Health can be applied in cooperation with other parties in local communities, municipalities, mental, social and youth care. It illustrates the cooperation between the social domain (community teams, welfare, youth care) and primary care (general practitioners, paramedics and pharmacists), also in the youth care, good collaboration is needed, as described in case no. 18.

Case no. 18: 13-year-old girl with behavioural problems

A 13-year-old girl with ADHD, impulse control issues and behavioural problems is causing her single mother and her younger brother a large amount of anxiety and worry. Because of COVID-19, the community day centre and special needs education have been unavailable. The situation at home has become untenable. The mother is distraught because her daughter is running away, daubing the walls, disobeying her and throwing things at her. The mother has been visiting the mental health practice nurse for herself, who advised her to make an appointment with her general practitioner.

Some time ago, the mother asked for help with her daughter, who was then placed on the waiting list for specialist youth mental health care. To bridge the period while she is on this waiting list (6 months), a multidisciplinary consultation was planned to discuss further support. The general practitioner has known the mother for years, and this is a trusted basis for her.

The general practitioner has held the *alternative dialogue* according to the Positive Health concept with the mother before, and started by asking what the mother considered to be important at that time. Despite the fact that the mother indicated to have problems sleeping and was suffering from headaches, she stated that the safety and care of her daughter came first. The level of urgency was clear and an intake was planned with the social community team for both parenting support and the mother's financial problems. The general practitioner asked the mother to let her daughter fill out the Children's tool of Positive Health. This in preparation for the intake, because the specialist youth mental health care recently also started working with the Positive Health concept.

The following week, the general practitioner discussed the daughter's insights into her own health and behaviour, using the results from the *Positive Health childrens' tool*. In this way, mother and daughter gained insight into the girl's perspective and what was of value to her. The daughter did not appear to be very troubled by her problems, she would however like to learn how to be less angry. At the youth mental health care intake, the specialist will be able to continue along the Positive Health lines already started by the general practitioners. The mother felt less pressure; she felt heard and supported during the multi-disciplinary meetings with the general practitioner, the mental health care specialist, mental health practice nurse and the social community team. The cooperation around her and her daughter has given the mother a sense of assurance. Although her daughter's problems could not be solved straight away, she felt confident that the care professionals around her would give her tools to cope better with the situation herself.

Case No. 18 shows how the general practitioner coordinates care, and, together with the *the other care providers, such as a mental health practice nurse*, she was able to create trust between mother and daughter. The following case – no. 19 on complexity – demonstrates the importance of cooperation within mental health care and assisted living, and the coordination between the various hospitals. In both cases, the Positive Health concept is able to provide support through its common language and working method.

Case no. 19: complexity– cooperation in the socio-medical domain

This case is about a 25-year-old woman who was staying in assisted living circumstances and who had a complex history. She was severely damaged in her youth, and in addition to post-traumatic stress, she was also suffering from serious psychological issues and severe adiposity. There were also regular complaints related to the musculoskeletal system, and because of reduced mobility and chronic pain, she would move around in a mobility scooter. In the beginning, the consultations with the general practitioner consisted mainly of referrals, feedback from psychiatry, obesity clinic, nephrologist, internist, gynaecologist and orthopaedic surgeon. The woman's days were completely filled with her medical circumstances, and hospital admissions.

The general practitioner was the woman's confidant. Because of her frequent visits to hospital and the surgery hour, the general practitioner was becoming frustrated, feeling powerless. During the next consultation, the general practitioner mentioned this to her and asked her about what she was hoping for or what she considered to be important. She indicated how she wanted a normal life and a job. At that moment, it was very difficult for her to participate in society, both physically and mentally. Slowly, and in consultation with her personal counsellor and psychiatrist, the care surrounding the woman became more focused on her perspective and what she found important, and more support was organised from within her own environment. Meanwhile, a psychosomatic physiotherapist was helping her to deal with chronic pain and to build up her physical mobility. The GP asked her to fill out the Positive Health spider web. The woman would set small goals with respect to nutrition and healthier eating habits, and once a week she would go with the personal assistant from the assist living group to buy healthier food products and cook healthier food and visited the community platform: *Indekerngezond* (see ▶ sect. 7.4.1).

Her health goals were also included in the psychiatrist's personal treatment plan and, step by step, the woman was gaining more insight into and control over her complex life. Together with the pharmacist and psychiatrist, a start was made on phasing out sleep and mental medication. Since then, she has become more cheerful, has occasional setbacks, but is on the right track. She is more aware of the things she cannot change and those she can. Everyone has experienced how working with various professionals around this patient in her own environment has been pleasant and they know how to find each other. Positive Health offers an effective common language and perspective, and, most importantly, the patient was feeling better. From powerlessness and hopelessness, to *manageability, comprehensibility and meaningfulness* (see ▶ Chap. 2). Positive Health helped her toward greater insights, better overview and prospects.

The case shows how cooperation between the medical and social domains is possible for patients with complex problems. It may seem rather time-consuming, at first. But both cases are examples of patients who were already requiring a large amount of time, as they used to be frequent visitors to the general medical practice. The time invested in the Positive Health approach, with its common language, in line with what such patients require, is ultimately a step into the right direction, for all parties involved. Incidentally, both patients have been coming to the surgery far less frequently, in recent months.

> **Reflection**
>
> *What were your answers to the reflection questions at the beginning of this chapter?*
> *If you know how to contact the professionals within your local community, how does this benefit you as a general practitioner?*
> If you are not used to working together with parties in the social domain, do you know where to find the social workers and other care providers in this domain?
> - *Are you aware of all the available care providers in the local community?*
> - *Do you have a social map?*
> - *How is the cooperation within the community with social and welfare partners, on the one hand, and those providing terminal palliative care, on the other?*
> - *How could cooperation with local residents and community professionals contribute to improving the health of these residents?*
> - *What could be the benefits of working according to the Positive Health concept for you and your colleagues?*

General practitioners could make even more use of the social domain. For example, by referring people with health-related and other support questions to the municipality. Municipalities offer support for many different problems. They have a role to play in all areas that are important for the promotion of health for people of all ages, from sense of purpose, loneliness, community day centres, housing, mediation, financial support and structure, to practical support such as a stair lift and a personal health budget. In addition, there are community sports coaches or community team members who also work at a community health centre. The way these things are organised varies per municipality. How is the care within the social domain provided in your local community, region or country? Are there possibilities for cooperation with primary care? Perhaps this has already been implemented on a large scale, which will vary from country to country.

Most municipalities in the Netherlands attach great importance to cooperation with general practitioners in the provision of services and support on areas mentioned in the text box. Cooperation is not an end in itself, but serves to promote the health of all members of a local community. The National Association of General Practitioners (LHV) has published a document and digital workbook on cooperation between general practitioners and municipality. This includes a handy checklist for the role of the general practitioner in such cases of cooperation (LHV, 2017b). The Dutch College of General Practitioners (NHG) supports this type of community cooperation with its publication of guidelines on this subject (Samenwerken aan gezondheid in de wijk (available in Dutch)). These guidelines address how local cooperation within local communities could be created and organised together with local residents. The cooperation between general practitioners and municipalities also has its challenges (NHG, 2018):

- Cooperation between general practitioners and social work is not always equally successful. Sometimes it becomes stuck on the differences in working methods and language use. General practitioners are open to such cooperation, but do not always know where to start. It helps if care providers all have a community-oriented focus and know each other.
- Data exchanges with municipal employees come up against privacy issues. Written reports on the approach and progress of support to the general practitioner are often lacking. As a result, general practitioners, the municipality and municipal health services do not know who is doing what, which leads to fragmentation of both support and health care. It often happens that different professionals are dealing with the same problem at the same time, and sometimes using conflicting approaches. There is a need for consultation on patient level, cooperation (agreements) and coordination.
- Working together in the community takes time, time that is not foreseen in primary care funding. For community management tasks, funding is now available for general practitioners from the budget on Organisation and Infrastructure (O&I), see ► Chap. 8.
- There are 288 municipalities in the Netherlands, all of which with their own policy on public health, sometimes in cooperation with other municipalities. The regional organisation between general practitioners (care groups), municipalities and municipal health services (GGDs), is not always in line with the O&I, which makes it difficult to secure initiatives at the various levels. This also hampers agreements on national preconditions for the cooperation between general practitioners (care groups), municipalities and municipal health services (GGDs).

How could the cooperation of the medical and social domains be made more sustainable? Who would be responsible for this effort? Answering these types of questions requires a critical look at the entire health care system and possible changes. Will an increase in referrals to the social domain translate into fewer referrals to medical specialists and hospitals?

The development of an integrated approach based on a shared vision would enormously benefit community-oriented harmonisation that is in line with the needs of local residents (see ▶ sect. 7.6). Positive Health has been found to be a very effective connecting factor. This applies to the concept's common language and vision, and is also very practical in the cooperation between various initiatives. When a person-oriented Positive Health conversation leads to certain patient questions that require a non-medical answer, the next step for the general practitioner may be to refer this patient to the appropriate services in the local community.

7.5.5 Social prescribing

Social prescribing is known e.g. in the UK as a way for local agencies to refer people to a link worker. Link workers give people time, focusing on 'what matters to me' and taking a holistic approach to people's health and wellbeing. They connect people to community groups and statutory services for practical and emotional support.

Social prescribing (*Welzijn op Recept* (in Dutch), as mentioned in ▶ Chap. 5 can be one of the courses of action following the *alternative dialogue*. It supports the required cooperation between parties to provide customised care. It can be used, for example, for complaints where underlying social problems play a role, such as the death of a partner, job loss or loneliness. In addition to explaining that no medical diagnosis or treatment is required, the general practitioner or other primary care provider can then refer such patients to a well-being coach. This is a social worker usually employed by a welfare organisation.

> **What is Social prescribing?**
>
> Social prescribing is a short-term intervention whereby people who go to a primary care provider for their psychosocial complaints are referred to welfare organisations. These complaints include worrying, sleeping badly, fatigue, back and shoulder complaints, and headaches. These people regularly visit their general practitioner with these complaints, and often they do not need any medication or referral to a physiotherapist, psychologist or medical specialist. In such cases, they are referred to a well-being coach who, together with them, will look for a suitable activity or other solution that provides positive experiences and social contacts. Something these patients used to enjoy in the past and that gave them energy. Social prescribing is aimed at bringing some colour back into people's lives. In the Netherlands, social prescribing started in 2011–2012 and the method has since spread throughout the Netherlands. At the time this handbook was published, social prescribing was being implemented in over 100 Dutch municipalities (◘ fig. 7.6).
> **Effects and results of social prescribing in the Netherlands**
> In the Netherlands, a number of process evaluations were carried out in Social Prescribing projects and a number of scientific studies. These were mainly conducted over the 2015–2016 period (▶ https://welzijnoprecept.nl/publicaties/). The largest study in the Netherlands was conducted in Nieuwegein (2015), where researchers looked at primary care consumption and the use of medications. A decrease in visits to the

surgery hour was shown after social prescribing was applied, but seeing the timespan of only one year and the small size of the trial group (172 patients), this outcome is not yet statistically significant. No significant difference was found regarding the use of medications between the periods before and after the application of social prescribing. The related qualitative sub-study (Heijnders et al., 2015) mainly provides information from the patient perspective, with participants in the social prescribing method saying that they felt healthier and more self-reliant, had more self-confidence, experienced greater well-being and had a more positive outlook on the future because of social prescribing. The final report on social prescribing (Vissers 2015) shows a clearly measurable increase in well-being and a sharp decline in the use of primary care related to psychosocial complains. However, no control group was used, which means that the scientific evidence is limited.

A cost–benefit analysis of the added value of social prescribing, conducted in the Netherlands by Van Gorp (2019), clearly shows the areas in life that are impacted by social prescribing and describes the cost-saving potential. Although this analysis was fully based on assumptions, the study does conclude that investing in social prescribing would avoid any additional high costs incurred in medical and social domains. The practice of social prescribing is growing steadily, throughout the Netherlands. A quick scan was done in 2019 amongst all Dutch municipalities that were working with social prescribing. The report contains the main findings on types of referrals, the target group, and the essential elements of social prescribing.

Via the Dutch national knowledge network on social prescribing, or the handbook on social prescribing (Heijnders and Meijs 2019), tools are available on how to organise this together with social welfare organisations and the municipality. Patients, general practitioners, well-being coaches and the municipality all have experienced the added

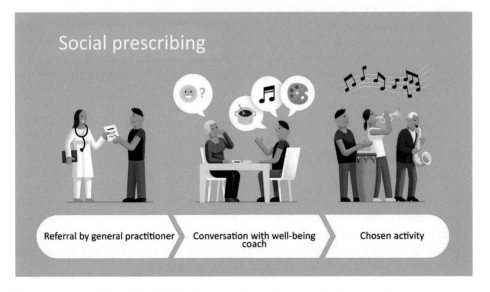

◘ **Figure 7.6**   Social prescribing (Heijnders and Meijs 2019). ▶ www.welzijnoprecept.nl

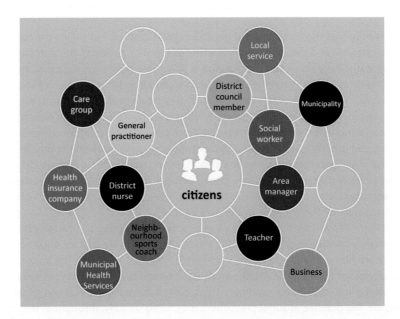

□ **Figure 7.7**   Cooperating partners from the Community Prevention programme. (Source: Infographic *Gezondewijkaanpak* (Healthy community approach), *Loket gezond leven* (healthy living desk) 2018)

value of social prescribing (for more information (in Dutch), scan the QR code at the end of this chapter).

Linking Positive Health and Social prescribing

A general medical practice in Hengelo together with the Dutch municipality of Hengelo and GGD-Twente are cooperating on improving the connection between the medical and social domains. In a pilot project, the spider web of Positive Health is used for patients with long-term unexplained complaints. The general practitioner conducts the Positive Health conversation and, where needed, patients are referred to the social domain with a type of 'prescription card' (*social prescribing*). The card has the spider web printed on it, with a link to ▶ https://my.positivehealth.com, and a referral to the well-being coach who works at the general practice once a week.
General Practitioner Martijn van der Waart of Medical Centrum Slangenbeek, Municipality of Hengelo and *GGD Twente.*
(▶ https://tinyurl.com/grip-op-klachten)

The *alternative dialogue* according to the Positive Health concept helps to gain insight into a patient's health situation. For many patients with psychosocial complaints – of which the cause does not appear to be medical – the social prescribing intervention is a next step. The examples will hopefully demonstrate that a good connection between the medical and social domains has added value (Van Wijck 2020).

In cooperation between various care professionals in primary care, Positive Health can also be applied very effectively as a common language. General practitioners are already working together with paramedics, such as dieticians, primary care psychologists, midwives, physiotherapists, remedial therapists and pharmacists. In the cooperation around a patient, it is useful when those primary care professionals are also familiar with Positive Health.

7.5.6 Application Positive Health paramedics

After the general practitioner has conducted an *alternative dialogue*, patients can, depending on the need for follow-up, also discuss their spider web results with, for example, a dietician, midwife, remedial therapist or physiotherapist. Patients are indicating that they like the fact that care providers all speak the same 'language'. For instance, when at the dietician, patients can elaborate on the Positive Health theme of lifestyle and nutrition. Here, two examples are described to illustrate that also these other care professionals, the people rather than their complaints form the central element. Positive Health can be applied broadly in many disciplines. Physiotherapists, for example, are reporting surprising results and increased job satisfaction when using the Positive Health concept, as is also shown in the example below.

> **Example from a physiotherapy practice: 'This is why I work with Positive Health'**
>
> Frederik Jaspers Faijer, of the De Haere practice in the Dutch town of Hellendoorn, has been working as a physiotherapist for 21 years.
> 'When you have just started out in your profession, your main focus is on people's physical complaints. Over the years, as your experience grows, you gradually become more intensely aware of the essence of your profession: this is why I am doing this. You begin to see the person behind the injured elbow – a human being who, for example, wants to be able to do his job, hug his partner and feed his children.'
> Since he attended a lecture by Machteld Huber on Positive Health, Frederik has been more successfully able to define what his practice is really about. Positive Health gave him the tools to conduct the *alternative dialogue*.
> He also believes that working together with other care providers is important, for example, when patients are young and overweight, or people who have medically unexplained physical symptoms (MUPS) or are suffering from chronic pain, as well as in caring for the elderly. Older people who are still living independently at home, and schoolchildren who are developing their motor skills. 'If we fail to do the right thing for them when they are young, they may well become chronically ill later on in their lives. This requires commitment from all those involved, such as the school, the municipality and us physiotherapists. The language used in the spider web helps us to understand each other better.'
> Frederik's tip:
> 'Stay true to yourself. Don't start working with Positive Health if it doesn't suit you. The method requires you to really engage in a conversation, and that you are sincere

in your intentions. It is not a clever trick. Because, if you are insincere, you can be sure that patients will see right through you.'
Source: iPH Newsletter (2019c)

Positive Health is also very suitable for remedial therapists. They often describe how it fits in very well with their way of working, as they already look at what people are still able to do. A quote of a remedial therapist from the Positive Health training: 'Positive Health can be an eye opener for all medical professionals so that they learn to look at things in the way remedial and occupational therapists do. It helps to see the total picture, the human being as a whole.'

Practical example of Positive Health at the remedial therapist

'Customised care is listening and watching intently, daring to let go of protocols and starting from what is needed.' By doing so, Estelle Schatorié, a remedial therapist from North Limburg, was able to make a young woman dance again after a cervical spine fracture. The woman was not cured as by a miracle, but she became motivated by the therapist who connected to the things she really valued. Estelle works according to the principles of Positive Health, just as the general practitioners and other care providers in her region. Together with her patients, she sets valuable treatment goals. Sometimes, patients have spent years battling physical complaints. These patients, some of whom have lost the courage to carry on, are referred to her by the general practitioners. As a remedial therapist, she listens intently to her patients and observes their body language. Therapy is nothing more than a tool to achieve a goal. It is about the patient regaining control.

Positive Health is thinking in possibilities rather than in limitations. How that can work out is illustrated by the story of Laila. When she was 21, Laila fractured a cervical vertebra and went into a coma. When she woke up, she was paralysed on one side of her body. The rehabilitation centre said she was not motivated to get better. Estelle: 'Before we started the first treatment session, we went to the ballet hall together where she used to dance.' Estelle noticed how hopeless and afraid of her future the girl seemed. That is something quite different from being insufficiently motivated! She asked Laila: 'Suppose that you wake up tomorrow and a miracle has happened, the unimaginable, what would that miracle be?' For Laila, this was being able to both dance and study again. Then, when Estelle put on some music, something miraculous did happen. Because of the rhythm of the music and by mirroring the movements of Estelle, Laila started to crawl. Something she had not been able to do before.

Even walking, which Laila had relearned in rehabilitation, was more successful. She had less focus on her disability, but was looking ahead towards her goal. That is the whole point – it is all about the possibilities that people are able to see for themselves. The final result, in this case, was that Laila returned to dancing again. She shines in her own dance performance, 'Catching Dreams', has graduated from university and is now also working. Estelle hopes to use the concept of Positive Health to provide even more customised care and to stimulate other people to change from focusing on their disease to looking at what they can do.

> A short film was made of Laila's rehabilitation process and the realisation of her dream. The Dutch film has English subtitles and can be accessed via the QR code at the end of this chapter.

The core value of 'together', thus, takes shape between various professionals around the care for individual patients. It can also be interpreted in a broader sense, more focused on the population as a whole, the local residents in the community in which a general practitioner works. Next, this handbook discusses the organisation of a broad cooperative network, for example in an integrated healthy community approach, with an outline of the role and added value of the general practitioner, in this regard.

7.6 Integrated cooperation within the community

Why is integrated cooperation within the community so useful to general practitioners? As described above, citizens' initiatives, informal care and social care offered by municipalities can be utilised even more effectively by general practitioners. They would also be more supported if there was a greater insight into which health topics occur most frequently amongst the local community. This could lead to a more efficient cooperation around themes such as loneliness, prevention and a healthy lifestyle, mental health care and vulnerable elderly people.

An article in the Dutch scientific journal for general practitioners, 'Huisarts & Wetenschap' explains the importance of community-oriented primary care. Using a community health profile, demographic data on community level are linked to data on lifestyle and health. In this way, health care can be addressed in a more targeted manner, which is becoming important for general practitioners. The great diversity in general practitioners in the Netherlands, both with respect to how their practices are organised and what their personal areas of interest are, means that various roles are possible and needs may differ.

Representatives from a local general practice who participate in a community-oriented approach can provide the general practitioner with more insight into the most important health themes of that community (based on the community health profile), supplemented by data from the electronic health records (EHRs). This then leads to the question of whether the general practitioner and other parties involved in the community recognise the resulting picture. From a shared vision about the community, the type of care offered can be customised to suit the local population. For this purpose, local initiatives are developed to outline what is needed and to formulate suitable health services. It is important that integrated services are designed in consultation with all stakeholders, in order to prevent the municipality or the Municipal Health Services (GGD) from offering health services that do not meet the needs of local citizens and professionals. For this reason, most municipalities attach great importance to the cooperation with general practitioners and other community stakeholders, in shaping an integrated community health approach. Subsequently, agreements can be made about population-oriented activities or about a more efficient cooperation focused on individual people. For general practitioners, it may be useful to get to know other professionals in the community and to know which other local services are available.

There are various possible roles for general practitioners in such integrated community cooperation. One may be actively involved as a representative of a general practice, health centre or care group, while another may only want to be kept informed. Active involvement may also include participation in healthy community meetings or taking on a leading role in the organisation.

Reflection

- *What were your answers to the reflection questions at the beginning of this chapter?*
- *Are there arrangements about cooperation within your municipality, village or local community?*
- *Has a joint agenda been drawn up? Are the frequently occurring health topics known?*
- *Are mutual expectations and common goals sufficiently clear?*
- *As a general practitioner, do you inform the municipality if you would like to address topics related to local public health policy?*
- *Is your team aware of the locally available welfare, care and support services, and where those can be found?*
- *Would you like to be actively involved in establishing such local public health policy?*

There are various methods for arriving at an integrated approach to public health within the community. The ABCD method has already been briefly addressed in relation to community strength (see ▶ sect. 7.3), a procedural method for a community approach. Two other examples are given below:

- Community-based prevention
- Improving community health via Positive Health

7.6.1 Community-based prevention

The Community Prevention programme is intended to optimise cooperation between primary care, welfare and prevention, to raise the level of health of the local inhabitants. The focus is on the local residents' own control over their health. It is a programme that was commissioned by the Dutch Ministry of Health, Welfare and Sport and was implemented by the Dutch National Institute for Public Health and the Environment (RIVM) and the Dutch College of General Practitioners (NHG). The methodology used in the healthy community approach, however, has been around for some time (Leemrijse et al., 2017). In the Dutch community Leidsche Rijn (Utrecht), this approach was organised through a community health coordinator (see text box).

Cooperation on health in the community can be facilitated by a work session from the Community Prevention programme. A toolkit is available for this purpose that can be used by everyone, at no cost (RIVM, 2018a). The programme took place in 20 different communities throughout the Netherlands, over the 2016–2018 period, involving 400 local professionals within the fields of prevention, health care and welfare (◻ fig. 6.8).

Health in the community

Health in the community is designed with cooperating partners from various disciplines. It can be applied in all settings, both rural and urban, in small villages or local communities with multiple problems. The villages or communities in which integrated cooperation is applied, all have their own local colour. The professionals involved will organise the cooperation together with and to the benefit of local residents.

◘ Figure 7.8 illustrates the steps in the cyclical process of cooperation. The script in the toolkit for a local work session about cooperation on health in the community is easy to organise, but there is also an NHG training course on the subject (NHG, 2018). It focuses on:

- view of the community;
- view of the network;
- jointly choosing priorities around health and prevention;
- making the proper arrangements to achieve good community-oriented goals;
- establishing a cooperative network (which is the next step).

Preconditions for organising integrated cooperation within the community:

- a local stakeholder who takes the lead in creating the cooperation and monitors the follow-up;
- agreements about process responsibility within the community;
- timely involvement of local residents and sufficient support amongst the professionals involved;
- sufficient financial means.

Drafting a cooperation agenda between health insurance companies and municipalities on prominent subjects, such as cooperation within the community and prevention, has proven to be important. It is also important that there is funding available to prevent initiatives from being financed as a pilot project, without structural funding for whatever comes next.

The added value of cooperation on health within the community under the Community Prevention programme is discussed in an e-magazine (RIVM, 2018b). The main lessons and benefits are:

- People meeting each other within a network environment is important.
- General practitioners were often surprised at the amount of care services available within their community.
- Having insight into the health situation in the community and being more aware of the importance of working together on prevention make arrangements within the network self-evident and desirable.
- Practice nurses and practice assistants are an indispensable link when it comes to both cooperation within the community and lifestyle coaching.
- The cooperation on health in the community has been given a clear impulse by the work sessions, which will continue to have an effect six months later.
- A start has been made on a joint approach and arrangements for cooperation.

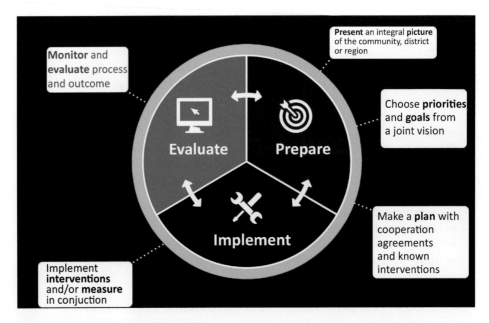

Figure 7.8 Getting started (Toolkit cooperation on health in the community (RIVM 2018a))

- Participants can see differences in pace, language and culture, with respect to health care and welfare.
- The principles of Positive Health and the resulting common language are beneficial for the cooperation.

General practitioners indicate that the most important reasons for participating in the Community Prevention programme is the better quality care they are able to offer their patients as well as the time-saving aspect, as it makes it easier to treat or refer patients.

Below, a list of other benefits, as experienced by general practitioners:

- *'Some patients require a different type of care than the one I'm able to offer them in my consulting room.'*
- *'Effective cooperation within the community saves me time. Patients can be treated or referred more efficiently.'*
- *'I can clearly see that many of the patients' questions transcend the general practice. Finding better solutions for those patients requires cooperation with other care providers.'*
- *'After having done the work session, general practitioners will tend to look for non-medical solutions earlier than they would have done before.'*
- *'Because of the work session, when I'm seeing patients, I now have a greater focus on physical exercise and nutrition. It's back on the agenda, and I also talked to colleagues about it right away.'*
- *'I have learned a lot, not only about the supporting services offered by the social community team and youth team, but also about what schools and street workers can do.'*

Example: Healthy community alliance Leidsche Rijn – Vleuten–De Meern

In Leidsche Rijn and Vleuten-De Meern (communities in the Province of Utrecht), where author Karolien van de Brekel-Dijkstra works in one of Julius Health Centers (LRJG) five health centres (▶ www.lrjg.nl), an integrated community approach is already being applied for years. The healthy community alliance between Leidsche Rijn and Vleuten–De Meern was set up with 14 health care and welfare providers, in cooperation with the municipality and residents' platforms (Van den Brekel, 2015). The cooperative network is based on the principles of the Positive Health concept. Meanwhile, meetings are being organised in all districts in the Dutch city of Utrecht, themed 'from community data to community effort' (van wijkdata naar wijkdoen). On the basis of data from the public health monitor of the municipality and data from the electronic health records (EHR), the main health themes of the community are formulated and primary issues are selected. In Leidsche Rijn, the themes are youth problems and social isolation. In addition, many care professionals in the cooperative network followed a training course about conducting an *alternative dialogue* according to the Positive Health concept (Oude Weernink, 2020). This has achieved a greater understanding of each other's working methods, the staff of the various health care and welfare organisations have gotten to know each other better, and cooperation is more easily accessible.

7.6.2 Improving community health via Positive Health

— Integrated cooperation on public health is often organised from the perspective of creating or maintaining a healthy local environment. Positive Health is a good foundation from which to organise this environment. A healthy community approach in a district in Amsterdam (*Zuidoost*) was organised from 2016 to 2019, in cooperation with the Louis Bolk Institute, which was evaluated using the integral model for Positive Health and environment concept as the guiding principle.

Seven steps of community-oriented solutions

The following seven steps will improve the chances of success for community-oriented solutions that are set up together with local residents and other stakeholders (Wietmarschen et al., 2019):

1. Involve local residents from the very beginning.
2. Ensure there is a multidisciplinary project team of active participants.
3. Talk with local residents; interview them.
4. Identify any shared interests.
5. Organise research to the benefit of local residents.
6. Use various media to communicate about the project.
7. Utilise the strong points of local residents and ensure that activities never depend on one person.

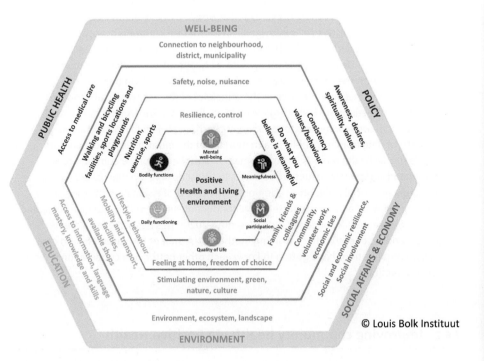

**Integrated model for
Positive Health and Environment**

◻ **Figure 7.9**   Integral model for Positive Health and environment (Louis Bolk Institute), source:
Van Wietmarschen 2019a)

In a local community in Amsterdam (Venserpolder), the physical environment was
reorganised on the basis of the dimensions of Positive Health. Local residents were
in charge and their interests came first, and a guidance document was published on
this subject. ◻ Figure 7.9 illustrates how such a process could be organised in practice,
based on the experiences in the Venserpolder community. An innovative and challenging part of the project was to investigate the concept of Positive Health on four themes
amongst citizens with a multi-ethnic background. In addition, organising the physical
environment according to the Positive Health concept, using the model in ◻ fig. 7.10,
had never been done before. In Limburg, the physical environment is also the central element around which Positive Health is organised within the community (Hesdahl et al., 2018). In Venserpolder, the main focus was on the needs of local residents,
whereas in Limburg the focus was more on policy. Both examples show how many
starting points there are for people to work in their own environment on promoting
everyone's unique health needs.

More and more initiatives are being developed around Positive Health and the
physical environment. In this way, when organising the layout of a community, such as
on the Dutch island of Texel (see ▶ sect. 7.4) or an urban village, the architecture can
be in line with how the Positive Health concept is being implemented within the local

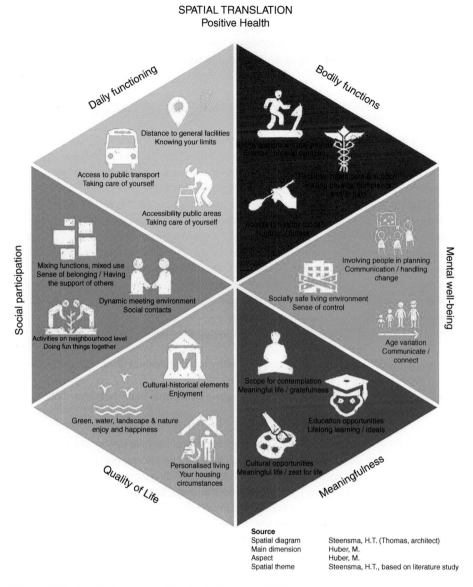

SPATIAL TRANSLATION
Positive Health

Source

Spatial diagram	Steensma, H.T. (Thomas, architect)
Main dimension	Huber, M.
Aspect	Huber, M.
Spatial theme	Steensma, H.T., based on literature study

Figure 7.10 Architecture and Positive Health (Steensma 2020)

community. Buildings can connect the physical environment to the social environment, creating a valuable living environment that meets the needs of local residents. As a result, the residents' well-being, health and overall quality of life will be greater (Ontroerend goed 2020).

General practitioners are not the only ones working with health within a community. For example, community initiatives may actively involve local residents in the reorganisation of the physical environment or the care and welfare around residents in such a way that they have a greater say in what happens. It pays off to pursue a type of cooperation based on these broad perspectives. Also in cases where you are, for example, starting or redesigning a new practice or a new health centre. It is then a good idea to always consider the broad perspective on health, which will provide insight into the social challenges and shed a light on where any support from general practitioners is needed.

Example Architectureand Positive Health

What is the relationship between Positive Health and architecture?
Architect Thomas Steensma investigated what impact the Positive Health concept could have on the way urban villages are designed. The six dimensions of Positive Health proved to be a useful instrument. Also useful for those who plan to start or redesign a new practice or health centre. Steensma noticed that architects are experienced in designing buildings with a medical function. However, he had not designed a building from the perspective of Positive Health before. 'The relationship with the community is much larger than we realise, after all it's about people's living environment.' That also applies to a general medical practice which, after all, is generally somewhere within its patients' environment. Steensma translated the spider web into spatial themes. He did so on the basis of a literature study. Instructions are given for each pillar in his spatial translation.

- *Daily functioning*: accessibility by public transport and walking distance to basic facilities are important.
- *Quality of life*: for example, access to healthy food and characteristic buildings that relate to people's personal history.
- *Social interaction*: having meeting places and being able to undertake activities together within the community.

Steensma then applied the colours of the spider web of Positive Health to a map of the centre of the Dutch city of Delfzijl, which he based on information provided by local residents about the locations of characteristic buildings, greenery and access to primary care. By doing so, he aligned himself with the basic principle of Positive Health that people's experience is the most important element. He went out into the community to interview people on the street.
It turned out that there were not many places where people could meet in an accessible way. They were no areas where they could grow their own healthy food. And the harbour – which was so very characteristic of the city – appeared difficult to access for certain inhabitants, because of a number of steps that needed to be navigated and a busy road that they would have to cross. On the basis of these findings, he defined a spatial development plan for the city and made certain changes to the harbour area. The dimensions of Positive Health were paramount to his plan and he incorporated the wishes of the local residents into his design. The local government authorities of Delfzijl thought Steensma's approach was an eye-opener, and they could see many opportunities for applying Positive Health in an integrated way, in both the physical and social domains.

> **Tips**
>
> For general practitioners who are looking to design or redesign a medical practice:
>
> - Postpone thinking about the design, for as long as possible. This prevents you from rushing into solutions. Perhaps the spatial spider web will lead you into another direction or change the emphasis you first had in mind.
> - Involve residents in the design or redesign of the medical practice by filling out the spatial spider web with them and discuss the results together. Their experience is paramount, because it is about the impact that the environment has on their health. This will tell you much about what they are thinking and participating in the process will also make them very enthusiastic. You will hear a lot about what is going on. And it generates a great deal of enthusiasm.
> - Use a scale model instead of a floor plan, which is often too abstract and one-dimensional for people to imagine the 'real thing'. In a scale model you can move objects, greenery or buildings around.
> - Use the integrated aspect: invite all your key actors to the table. Preferably at the same time, in order to have a good conversation. This provides valuable input for the designer or architect.
> - Call on the representatives of the community to provide you with information. Or hold a central meeting or street interviews.
> - Take the time to report your findings back to everyone involved, including the local residents.
>
> **Like to read more? (iPH,** 2019c)

In addition to the integrated cooperative networks that are being set up in many places in the Netherlands, there are already more medical science networks, as described in ► sect. 7.5. Such networks can be organised around an individual patient from a specific target group, for instance the elderly, people suffering from dementia or Parkinson's disease. This may also involve an increased use of technology, in the search for the right type of care in the right place. In addition to network care around a patient, there are also networks of care professionals within the community who, for example, are all working on the basis of the Positive Health concept. Positive Health is the common language and vision, with a broad perspective on health. Many networks based on Positive Health work on a regional level. This is further discussed in ► Chap. 8.

7.7　Prevention and lifestyle in the community

Chapter 5 describes the core task of '*preventive care*' in relation to Positive Health and the individual patient. In the recently published elaboration of the core tasks (► www.toekomsthuisartsenzorg.nl (only available in Dutch)), a more specific explanation was given, namely that *general practitioners limit themselves to indicated and care-related prevention* (for people who are at risk of developing or already have a chronic disease). In principle, they bear *no responsibility* for population-oriented prevention (universal and selective prevention). An exception is the role of general practitioners in medical-preventive care arising from national prevention programmes (such as flu vaccinations or follow-up care related to breast cancer screening). The reason for this exception is that the contribution of general practitioners in these areas provides added value, as they know the circumstances of their patients the best (follow-up screening) or because the primary care offered by general practitioners is to most effective and efficient and the turnout is likely to be higher than when organised by public health officials (i.e., in the case of vaccinations). Municipalities and government authorities are mainly responsible for universal and selective prevention. However, public prevention takes place on the interface between the municipal and medical domains. Here, again, cooperation is important, and is being organised from within the local community and people's own physical environment.

The starting point for determining the preventive care offered by general practitioners is the contact with the patient in the consulting room. The most important task of general practitioners is to *identify* and *openly discuss* the possibilities of prevention. This can all be done on the basis of Positive Health. Any follow-up steps may either be within or outside the general practice. For people who are at risk of or already have a chronic disease, the practice nurse can offer lifestyle coaching or counselling to help people quit a smoking habit. They may refer people to GPinfo.nl, for lifestyle advice, dieticians, physiotherapists, *combined lifestyle intervention* (CLI) or, for example, initiatives such as the *walking challenge for diabetes* or the *reverse diabetes programme* (▶ www.keerdiabetesom.nl). Some general practices choose to offer a supplementary type of service by inviting specific target groups to the practice themselves, on a regular basis.

In addition, various health and lifestyle programmes, fitness tests and health checks are sometimes available organised by the municipality in cooperation with community sports coaches. With regard to lifestyle, physical exercise is a low-threshold option that can easily be applied in the community. In general, people are all able to walk or cycle by themselves, they can be encouraged to do so by providing them with a pedometer and they can be referred to all kinds of formal and informal walking clubs. It is important, as general practitioner, to know where such sports-related information can be obtained – usually via municipal sport services and community sports coaches. The *Diabetes Challenge* is being organised in more and more municipalities in the Netherlands (▶ www.nationalediabeteschallenge.nl). Every year, thousands of people in the Netherlands walk along with the National Diabetes Challenge. It is intended for people with or at risk of type 2 diabetes and anyone who wants to walk with them.

The preparation for the national challenge covers 16 to 20 weeks, where people are encouraged to structurally increase their level of exercise, in cooperation with professionals working in the care, sports and municipal domains. Often, at least one group walk per week is offered, organised by the local general practice or other central community organisation. Practice staff, volunteers and walking coaches take turns in participating in those walks. In addition to walking together as a group, once a week, participants also walk independently at least once a week and try to get to 5,000 or even 10,000 steps per day. Participants work towards the National Diabetes Challenge, which is a four-day walk, with all participants walking together from one central location on the final day. This final day is organised by the Bas van de Goor Foundation. Research shows that this helps people to feel fitter and their quality of life improves. The social aspect of walking together also appears to be highly appreciated (National Diabetes Challenge 2019). There is also active walking in nature, for example, in the form of biowalking (see text box).

Case no. 20 Biowalking and diabetes

Biowalking is walking in nature for people with a chronic disease or impairment, under guidance of a nature guide and general practice assistant. A biowalk takes about two hours. Participants start by walking for half an hour to improve their physical condition. After that, the nature guide shown the various natural and landscape elements along the way. Participants can rely on the practice assistant for any questions about their health. And blood sugar levels are measured before and after the biowalk. In this way, participants are able to immediately see the effect of the physical exercise on their body. The biowalk ends with an informal talk afterwards.

In 2015, Fred went to see his general practitioner. Fred (then 63) had become unwell. His blood pressure and blood sugar levels were found to be dangerously high. Medication was used to bring down his blood pressure, and, to lower his blood sugar levels, the practice assistant suggested he would follow the biowalk programme organised by the general practice.

The practice assistant explained: 'We can measure the effect of exercise on blood sugar levels with great precision. Before every walk, we will measure your blood sugar by piercing the tip of your finger to draw a little blood. And we do this again after the walk. This shows participants the beneficial effect of exercise.' This visible effect motivated Fred to take charge of his health.

But biowalking does more than that. Walking with like-minded people in a relaxing environment makes it easier to talk about living with diabetes. Exchanging experiences also helps to put things into perspective. And the effects can be long-lasting. Fred has stopped smoking and drinking, for years now. He feels fit, has lost weight, his blood pressure has gone down and his blood sugar level has become normal without him having to take medication for it. Fred walks an hour every morning in the beautiful national park De Maasduinen (Planet Health 2019).

7.7.1 Combined lifestyle intervention (CLI)

In the Netherlands, there are several accredited combined lifestyle intervention (CLI) programmes, with group meeting ever week for an initial period of six months, followed by community care offered over another 18-month period. The aim is to achieve sustainable behavioural change. At the time of publication of this handbook, there were three recognised interventions in the Netherlands: *Slimmer, Beweegkuur* and *Cool*, with contracts organised by the health care groups. There is national debate about who should organise CLI programmes, which has so far not resulted in a final decision. It is important that insurance companies know which GLI programme is available per region, and for general practitioners to be able to refer patients to participate in such CLI programmes. The combined lifestyle intervention (CLI) 'HealthyLIFE' is a good example of a joint lifestyle project based on Positive Health that is financed by both the province, the municipality and general practitioners (see text box).

HealthyLIFE

HealthyLIFE is a programme for adults with the aim of promoting an active lifestyle and a healthy diet. The programme is available in various municipalities in Limburg. By 2020, 850 people had already started, with half of them having been referred by their general practitioner and practice assistants. The effects of HealthyLIFE are being investigated by the Ecsplore Foundation, in cooperation with Maastricht University and Fontys Sports University.

Positive Health is at the centre of the whole programme. Participant fill out the Positive Health questionnaire three times and the results are discussed on the basis of the spider web. Project manager Jorn van Harwegen den Breems: 'Positive Health gives a much broader picture of the participants. Personal motives come to the surface during conversations. The lifestyle coaches see great added value in the application of Positive Health to find elements that may be used to achieve behavioural change.' Based on the positive experiences, so far, the programme will be extended from 32 weeks to 24 months and from a single focus on physical exercise to attention for all the dimensions of Positive Health.

► healthylife.ecsplore.nl

Current lifestyle advice is briefly discussed in ► Chap. 5 and can be extensively studied from the practice guide on cooperation related to health within the community (Samenwerkenaangezondheid in de wijk), the NHG lifestyle module ('*Leefstijl*') about alcohol, exercise, smoking and nutrition (NHG, 2015) and the handbook on lifestyle medical science (Handboek leefstijlgeneeskunde) (De Vries and De Weijer, 2020).

Lifestyle advice is an important part of general medical care. In a recent study for a congress organised by 'Arts enLeefstijl' in 2020, half of the attending general practitioners appeared unfamiliar with the NHG lifestyle module (see ► Chap. 5), and only about one sixth of them were actually using the module. It also appeared that about a third of general practitioners and practice assistants were not charging for lifestyle consultations.

Coming back to the reflection questions at the beginning of Chap. 7

What are your insights after reading this chapter?
What had you written down and considered at the beginning of the chapter?
How could Positive Health contribute, in the context of community cooperation, promotion of health and offering appropriate care services for your patients?

The Positive Health philosophy turns out to be very applicable in a community setting. On the one hand, from a shared vision and language, and on the other, for stimulating people's level of self-reliance and self-management and the design of community cooperation and citizen networks. ► Chapter 8 describes how Positive Health could be applied on regional and national levels and how it could be included in medical education.

7.8 Conclusions

Taking health as a starting point, with people and the local community in central position, what does this mean for the roles and tasks in primary care? What is important for people to be able to live together in a healthy way in their community? With Positive Health as a common language, local residents appear to be taking more control of their community. Informal care, citizens' initiatives and other community and prevention initiatives can be of greater significance for general practitioners than is currently recognised. Although care providers are used to look for medical solutions, many health care questions do require a broader answer. There are many possibilities for patients to take better care of their own health on the one hand, while making use of social and lifestyle services in the community, on the other. Integrated cooperation in local communities is crucial, in this respect. Knowledge of community networks that relate to the health care questions of their patients may support general practitioners. It is not without reason that the new core value of 'together' and core task of 'care coordination' have been added to the core values and core tasks of primary care.

Appendix 7.1

Definitions and explanations

Informal care
    The people closest to patients are, in first instance, their family, friends, neighbours and volunteers. Informal care is defined by the three pillars of fellow sufferers, informal caregivers and voluntary caregivers. Citizens' initiatives, citizen participation and self-reliance are organised in close proximity to and around local residents (Struijs, 2006) (see the text box in Chap. 7).

Citizens' initiatives
Citizens' initiatives are set up by one or more citizens without obligation, for the benefit of others or society as a whole (Rijksoverheid 2010)

Community strength
Community strength is the positive energy that is released when people help each other to achieve an increasing number of goals by sharing their resources. For more information, see the brochure on community strength ('*Samen recht doen aan gemeenschapskracht*' (Van der Aa 2018)).

Municipality
A municipality is a group of residential areas (i.e., villages, cities) that are jointly governed by a political administration. In most countries, municipalities are the smallest administrative unit of the political administration structure. In the Netherlands, the layers above the municipal level are that of provinces and the national government.

Municipalities play an increasingly important role in local health care and support for citizens, which means that general practitioners and municipalities are in frequent contact and need to work together.

Well-being and welfare
Under the current Dutch health care system, a distinction is made between health care and well-being/welfare. Health care encompasses the totality of activities aimed at improving public health within the country. In everyday life, the term *well-being* primarily refers to the wide range of health-related aspects. From the perspective of the social domain, the term *welfare* refers to the organisations that support participation and sense of purpose within local communities.

Social domain
The social domain includes all municipal efforts in the areas of employment, participation, self-reliance, health care and youth, based on the Social Support Act (Wmo) 2015, the Participation Act, Youth Act and the Municipal Debt Counselling Act.

Community Health Services (GGD)
The Community Health Services (GGD) of the Netherlands protect, monitor and promote the health of Dutch citizens. This is also referred to as public health care. The GGD departments have a number of legal tasks, described in the Public Health Act. These tasks include youth health care (child health centres and school doctors), medical environmental science, combating infectious diseases, population screening and health education. In addition to the statutory tasks, each GGD also carries out supplementary tasks for the municipality, described in the municipal policy documents on local health care policy.

District nursing
District nurses can be seen as a link between the medical and social domains. It is the ambition of many of their clients to remain living at home, as independently and long as possible. This means more care being provided by, amongst others, the general practitioner, district nurse and informal caregivers.

Medical domain
The medical domain refers to the care provided by integrated primary care (e.g., general practitioners and paramedics) and secondary care (i.e., specialist care). This concerns all treatments that are reimbursed from the Dutch Health Insurance Act (Zvw).

Geographic demarcation: region, district, rural village, urban village, neighbourhood
Regions cover at least 100,000 inhabitants. District/community health refers to a scale of about 10,000 to 15,000 inhabitants. This could be, for example, several villages together, or a district/city area that usually consists of a number of neighbourhoods.

For more background information on cooperation within the community, there is a Dutch e-magazine available: ▶ https://tinyurl.com/samenwerken-aan-gezondheid. Furthermore, there is also a digital NHG refresher course on health-related cooperation within communities, a free e-learning environment about prevention, with inspiring examples and videos about lifestyle coaching and how to organise cooperation on health in the community.

For more information, background or videos about this chapter scan the QR code.

SCAN ME

References

Beter oud (2019). *Kwetsbare ouderen thuis handreiking voor integrale zorg en ondersteuning in de wijk.* Accessed in in oktober 2020 van ▶ https://www.beteroud.nl/beteroud/media/documents/handreiking-kwetsbare-ouderen-thuis-mei-2019_2.pdf.

Bruijn, D. (2016). *Wat knelt. Knelpunten bij burgerinitiatieven in zorg en ondersteuning.* Accessed in October 2020 of ▶ https://www.movisie.nl/publicatie/wat-knelt-knelpunten-burgerinitiatiev-en-zorg-ondersteuning.

Burgerkrachtlimburg (2020). *Impactmeting workshops Positieve Gezondheid en IK Positief Gezond.* Accessed in October 2020 of ▶ https://www.burgerkrachtlimburg.nl/nieuws/workshop-positieve-gezondheid-en-ik-positief-gezond/.

Drenthen, T. (2020). *Samenwerken aan gezondheid in de wijk loont, e-magazine.* Accessed in October 2020 of ▶ https://www.nhg.org/preventieindebuurt.

Federatie medisch specialisten (2015). *Visiedocument Medisch Specialist 2025.* Accessed in October 2020 of ▶ https://www.demedischspecialist.nl/sites/default/files/Visiedocument%20Medisch%20Specialist%202025-DEF.pdf.

Gemeente Utrecht (2019). *Nota Gezondheid voor iedereen, gezondheidsbeleid Utrecht 2019–2023.* Accessed in October 2020 of ▶ https://omgevingsvisie.utrecht.nl/fileadmin/uploads/documenten/zz-omgevingsvisie/thematisch-beleid/gezondheid/2019-10-nota-gezondheid-voor-iedereen-volksgezondheidsbeleid-2019-2023.pdf.

Guldemond, N. (2015). Accessed in October 2020 of ▶ http://intelligence.agconnect.nl/content/het-iot-de-zorgsector.

Heijmans, M., Waverijn, G., Van Houtum, L. (2014). *Zelfmanagement, wat betekent het voor de patiënt?* Accessed in October 2020 of ▶ https://www.nivel.nl/nl/publicatie/gezondheidsvaardigheden-van-chronische-zieken-belangrijk-voor-zelfmanagement.

Heijnders, M.L., Meijs, J. J. (2015). *Welzijn op Recept. Bijblijven,* (31), 926–934 and ▶ https://welzijnoprecept.nl/publicaties/.

Hesdahl, B. (2018). Positieve Gezondheid helpt de huisarts naar mens en omgeving te kijken. *Bijblijven, 35,* 39–48.

Ineen (2020). *De blik vooruit, veranderen kan alleen samen.* Accessed in October 2020 of ▶ https://ineen.nl/actueel/de-blik-vooruit-veranderen-kan-alleen-samen/.

iPH Institute for Positive Health (2019a). Accessed in October 2020 of ▶ https://iph.nl/staatssecretaris-paul-blokhuis-over-de-landelijke-nota-gezondheidsbeleid-2020-2024-met-positieve-gezondheid-kunnen-we-vraagstukken-in-onze-samenleving-in-een-ander-licht-bekijken/.

iPH Institute for Positive Health (2019b). *Samen werken aan Positieve Gezondheid*. Accessed in October 2020 of ► https://iph.nl/boek-samen-werken-aan-gezondheid/.

iPH Institute for Positive Health (2019c). Accessed in October 2020 of ► https://iph.nl/uit-de-fysiotherapie-praktijk-daarom-werk-ik-met-positieve-gezondheid/.

iPH Institute for Positive Health (2019d). *Positieve Gezondheid op de tekentafel van architecten*. Accessed in October 2020 of ► https://iph.nl/positieve-gezondheid-op-de-tekentafel-van-architecten/.

iPH Institute for Positive Health (2019e). *Positieve Gezondheid prominent in landelijke nota gezondheidsbeleid*. Accessed in in augustus 2020 van ► https://iph.nl/positieve-gezondheid-prominent-in-landelijke-nota-gezondheidsbeleid/.

iPH Institute for Positive Health (2019f). *Handreiking Positieve Gezondheid en ouderen*. Accessed in October 2020 of ► https://iph.nl/wp-content/uploads/2019/08/iph-def-versie-korte-handreiking-positieve-gezondheid-en-ouderen.pdf en ► https://iph.nl/hoe-je-positieve-gezondheid-kunt-inzetten-bij-ouderen/.

Iresearch (2018). *Positieve Gezondheid in Gemeentelijke beleidsnota*. Accessed in October 2020 of ► https://www.iresearch.nl/projecten/positief-gezonde-gemeenten-27-11-2018.

Jung, H. P. (2019a). Uitkomsten van het hanteren van Positieve Gezondheid in de praktijk. *Bijblijven, 35*, 26–35.

Jung, H. P. (2019b). Zinnige zorg dreigt utopie te worden. *Medisch Contact, 47*, 18–20.

Kaljouw, M., Van Vliet K., (2015). *Naar nieuwe zorg en zorgberoepen: de contouren. Commissie Innovatie Zorgberoepen en Opleidingen*. Accessed in October 2020 of ► https://docplayer.nl/329738-Naar-nieuwe-zorg-en-zorgberoepen-de-contouren.html.

Landelijke Huisartsen Vereniging (LHV) (2017a). *Meer tijd, welke oplossing past bij uw praktijk?* Accessed in October 2020 of van ► https://meertijdvoordepatient.lhv.nl/.

Landelijke Huisartsen Vereniging (LHV) (2017b). *Werkmap huisarts en gemeente, samenwerken in de wijk*. Accessed in October 2020 of ► https://www.lhv.nl/service/werkmap-huisarts-en-gemeente.

Leemrijse, C. et al. (2017). *Rapport Overvecht Gezond Krachtige basiszorg. Theoretische onderbouwing van de 'krachtige basiszorg' in de Utrechtse wijk Overvecht*. Accessed in October 2020 of ► https://nivel.nl/sites/default/files/bestanden/Rapport_Overvecht_gezond_NIVEL.pdf.

Loketgezondleven (2018). *Infographic gezonde wijk aanpak*. Accessed in October 2020 of ► https://www.loketgezondleven.nl/integraal-werken/gezonde-wijkaanpak/infographic-gezonde-wijkaanpak

Nederlands Huisartsen Genootschap (NHG) (2018). *Praktijkhandleiding samenwerking aan gezondheid in de wijk*. Accessed in October 2020 of ► https://www.nhg.org/sites/default/files/content/nhg_org/uploads/nhg-praktijkhandleiding_samenwerken_aan_gezondheid_in_de_wijk_web_1.pdf.

NHG (2020). *Dossier e-health*. Accessed in October 2020 of ► https://www.nhg.org/actueel/dossiers/dossier-e-health.

Oude Weernink, T. (2020). *Een persoonsgericht gesprek in de Huisartsenpraktijk – Een Haalbaarheidsstudie*. Accessed in October 2020 of ► www.lrjg.nl/nieuws/ander-gesprek.

Pharos (2020). *Handen ineen voor toegankelijke en betrouwbare e-health voor iedereen*. Accessed in October 2020 of ► https://www.pharos.nl/over-pharos/programmas-pharos/ehealth4all/.

Polder, J. J., et al. (2011). *De gezondheidsepidemie, waarom we gezonder en zieker worden*.

Rademakers, J. (2014). *Kennissynthese Gezondheidsvaardigheden, iet voor iedereen vanzelfsprekend*. Accessed in October 2020 of ► https://www.nivel.nl/sites/default/files/bestanden/Kennissynthese-Gezondheidsvaardigheden-2014.pdf.

Rijksoverheid.nl. (2018). *Nationaal Preventieakkoord*. Accessed in October 2020 of ► https://www.rijksoverheid.nl/documenten/convenanten/2018/11/23/nationaal-preventieakkoord.s

Rijksoverheid.nl (2020a). *Landelijke Nota Gezondheidsbeleid 2020-2024*. Accessed in October 2020 of ► https://www.rijksoverheid.nl/documenten/rapporten/2020/02/29/gezondheid-breed-op-de-agenda.

Rijksoverheid.nl (2020b). *Zorg goed voor jezelf*. Accessed in October 2020 of ► https://www.rijksoverheid.nl/onderwerpen/coronavirus-covid-19/documenten/publicaties/2020/07/15/poster-zorg-goed-voor-jezelf.

Rijksoverheid (2020c). *Werkboek help een burgerinitiatief*. Accessed in October 2020 of ► https://www.rijksoverheid.nl/documenten/brochures/2010/11/08/werkboek-help-een-burgerinitiatief.

Russell, C. (2020). *Cormac Russell over corona communities*. Accessed in October 2020 of ► https://www.wedoenhetsamen.nu/cormac-russell-over-corona-communities/.

Schers, H., De Maeseneer, J. et al. (2014). Wijkgerichte aanpak in de eerste lijn werkt. *Medisch Contact* 01-07-2014.

Smeets et al. (2019). *De IJslandse aanpak van middelengebruik onder jongeren Een verkenning van de wetenschappelijke literatuur*. Based on web: ► https://www.trimbos.nl/docs/30a578c4-0be7-4c6e-924d-9ce7b3b2d8c1.pdf.

Spoelman, W., Bonten, T., De Waal, M., et al. (2017).*Effect of an evidence-based website on healthcare usage: An interrupted time-series study*. ► https://bmjopen.bmj.com/content/6/11/e013166; BMJ Open. 2017. ► https://doi.org/10.1136/bmjopen-2016-013166corr1.

Struijs, A. J. (2006). *Informele zorg. Het aandeel van mantelzorgers en vrijwilligers in de langdurige zorg. Raad voor de Volksgezondheid en Zorg*. Accessed in October 2020 of ► https://cdn.atria.nl/epublications/2006/Informele_zorg.pdf.

Terluin, B. (2013). Weg met de poortwachter! *Huisarts en Wetenschap*, p. 127. Accessed in October 2020 of ► https://www.henw.org/artikelen/weg-met-de-poortwachter-0.

Texel samen beter (2020). Accessed in October 2020 of ► https://www.texelsamenbeter.nl/application/files/6515/3789/7886/texel-samen-beter_flyer_A4.pdf and ► https://www.zonmw.nl/nl/onderzoek-resultaten/geestelijke-gezondheid-ggz/programmas/project-detail/juiste-zorg-op-de-juiste-plek/programma-gezond-texel-2030/.

Van den Brekel-Dijkstra, K. (2015). Persoonlijke preventie in de wijk, een voorbeeld van implementatie in Leidsche Rijn. *Bijblijven, 31*(10), 877–888.

Van den Brekel-Dijkstra, K., Cornelissen, M., & Van der Jagt, L. (2020). De dokter gevloerd. Hoe voorkomen we burn-out bij huisartsen? *Huisarts en Wetenschap, 63*(7), 40–43. ► https://doi.org/10.1007/s12445-020-0765-8.

Van den Brekel-Dijkstra, K., & Van Rixtel, B. (2020). Positieve gezondheid. *Nurse Academy, 2*, 25–31. Accessed in October 2020 of ► https://iph.nl/publicatie-in-nurse-academy-over-positieve-gezondheid/.

Van den Muijsenberg, M., Schers, H., & Assendelft, P. (2018). Huisarts werkt in de toekomst wijkgericht. *Huisarts en Wetenschap*, 1–3.

Van der Aa, A., & De Jager, M. (2020). *Sociale basisinfrastructuur voor vitale en gezonde gemeenschappen*. Accessed in October 2020 of ► https://www.allesisgezondheid.nl/wp-content/uploads/2020/06/Sociale-basisinfrastructuur-online-def.pdf.

Van der Aa A., & Smelik J. (2018). *Dialoog gemeenschapskracht. Samen recht doen aan gemeenschapskracht*. Accessed in October 2020 of ► https://www.dialooggemeenschapskracht.nl/p/12/Gemeenschapskracht.

Van Gorp, J. (2019). *Publiekssamenvatting maatschappelijke business case sociaal makelen/welzijn op recept*. ► https://welzijnoprecept.nl/wp-content/uploads/2020/02/Publiekssamenvatting-maatschappelijke-Business-Case-sociaal-makelen-2019-def.pdf.

Van Tuyl, L., Batenburg, R., Keuper, J., Meurs, M., & Friele, R. (2020). *Toename gebruik e-health in de huisartsenpraktijk tijdens de coronapandemie. Organisatie van zorg op afstand in coronatijd*. Nivel.

Van Wietmarschen, H., & Staps. J. J. M. (2019a). *Positieve Gezondheid de wijk in!: Handleiding Integrale Wijkaanpak op basis van Positieve Gezondheid en Leefomgeving*. Brochure Accessed in October 2020 of ► https://iph.nl/wp-content/uploads/2019/11/positieve-gezondheid-de-wijk-in-web.pdf.

Van Wietmarschen, H., & Staps J. J. M. (2019b). *Positieve Gezondheid de wijk in!: Handleiding Integrale Wijkaanpak op basis van Positieve Gezondheid en Leefomgeving*. 6 p. *Brochure (klein)*.

Van Wijck, F. (2020). Paul blokhuis over welzijn op recept. Meer inzetten op collectieve preventie. *De Eerstelijns*, 37–39. Accessed in October 2020 of ► https://www.de-eerstelijns.nl/wp-content/uploads/2020/04/DEL_3_APRIL_2020-pag_36-39_Blokhuis-DEF.pdf.

Vissers, D. (2015). *Eindrapport welzijn op recept Delft. Pilot in twee huisartsenpraktijken in Delft 2013-2015*. Delft: Zorgorganisatie Eerste Lijn.

Welzijnoprecept.nl (2019). *Rapport quickscan welzijn op recept*. Opgehaald van het web in november 2020 van ► https://welzijnoprecept.nl/welzijn-op-recept-quickscan-2019/.

Wind, A., & Te Velde, B. (2019). *Kwetsbare ouderen thuis. Handreiking voor integrale zorg en ondersteuning in de wijk*. Accessed in October 2020 of.

Zelfregietool (2020). Based on web ► https://zelfregietool.nl/wp-content/uploads/2020/03/von-2010-Nutzen-der-Selbsthilfe-Wertgutachten-BayernZusa-.DKGKwh.pdf.

Zelfzorgondersteund (2019a). *Infographic samen gezonder worden*. Accessed in October 2020 of ► https://zelfzorgondersteund.nl/wp-content/uploads/Infographic-Samen-gezonder-worden.pdf.

Zelfzorgondersteund (2019b). *Infographic haal het gezondste uit jezelf*. Accessed in October 2020 of ► https://zelfzorgondersteund.nl/wp-content/uploads/Infographic-haal-het-gezondste-uit-jezelf.pdf.

Zorginstituut.nl (2016). *Innovatie Zorgberoepen & Opleidingen*. Nieuwe kijk op beroepen en opleidingen in zorg en welzijn.

Chapter 8

Macro
Regional /
national

Meso
District / community

Micro
Practice / organisation

Nano
Patient / citizen

I swear/promise to practise the art of medicine to the best of my ability for the benefit of my fellow man.
I will care for the sick, promote health and relieve suffering.

I will put the patient's interests first and respect his/her views. I will do no harm to the patient. I will listen and inform him/her well. I will keep secret what has been entrusted to me.

I will advance the medical knowledge of myself and others. I will recognise the limits of my possibilities.

Positive health from a broader perspective

© Bohn Stafleu van Loghum is an imprint of Springer Media B.V., part of Springer Nature 2022
M. Huber et al., *Handbook Positive Health in Primary Care*,
https://doi.org/10.1007/978-90-368-2729-4_8

> **Main messages**
> – Positive Health can be one of the answers to the current problems in the health care sector.
> – In the Netherlands, Positive Health has been laid down in national policy and is increasingly being implemented on local and regional levels. It is proving to be a universal philosophy that can also be applied internationally.
> – The Institute for Positive Health (iPH) can support professionals to implement Positive Health in policy, practice, research and education and to achieve a turning point in health care.
> – Certain preconditions are required with regard to cooperation, financing, substantiation and training to ensure the sustainable implementation of Positive Health.
> – In the Netherlands, there are other concepts with a similar broad perspective on health working with the same objective, as there appears to be a need for such broad concepts of health.
> – Positive Health will be included in the training of future health professionals.

The aim of this chapter is to look at Positive Health from a broader perspective. Part I of this handbook describes the future challenges in addressing universal health care problems around the world, the origins and development of Positive Health and how the concept may contribute to the transition from disease-oriented to health-oriented health care. Here, the future of primary care in the Netherlands serves as an example. Part II focuses on applying Positive Health in practice in the Netherlands. In the consulting room and in the general medical practice as an organisation, as well as in local communities, regions and nation-wide. Meanwhile, interest in the concept is also growing, internationally. A number of developments support the turning point in health care:
– Politics and national policy are paying more attention to prevention and a healthy lifestyle.
– There is a shift towards more regionalisation, network medicine and integrated cooperation.
– There is a new framework plan for medical training with, amongst other things, a focus on Positive Health.

In addition to the increasing examples of best practices in the Netherlands, with respect to the implementation of Positive Health, there are also great challenges in the shift from disease-oriented to health-oriented care. This chapter discusses the preconditions that are required to achieve this, as well as the bottlenecks to arrive at affordable health care systems (Christensen 2017). The development of sustainable economic models that allow preventive approaches in new concepts of health care is also embraced by the International Consortium for Personalised Medicine (ICPerMed 2020). Positive Health not only fits well with the international shift from one-size-fits-all to person-oriented health care (see ► Chap. 4), but also, and especially in the COVID-19 pandemic, we learned the importance of strengthening resilience and promoting health.

The challenges related to a true shift in health care are described below, based on the work of inspiring author Christensen on innovation, with a focus on the situation in the Netherlands. The Institute for Positive Health, Positive Health networks, regional care groups and national organisations contribute, each in their own way, to the further development of Positive Health.

This chapter will also briefly talk about other broad perspectives on health, describing their mutual differences and how they strengthen each other. Attention is also paid to research and the substantiation of Positive Health, as well as to the importance of including it in the medical training and education of future health professionals. In this way, physicians can advance the medical knowledge of themselves and others. The Institute for Positive Health is the catalyst, the driving force behind the movement of Positive Health in the Netherlands and its international expansion.

> **Reflection**
>
> Please take a moment to reflect on the challenges in your situation. Addresses the reader:-What are your challenges in health care?- Which comparable developments are taking place within your community, region or country?- What would be needed with regard to health-related transformations and how can Positive Health contribute to that? All this and more can be found in this chapter, starting with the challenges of the transformation in health care.

8.1 The challenges related to the turning point in health care

The Positive Health movement in the Netherlands is well on its way. However, a true turning point in health care, from a disease-oriented to a broad health-oriented perspective, requires more than that. The authors of this handbook became inspired by the book titled 'The Innovator's Prescription: A Disruptive Solution for Health Care', by Harvard Business School Professor Clayton Christensen, (Christensen 2017). In his book, he describes a disruptive solution for health care after analysing the health care problems in the United States.

This handbook was written in the middle of the COVID-19 crisis. A greater disruption cannot be imagined. What insights can be obtained from Christensen's theory of disruption? What insights have already been gained from the changes in working methods, as a result of the COVID-19 outbreak? What are the preconditions for a broader implementation of Positive Health in health care?

8.1.1 The Innovator's Prescription

In his book, Christensen describes what he considered to be the root of the health care problem: the business model of health care is based on the diseases of patients, rather than on their health – on chronic disease instead of chronic well-being. In addition, the reimbursement system ensures that health care providers do not provide the required amount of care, but rather as much care as possible. Health care is also organised in

such a way that empirical medical-analytical care is provided to all patient groups – despite the fact that it would be better to distinguish between patient groups. There are various needs and patient groups:
- those who benefit from a good medical analysis of their complaint (*solution shops*)
- those who mostly need simple protocol-based treatment (*value-adding processes*)
- those with chronic diseases who particularly are in need of person-oriented care (*facilitating networks*)

Christensen studied innovations in other areas of society and found that changes would all come about in a disruptive manner. Disruptive, because those changes had all drastically altered existing technology and entire economic markets, or even destroyed large organisations. Some examples of the developments and innovations studied by Christensen:
- Letter → telegraph → telephone → mobile device
- Slide rule → mainframe computer → desktop → notebook
- Shop → supermarket → shopping centre → web shop
- Carbon copy → copy shop → matrix printer → inkjet printer
- Stage play → movie theatre → video → DVD → online streaming
- Village musician → concert hall → turntable → CD player → portable media player → online music streaming
- Money under the matrass → local bank branch office → cash machine → online banking

These innovations led to accessible and affordable products. How could the related insights be applied to health care? How could health care be organised more efficiently, thus making it more affordable and accessible? Christensen argues that real changes in health care can only come about through disruptive innovation. In order for disruptions to occur, three conditions must be met:
- a technology needs to be available as a simple substitute for complex technology
- a business innovation model needs to be available
- a disruptive network needs to be available.

According to Christensen, the technology that would be most suitable for a particular disruption depends on the diagnostic process (e.g., telemedicine, point-of-care testing and ICT diagnostic programs and electronic health records). There are increasing opportunities for modernisation of primary care through digitisation and assisted self-care, also in the diagnostic process.

A disruptive business innovation model consists of the following elements:
- Substitution: general practitioners conducting the tasks of specialists
- Transfer of tasks: Practice assistants, district nurses and nursing assistants conducting the tasks of general practitioners
- Citizens conducting the tasks of nurses, nursing assistants, welfare workers

The third element requires a regional or district network of care providers, patients and citizens' initiatives that is prepared to invest in this substitution chain and is also capable of organising continuous, person-oriented care for chronic patients.

Christensen describes the focus and disruption of general medical practice, with a shift in the role of general practitioner away from that of gatekeeper. In the Netherlands, as described in Sects. 1.5 and 7.5, the role of gatekeeper is shifting more towards that of intermediary, liaison and coach. Relating this to the situation in Dutch primary care, leads to the following possibilities (see ◻ fig. 8.1):

1. Diagnostic and therapeutic procedures performed by general practitioners that were previously performed by medical specialists (substitution, solution shop). Billing the patient for the procedure could be appropriate here (*fee-for-service*).
2. Simple medical-analytical procedures (rules-based precision medicine, value-adding processes), which can also be performed by nursing assistants (e.g., in addition to unblocking ears, they could also do stitches, wound treatment, contraception and an STD surgery hour), and online and telephone queries that can be answered in a standardised manner increasingly often via e-health (e.g., patients sending photos) or by telephone. Payment for the requested treatment outcome is then most appropriate (*fee-for-outcome*).
3. Continual, person-oriented care for the chronically ill, provided by practice nurses in consultation with the general practitioner, with the practice being part of a health network of which these patients are also a member. The appropriate payment system is a fixed subscription amount per year for the patient's membership of the health network (facilitating networks) (*fee-for-membership*).

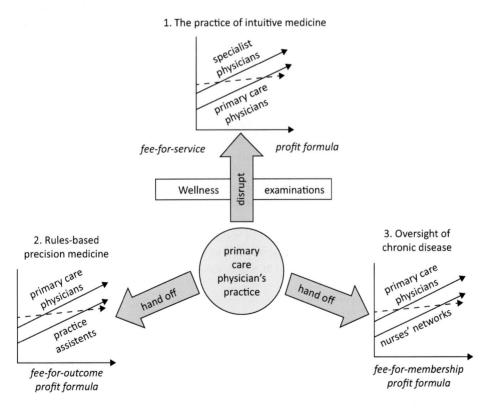

◻ **Figure 8.1**   Focus and disruption in the business models of primary care, based on (Christensen et al., 2017) and used with the consent of the publisher

In this way, general medical practices are able to create more time and attention for person-oriented care with the help of Positive Health. Sometimes, a medical diagnosis is still needed to demonstrate or exclude a disease. During consultations, general practitioners focus not only on disease but also and much more on health and meaningfulness. Based on shared decision-making, patients can be referred either to a hospital or specialist, or to other professionals or support from within the community. This is a form of customisation, for which a subscription fee (capitation) is appropriate, see ◘ fig. 8.1. One can think of projects in the context of more time for patients or a capitation system, with a fixed amount per patient, as was done in the practice in Afferden.

The theory of *The Innovator's Prescription* can be considered refreshing. It endorses the envisaged changes in future primary care, including substitution and a shift in tasks. New, in this respect, are the insights gained from the day-to-day practice of primary care, since the outbreak of COVID-19. This has been quite a disruption. On the one hand, cooperation was very efficient and effective within the teams, care groups and regional networks. Crisis appointments were made and policies were developed for helping people with or under suspicion of having the COVID-19 virus, in the safest possible way. On the other hand, usual care methods could not be applied in general medical practice and hospitals, and both patients and professionals were facing these types of changes. In the Netherlands, this situation meant that practices were set up with special respiratory surgery hours and there was more pressure on out-of-hours services following the outbreak of COVID-19. After a while, the pressure became somewhat less with health care questions often being dealt with by telephone, through patients sending electronic photos, or in video calls and e-consultations. Developments in e-health and innovations accelerated at an enormous pace. Where needed, more time for longer conversations between physicians and patients was created in an almost natural process. Most general practitioners experienced a sense of relief when this was happening. The newly developed forms of health care will continue to be offered also after the COVID-19 crisis has been dealt with. For patients, the new situation has meant initially more self-determination and seeking and offering support within their own network and local environment. People discovered that, for many complaints, a visit to their general practitioner was not really necessary if the practice provided good explanations and information, for example, by referring them to ▶ GPinfo.nl. There are also consequences related to conventional care processes having to be delayed, but, at the time of publication of this handbook, those were still insufficiently known.

In addition to the business model that is based on disease rather than health, Christensen describes what is wrong with medical training. In essence, the types of health care professionals who will be needed in the future are not being trained as such, today. This is further elaborated in ▶ Sect. 8.6.

Reflection

Which elements from Christensen's book do you recognise as having happened in your practice at the time of the COVID-19 crisis?
What are your own insights, what – if anything – have you learned in relation to COVID-19?
What, if any, are the new things you would like to maintain? Which would you abolish again? And are there things that are still missing?
What do you need?

What could be the impact of such a changing business model, as described in Christensen's book, on your situation and in your country? Turning points in health care are complex and prove to be difficult in practice. What does the transition from disease-oriented to health-oriented care mean for the way health care is currently financed? How complicated this can be is illustrated by an example of the general medical practice of Hans Peter Jung, one of the authors of this book. Jung wrote an article about this, titled 'catch-22', in the widely read Dutch medical journal *Medisch Contact*, describing how various interests can become too intertwined to disrupt. These catch-22 situations are a barrier to the implementation of changes in health care. Following the examples of such situations, a number of possibilities and current examples are elaborated with respect to financing the application of Positive Health in practice, in the Netherlands.

8.1.2 Sensible care is threatening to become a utopia – Catch-22

The general medical practice at Afferden is wedged in-between opposing demands.

> **Catch-22**
> The term catch-22 comes from the novel by the same name, written by US author Joseph Heller (1961) about bomber crews in World War II. It describes the following dilemma: People who fly their aircraft on incredibly dangerous missions must be crazy. But, if they are crazy, they would not be allowed to fly those aircraft. However, getting out of having to go on those missions by having themselves declared insane is considered a rational and sensible thing to do, ego not crazy... and by definition they would subsequently be considered fit to fly. 'If he flew them, he was crazy and didn't have to; but if he didn't want to, he was sane and had to'
> Catch-22 has become a widely used expression for a situation from which there appears to be no escape. The article 'Catch-22, Sensible care is threatening to become a utopia' published in the Dutch medical journal *Medisch Contact* (◻ fig. 8.2) clearly explains the intractability of innovation, in practice. In the Netherlands, innovations and reforms in health care are facing various interests within a complex financing system, such as in the case of agreements between health insurance companies and general practitioners. Certain catch-22 situations seem to stand in the way of the much-needed turning point in health care.

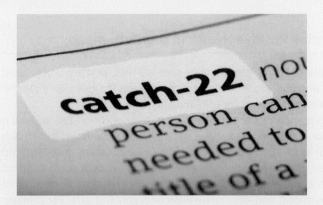

◻ **Figure 8.2**   Catch-22, sensible care is threatening to become a utopia (Jung et al. 2019)

More time for each patient

The fact that the workload in Dutch primary care has been increasing enormously, over the past decade, has already been extensively discussed in previous chapters. More time for each patient is also described in ▶ Chap. 3 and ▶ Sect. 6.5 and forms an important focal point for the Dutch National Association of General Practitioners (LHV). Together with health insurance company VGZ, the general medical practice in Afferden (of author Jung, see also ▶ Chap. 1) who has been pioneering by working in this way since 2015, reduced its number of patients per general practitioner FTE from 2,330 to 1,800. An additional 0.4 FTEs in general practitioner hours were implemented, for which VGZ has been footing the bill. Positive Health has become the starting point for the patient–physician relationship. As a result of these changes, the practice has been referring patients to hospital 25 % less often, the number of medical prescriptions has declined and patients say they are experiencing a higher quality of care. The level of job satisfaction of the general practitioners and other practice staff members also increased. Similar results were achieved in three other general medical practices in the same region. In 2017, the health care-related costs for the total practice population in Afferden were almost half a million euros lower than expected, and the local hospital narrowly escaped having to close down (Jung 2018).

The *right care in the right place* (in Dutch: Taskforce juiste zorg op Juiste plek (2019), *JZoJP: Juiste Zorg op de Juiste Plek*) – this sounds nice and there is widespread support for how important this is. The general medical practice in Afferden, however, shows how contradictory its effect can be: an insurance company finances a project so that the number of referrals to hospital will decrease, while also expecting that same hospital to increase its revenues.

There are plenty of arguments in favour of investing in *right care in the right place*, which ensures that people receive the appropriate care. This notion has been embraced by the Dutch Minister of Health and calls for a real transition in health care. Without the right stimulus, however, the *right care in the right place* will remain a utopia. This is shown, for example, in the search for the right format for this type of care, in the Catch-22 example above.

Following a description of the challenges of innovation, it is explained how Positive Health is able to contribute to reducing costs.

8.1.3 Financing Positive Health in the Netherlands

General practitioners who are changing the way their practice is organised will first face certain costs. If you would like to start working with Positive Health, in the Netherlands, there are several possibilities for obtaining financial support:

— *From innovation projects to embedding in regular care.* Most general medical practices or care groups that have started working with Positive Health received funding for innovation from a health insurance company and/or subsidy fund. In the Netherlands, insurance companies facilitate innovation by supporting projects, such as those related to personalised care, digital transformation, efficient working methods, and alternative ways of organising care. For primary care that is future-proof, various insurance companies (in their supplementary care policy) offer reimbursement of implementation of person-oriented care, as a logical and integral part of the provided health care (Zilveren Kruis 2020).

- The Dutch Healthcare Authority (NZa) has a policy whereby regional financial support for primary care and quality development is offered (NZa 2020, Nederlandse Zorg Autoriteit 2020). For example, through the platform in support of primary care in the Netherlands (▶ www.versterkingeerstelijn.nl), which is also cooperating with the 'Robuust', a regional support structure (ROS) (▶ www.rosrobuust.nl).
- These Regional Support Structures (ROS), which are active in all regions of the Netherlands, for example, provide support in training courses (▶ www.ros-netwerk.nl) (ROS network 2020).

In order to sustainably embed the financing of Positive Health in Dutch health care, the Institute for Positive Health (iPH) has started a consultative structure with health insurance companies. Elements of discussion are the connection between Positive Health, the policy of insurance companies and the reimbursement system to professionals, as this often appears to be a bottleneck, in everyday practice. iPH also thinks along with pilot projects of health insurance companies with population costing. iPH is also in discussion with the Dutch professional organisations of general practitioners about the application of Positive Health in relation to the future vision of primary care and translating this to general medical practice.

8.1.4 Preconditions of implementation

The previous sections describe the challenges of implementing changes in health care. Below, the preconditions for implementing and embedding the Positive Health concept are provided. These preconditions cover all four levels: the consulting room, the practice organisation itself, the local community, and both national and regional levels.

- First and foremost, the more person-oriented care in the Positive Health concept requires a different mindset. Do you work from the diagnosis-prescription model, disease-oriented, or is the care you provide more person-oriented, whereby patients are in central position and regarded from the perspective of health?
- General practitioners who want to implement Positive Health in their medical practice will need financing, capacity and time to start. Financing (as described in ▶ Sect. 8.1.3) for the initial start-up and training of staff members with respect to conducting the *alternative dialogue*. Initially this will cost time, but eventually it will save time. As described in *The Innovator's Prescription*, it is about reorganising the usual care and allowing more time and opportunity for person-oriented care for the people who need it. Ultimately, this will save time.
- Chapters 5, 6 and 7 describe what is needed in order to implement the Positive Health concept in actual practice, at different levels in the Netherlands. There are also other broad concepts of health; how do they relate to each other and how could they strengthen each other?
- It is important to connect to what is already happening within the community, in networks and on a regional level. Here, it is important for care providers to be familiar with citizens' initiatives and participation from within the community.

- It is also important to connect to national policy (also see ▶ Sect. 8.3). Positive Health has been included in the National Policy Document on Public Health 2020–2024 (◘ fig. 8.5), which represents an important endorsement by the Dutch Ministry of Health, Welfare and Sport (VWS) in stimulating the broad perspective on health care.
- To demonstrate the scientific basis and added value of Positive Health, health care innovations and projects need to be monitored and evaluated. Process and effects are both studied; are patients and professionals happy, have health levels improved and what are the effects on costs? (Quadruple Aim: (1) The health of the target group; (2) The experienced quality of health care; (3) The costs; (4) The well-being of professionals)
- It is also necessary to embed the care innovation in the education and training of care professionals of the future, in general medicine training courses, as well as in intermediate and higher vocational training and for well-being coaches, nurses and paramedics.

The question is how. For this purpose, the Institute for Positive Health (iPH) was founded in 2015 in the Netherlands, to boost the implementation of the Positive Health concept and has become a source of inspiration and authority in the field of Positive Health. iPH guarantees quality and is one of the driving forces behind knowledge development and best practices, and the developer and owner of practical Positive Health tools and products. iPH is a catalyst in the implementation of Positive Health in policy, practice, research and education.

8.2   Institute for Positive Health (iPH)

The mission of the Institute for Positive Health (iPH) is for the philosophy to penetrate all areas of Dutch society, in general, and health care, in particular. In addition, iPH aims to further develop and deepen the knowledge about Positive Health and, wherever possible, promote the implementation of Positive Health in actual practice. All this serves the realisation of a real paradigm shift in health care.

iPH works on further increasing the societal value of Positive Health on all levels: from consulting rooms (nano level, see ▶ Chap. 5), to the general medical practice as an organisation (micro level, see ▶ Chap. 6), to the local community (meso level, see ▶ Chap. 7) and the systemic, macro level (▶ Chap. 8). On each level, iPH distinguishes the domains of *policy, practice, research* and *education* and also stimulates in these areas.

iPH's strategic objectives for the various domains are:
- Embedding Positive Health in the everyday practice of health care institutions and organisations.
- Implementation of Positive Health in national, regional and local policy by talking with the ministry (VWS), provinces, municipalities, insurance companies and professional organisations.
- Researching the effects, applications and implementation of Positive Health and further anchoring its scientific foundations.
- The application and quality assurance of Positive Health in education on all levels of medical curricula, training courses and eventually also in primary education.

iPH is not the only organisation engaged in transforming health care. Together with others, iPH is moving into a new direction. For example, iPH cooperates with various training, implementation and network partners. The iPH Academy works with a hundred iPH-certified trainers around the country to meet the great need for lectures, workshops and training working with Positive Health. Follow-up modules are being developed for implementation in health care, and depending on the need, modules can be customised or offered on an in-company basis. The training working with Positive Health is also available in English, online, via the iPH Academy (▶ https://www.iph.nl/en/participate/training).

iPH offers citizens and patients the Positive Health digital spider web tool (and its further elaborations) as well as a link to the Dutch AppStore of the Municipal Health Services (GGD), with courses of action per dimension, which are under continual development. Amongst other things, there are also informative videos.

For the implementation in actual practice, iPH focuses primarily on health care and welfare, and especially on the quality of the interaction between professionals and patients/citizens, on the organisational consequences for the practice, interdisciplinary cooperation and the preconditions at the system level. Implementation is also taking place in other domains, such as for children and young people in education, Positively Healthy employment in businesses, Positive Health in policy and public health. Hospitals are also increasingly interested in working with the concept. iPH is cooperating with various universities on research and implementation projects, and with national organisations such as *All about Health (Alles is Gezondheid)*, association of lifestyle physicians (*Arts en Leefstijl*) and the student lifestyle foundation (*Student en Leefstijl*).

8.3 Positive Health from a regional and national perspective

8.3.1 Positive Health in regional networks

Why is there a need for more regional cooperation? There will be increasing centralised cooperation on a regional level, for many issues in primary care, such as ICT infrastructure, the increasing complexity of the demand for health care due to elderly people living independently for longer and people with mental health problems. To this end, far-reaching structural cooperation and organisation is taking place, on regional levels, within Dutch primary care and between care professionals (InEen 2020). General practitioners who are members of a regional alliance will receive a basic level of service provision from the regional organisation (e.g., use of data, organisation and implementation of training courses, administrative organisation). Labour market problems and workload management in general medical practices can also be addressed more effectively and sustainably by doing so together. A regional organisation that is mandated to speak on behalf of its members is able to unburden general practitioners by tackling issues on the most effective and logical levels (i.e., practice, local community or region).

The previous chapter (▶ Sect. 7.4) describes the importance of integrated cooperation on health on a community level. In the Netherlands, this is mainly regionally driven. Regional policies are also supported by data and certain online tools (e.g., ▶ regiobeeld.nl) that provide insight into the use of health care, health care provision, health and lifestyle, population development, and the social and physical environment. On the basis of such joint insights into data and health problems, the parties involved

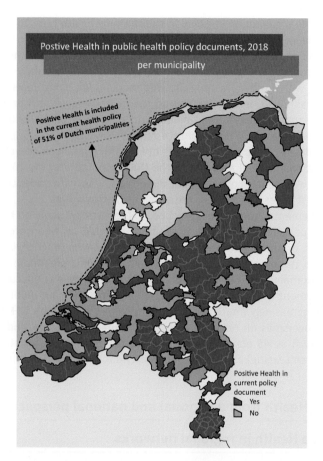

□ Figure 8.3 In the purple regions, Positive Health is included in the municipal policy documents on public health. Source: Iresearch (2018)

are able to formulate integrated public health policy. This integrated regional approach was also applied during the COVID-19 pandemic. Regional alliances and cooperations, with care groups and care networks, support general practitioners in their general medical practice as well as on a community level. Many regions and municipalities are already either applying the Positive Health concept or mention the concept in their policy documents (□ fig. 8.3). In these regions, more and more Positive Health networks are emerging.

Positive Health networks

A Positive Health network consists of various organisations or partners who work together from a common vision with Positive Health as a starting point. On local and regional levels, in particular, they cooperate on health issues and a healthy local environment. A Positive Health network involves close cooperation with municipalities, provinces, care institutions and employers. Regional networks may vary in population scale, with sometimes up to as many as 600,000 inhabitants.

Their shared objectives include:
- addressing regional health issues, each in their own way;
- connecting and supporting regional stakeholders;
- setting up joint activities to stimulate public health;
- sharing mutual experiences;
- implementation;
- exchanging best practices;
- learning together.

Positive Health first starts from a broad perspective on health, with inhabitants and social partners. The concept contributes to integrated cooperation across various domains. Many initiatives take place on different levels (from citizens (nano) to regional and national levels (macro)). It does not matter at which level the implementation starts, as long as it is realised that all levels are important and interrelated.

Such regional networks are necessary to shape national policy – with more attention for prevention and health – and as local as possible, in regions and local communities.

The text box describes lessons learned and the tools for successful regional cooperation, based on a broad perspective on health.
- Organisations can be enthused to participate if their mission and vision are in line with the broad view of health and they are willing and able to work in a network setting. Talking to one another across domains and not being afraid to give local residents an important voice.
- Network partners, together, can draw up a plan that includes targets which enable tracking progress and results of the cooperation. From a practical perspective, agreements should be made in advance about who does what within the network (e.g., data collection).
- At the beginning of such initiatives, partners should discuss how they would like to safeguard and sustain them; different working methods may require different types of funding. Administrative embedding will help, in this respect.
- Starting an initiative will require some capital, such as for project leading and management, which may be obtained from health insurance companies or through subsidy schemes (this may differ per country). One person from within the network should take responsibility for the communication and consultation around the various themes of the network, and a portfolio manager should be appointed.
- On a regional level, development of expertise and training courses are also needed, and business interests and social interests should be well aligned.
- Cooperating across domains will only have an impact if network partners, together with insurance companies and municipalities, join forces and make joint investments.

Zooming in on the provincial level, the foundations for Positive Health were first established in Limburg, the Netherlands' most southern province.

Limburg is a front runner and trendsetter, as it has embraced the Positive Health concept throughout the province. It all started after Machteld Huber and Hans Peter Jung gave a number of lectures on Positive Health. Various people in strategic provincial positions were inspired, after which the Province of Limburg commissioned iPH to conduct a three-year project to help Limburg become the first 'Positively Healthy' province of the Netherlands. Large groups of people were mobilised, with the Limburg Positive Health Movement and various other parties in Limburg, initially coordinated by iPH. After three years, the coordinating task was transferred to the Limburg Positive Health Movement. An informative brochure was published, as well as a video in which best practices are shared (*'Leren van Limburg'*). The QR code at the end of this chapter provides the related links.

Learning from Limburg

Just imagine having to implement a whole new movement in the region, to reduce health inequalities – and all without any proven results, without well-defined working methods, without a team. A deliberate choice was made for an approach where the movement itself is the yield and the outcome of the process the most important measurement result.

The lessons that can be learned from Limburg as the first Positive Health province of the Netherlands are explained in a magazine, in three categories:

1. The start and the initiative
2. Action plan and its execution
3. Transfer, results and start of the Limburg Positive Health Movement

The magazine is filled with people from Limburg who talk about the changes, the improvements and the new insights that were achieved due to Positive Health. They also discuss the importance of speaking the same language, of connection and the *alternative dialogue*, and how Positive Health is a catalyst for transformation. In areas where stakeholders are all responsible for their own share, Limburg shows how this contributes to the promotion of health, sustainable employability of the local labour force, less loneliness, greater self-reliance, and healthy schools. It is about the administrative courage of the Province of Limburg, the strength of Limburg and the Limburg Positive Health Movement who are now continuing with the health concept. People are at the centre of cooperation, knowledge sharing and networks, which are coordinated by the Limburg Positive Health Movement. In the coming years, the focus will be on the further development, deepening and sustainability of the concept, from three areas of attention – network, knowledge & expertise, training – for an even more positively healthy Limburg.

(Source: IPH newsletter 2019c (in Dutch)).

The approach is pragmatic, largely bottom-up and demand-oriented. Implementation is stimulated in areas that show potential. The support base is continually being expanded, with ambassadors in various domains. ■ Figure 8.4 shows some initiatives where vitality, participation and sense of purpose is created by working together within local communities and on regional levels. To illustrate what this can mean in practical terms, the text box describes an example from the Positive Health network in the region of the northern Meuse valley. It is a good example of shifting from aftercare to prevention, with health-related information being provided, for example, through a local public library rather than by care providers.

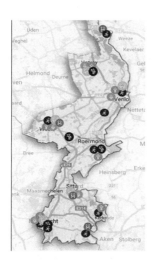

Limburg
Positive Health
Movement

Ambitions Limburg
Positively Healthy

🔲 **Figure 8.4**   Cooperation within the province (▶ www.limburgpositiefgezond.nl)

The Positive Health network northern Meuse valley
This network was first started by Syntein, a group of general practitioners (▶ www.syntein.nl). To achieve a healthier lifestyle in the region of the northern Meuse valley, Syntein works closely together with care providers, such as welfare organisations, health insurance companies, municipalities, municipal health care services (GGD), education and the business community. Syntein has created a programme for the implementation of Positive Health in general medical practices (available (in Dutch) from ▶ www.netwerkpositievegezondheid.nl).
Positive Health at public libraries is an example of a network activity.
Specifically for citizens, since 2018, the Positive Health network northern Meuse valley is organising thematic workshops, which are held at all the public libraries in the 'Land van Cuijk' region and in northern Limburg. The workshops are intended to show citizens how they could be more in control of their own health and help others to do the same, based on the concept of Positive Health. Workshop themes are determined on the basis of regional citizen focal groups and include: sleeping well, feeling energetic, healthy food and the final stage of life. Participation in these workshops is free of charge, they are facilitated by a discussion leader and the speakers are general practitioners.
The number of participants per workshop has increased over time, with each series of workshops. Participants were surveyed afterwards and their reactions have been very positive. At the end of a workshop, nearly all participants said they had formulated a personal health goal! The series of workshops have been so successful in the northern Meuse valley that they are likely to be repeated. The initiatives are also being scaled up to other locations in the region, where similar workshops are currently being organised in local public libraries. And there appears to also be some international interest in these initiatives, such as by a Belgian general practitioner (in Genk), who has set up language lessons at local primary schools, for female immigrants.

Positive Health network northern Meuse valley is one of the regional networks affiliated with All about Health.

All about Health (▶ https://tinyurl.com/allesisgezondheid) is a government-funded organisation that promotes the creation and expansion of local health-related networks. It stimulates regional partnerships and cooperatives that create new opportunities for working together on a healthy environment. For example, this has led to the emergence of a self-regulating network of over 3,000 stakeholders, representing the movement towards a more vital Netherlands. iPH works closely with All about Health, amongst other things, to create an overview of regional networks, support them with knowledge where necessary, and connect these networks. In addition to the networks in Limburg, many other examples of regional networks of Positive Health can be found on the All about Health website (e.g., Coalition Positive Health Texel, ▶ www.texelsamenbeter.nl/, see ▶ Sect. 7.4; and WEL, ▶ www.welinflevoland.nl). The networks have set themselves the goal of becoming a Positive Health region, and each network determines for their local environment what this means in actual practice. This is also relevant for general practitioners, as such networks may support regionalisation within the care groups.

8.3.2 Positive Health from a national perspective

The fact that national policy on public health has embraced Positive Health in its National Policy Document on Public Health 2020–2024 is of great added value for the application of Positive Health in the Netherlands (◻ fig. 8.5). This has created national support, on the one hand, while stimulating the government to apply Positive Health more broadly in various domains, on the other. In actual practice in the Netherlands, this is still difficult, because it means that various government departments are responsible for this. This National Policy Document on Public Health focuses on three pillars: underlying problems, cooperation and Positive Health. The theme of health features in a broad sense on the Dutch policy agenda. Health problems often do not exist in isolation, but are linked to problems in other areas. Therefore, an approach outside the health domain may also deliver health gains. 'A healthy physical and social environment can have a positive impact on the participation, well-being and health of citizens', according to the Dutch State Secretary of Health, Welfare and Sport (iPH 2019a). Positive Health, thus, is gaining a foothold on a macro level, as an umbrella and binding element for a strong and resilient society.

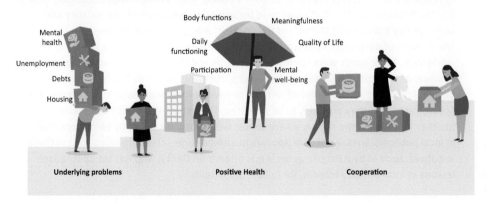

◻ **Figure 8.5**   Visualisation of the National Policy Document on Public Health 2020–2024. Source: Rijksoverheid (2020a)

8.3.3 National organisations

In the Netherlands, general practitioners are being represented by three organisations, each with their own role to play. The three umbrella associations, the Dutch College of General Practitioners (NHG), the National Association of General Practitioners (LHV), and InEen (association of primary care organisations), have jointly expressed their views on the future in the new core values and core tasks in primary care (see ▶ Chap. 4). Each organisation has its own objectives in this respect with regard to implementing and supporting person-oriented care and promoting health on the level of general medical practices and local communities. NHG maps out the scientific knowledge and translates this into practical recommendations and education for general practitioners. The necessary preconditions are regulated and established by the LHV, while InEen supports and facilitates the organisation of care, especially the structured, integrated approach in primary care.

As described in ▶ Chap. 4, the core values and core tasks for general practitioners have recently been reviewed and clarified on a national level. At the core of the profession are the aspects of providing care that is *person-oriented, medical generalist, continuous* and done in cooperation with others (i.e., *together*). Facilitating this type of care requires the right preconditions. InEen and NHG embrace person-oriented care. At the time this handbook was written, support was being developed for general practitioners and care groups in the areas of training, communication and an action plan for the implementation of person-oriented care. This is facilitated by webinars, inspiration and information for the regional cooperation amongst care groups. Professionals need training with respect to the application and embedding of person-oriented care. More information on this subject can be accessed via the QR code at the end of this chapter. In addition to the basic and follow-up modules via training partner Visiom, training courses were recently started specifically for general practitioners via the LHV Academy. One of the preconditions is also that more time and funding will be made available for conducting the *alternative dialogue*. Sections 6.5 and 8.1 describe the initiatives that have already been developed by the LHV in this area.

The Foreword in the Dutch version of this handbook, by Ella Kalsbeek, former chair of the Dutch National Association of General Practitioners (August 2020).
Furious, he stands at the front desk of the general practice. 'What do you mean, I don't get sleeping pills? Wasn't I clear enough on the phone?' His general practitioner eventually manages to calm him down. She listens to his complaints and rules out certain medical causes. Sleeping pills are not going to fix his symptoms, she tells him. But isn't there anything else that would help him right now, though? This question appears to open the door for him to start talking about his real problems. He has been unemployed for six months, drinks far too much and his relationship is about to fail. He wants help, but does not know how to get it.
'Putting the person first, rather than the disease.' Is that really such an innovative starting point for a general practitioner, I hear you think? Positive Health looks beyond the medical, it considers all health-related facets of life, with the patient being the one in charge. As obvious as this may sound, this is not easy to do in the day-to-day practice of medical analytical health care.

This handbook inspires care professionals to get started with a solution-oriented approach that lets physician and patient jointly discover what works, at a particular time, within the patient's personal context. This method of working not only suits the general practitioner, but also the practice assistant and the nursing assistant. Your strength lies in the fact that you know your patients, build a relationship with each of them and create trust. This is a solid basis for reaching appropriate personal advice together. An advice with room for other types of help, outside the medical domain, without you having to organise this help from your own practice.

At first glance, the *alternative dialogue* method seems a time-consuming effort. However, I speak with experience experts, general practitioners, who are actually very pleased with the results; patients learning that they do not need to see their general practitioner for every complaint and that the general practitioner is there mostly for medical problems. Positive Health produces more interesting conversations, more creativity and patients who are more satisfied. The different working method combined with extended consultation times, in the Dutch Province of Limburg, shows that fewer medications are being prescribed and hospital referrals have been reduced. Moreover, the concept is about more than just having the alternative type of doctor-patient conversation. General practitioners and the other people working in the practice also see a more equal cooperation with professionals in the social domain, because they use each other's expertise to look at the patient's best interest. For a general practitioner, it is normal to know the specialists in the hospital by name, and with this new approach they will soon know the care providers outside the medical domain equally well.

Positive Health is a stimulating method for tackling the problems of patients in the present time – and for keeping the profession of general practitioner attractive, both now and into the future. Here, I would like to express the wish that the motivational concept of Positive Health be widely adopted in primary care, so that general practitioners can continue to practice their wonderful profession with pleasure.

In the Netherlands, there are many national organisations for the wide variety of health care providers working in primary care: the *NVDA* (Dutch association of nursing assistants; ► www.nvda.nl), the *NVvPO* (association of practice nurses and nurses; ► www.nvvpo.nl) and the *Landelijke Vereniging POH-GGZ* (the national association for mental health practice nurses; ► www.poh-ggz.nl). All have their own educational system, lectures and training courses on the concept of Positive Health. The same applies to paramedical professions, nursing training programmes (Laurant and Vermeulen 2018) and, for example, to lower vocational education in the areas of sport and welfare. For example, in 2020, *ROC Midden Nederland* (the Central Netherlands Regional Education and Training Centre) opened a vitality lab at its Utrecht location, based entirely on the Positive Health concept (► www.rocmn.nl/vitaliteitslab). Incidentally, Positive Health-related training programmes in the regional networks are often provided in a multidisciplinary way, which directly strengthens the mutual cooperation and common language, more and more towards 'One Health'.

8.4 Positive Health in relation to other health concepts and working methods

The various examples and initiatives of tools and methods that are available show that many people are already working with broad concepts of health. So, there is a need to look from a wider perspective. Positive Health can be a connecting philosophy, as also intended in the National Policy Document on Public Health. The person-oriented, health-related perspective is at the centre of all broad health concepts, as it is in the horizontal bar of the T-shaped professional (see Sects. 2.6 and 8.5). When comparing the Positive Health concept against other widely used broad health-oriented methods and visions in the Dutch health care system, they all seem to consider similar themes important, such as daily functioning, self-reliance and self-management. There are differences with regard to objectives and target groups, approaches, directions and types of questions. In the Netherlands, other health concepts have been described and researched that differ slightly in their nuances of use. Some are theories, visions or approaches, while other examples include conversational tools or classification systems. Target groups also differ, from being specifically intended for a certain group, to broader holistic approaches. Some are more solution-oriented while other approaches focus more on problems. Other differences concern style (who is in charge, the patient or the care provider) or circumstances (is it a one-off intervention, or is follow-up required?). Choosing a certain concept sometimes seems to be based on the objective, but considerations also seem to be mainly pragmatic. Thus, organisations tend to choose a concept that fits their ambitions – for example, those who wish to provide citizens with more control, or who want to contribute to becoming the healthiest region in the Netherlands. There are various tools, methodologies can also co-exist, depending on the level where cooperation takes place. Organisations or initiatives choose the concept that interconnects them or their cooperating partners (e.g., health and welfare organisations, health insurance companies, educational institutions, or citizen representatives). This, for example, depends on the municipal procurement policy, contracting of insurance companies, or the experience of various front runners within the community or region.

For care providers, it is important to know about the various concepts and tools that are available and, for some of them, to discover the elements that may help to apply them. In actual practice, the various methods also appear to complement and enhance each other. The Positive Health philosophy appears to be the basis, the common vision or language, which is now also reflected in the National Policy Document on Public Health (▶ Sect. 8.3) and in the framework plan for medical training programmes (▶ Sect. 8.6). The common goal, shared by all health concepts, is that of wanting to provide insight for people and support them to live a healthy life.

Positive Health, as described in this handbook, is a broad basis and common language for providing *person-oriented care* and the *alternative dialogue*. The various concepts all have the same goal, namely to promote good health in citizens, with the right care in the right place, as much as possible.

In the Netherlands, there are various methods for conducting patient–physician conversations that have a broad perspective on health and are person-oriented. Dutch examples include: the 4-domain model (▶ https://tinyurl.com/4Domein-model); an app 'from disease to good health' (▶ www.bettery.nl/app), Bettery.nl (2020); vitality and lifestyle with the lifestyle tool (see ▶ Sect. 5.7); solution-oriented approach (see ▶ Sect. 5.5), and those for people with a chronic disease, such as diabetes mellitus, there is the Diabetes Conversation card from the NDF, the Dutch diabetes federation (▶ www.ndf-toolkit.nl), just to name a few.

Here, two concepts are highlighted that are also widely used, internationally: the International Classification of Functioning, Disability and Health (ICF) and Value-based health care (VBHC). ICF is a conceptual framework created by the World Health Organization and its partners, which can be used to classify the functioning of people and any problems they experience while functioning. VBHC is specifically disease-oriented, but with an emphasis on value-driven care. Positive Health concerns the well-being of the whole person. Although there are differences between them, the concepts nevertheless all complement each other. How they relate to each other is described in Sects. 8.4.1 and 8.4.2.

8.4.1 Value-based health care (VBHC)

Value-based health care (VBHC) was first introduced in 2010, by Michael Porter (Harvard University) in the New England Journal of Medicine (Porter, 2010). The VBHC concept arose from the need to make health care more sustainable. The focus of VBHC is on increasing the value of health care for patients, while trying to reduce the costs of that care. The core of VBHC is good communication with the patient (person-oriented care) and good communication with the health care network in *Integrated Practice Units*, whose members include health care professionals. According to the VBHC concept, financing care ideally takes place by means of a subscription system (Bundled Payments, Capitation System or Fee for Membership). VBHC particularly seeks solutions to prevent unnecessary or even harmful care (Van Stratum 2019). With Positive Health, by having alternative-style, person-oriented conversations with patients, better, customised care can be provided. In 2020, Jung's practice won the 'Afferden initiative on Positive Health' – the international Value-Based Health Care Primary Care Excellence Award – for its efforts to combine the ideas of Positive Health and VBHC.

Another example of a broad approach to health is the use of ICF, also referred to in ▶ Chap. 2.

8.4.2 International Classification of Functioning, Disability and Health (ICF)

The ICF model looks at human functioning from three perspectives:
- Bodily functioning
- Human behaviour
- Participation in society

The three perspectives are interrelated and influenced by external and personal factors. Although the model mentions the disease or disorder, this is of minor importance.

ICF describes how people perceive their own level of health. It is a classification system that provides a standard terminology for functioning and external factors and a scheme that represents the conceptual model of health. ICF distinguishes the

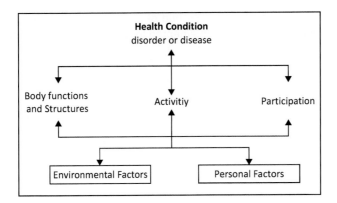

Figure 8.6 ICF classification (▶ whofic.nl, 2020)

following six domains: (1) diseases and medical complaints, (2) functions and anatomical characteristics, (3) activities and related limitations, (4) participation, (5) external factors and (6) personal factors. The domains are subdivided into around 1,500 categories, with the exception of the personal factors, for which no sub-categories have yet become available. ICF creates a common language to describe a person's functioning that improves communication between health professionals and other sectors as well as people with functioning problems. Huber's research (▶ Sect. 2.4), which led to the philosophy of Positive Health, closely studied the ICF classifications when categorising the various concepts. However, there seemed to be insufficient overlap with what people had been saying in the interviews held during the study. In the first place, because ICF lacks a classification of personal factors and, secondly, because a relatively free narrative was a better fit for the interviews, compared to a classification system (▢ fig. 8.6). Cooperation between Positive Health researchers and those from ICF has led to a proposal whereby the ICF model focuses even more on health (Heerkens & Stallinga, 2021, Heerkens et al., 2017).

In order to substantiate the nationally envisaged transition in health care, from a less disease-oriented to a more health-oriented mindset and approach, it is important to also look at the results from the above-mentioned interventions.

A report by RIVM (the Dutch National Institute for Public Health and the Environment, RIVM 2020; Lemmens et al. 2019) on the evaluation of the various broad concepts of health (including Positive Health) shows similar goals between concepts (irrespective of method):

- Improving people's health, and how it is perceived, as well as their well-being (90 %);
- Stimulating cooperation and coordination between health care and welfare professionals (62 %);
- Improving the well-being and job satisfaction of professionals (45 %);
- Improving people's access to care and support (38 %);
- Managing health care costs (28 %);
- Other goals, including perception of better quality of care, speaking a common language, and greater patient involvement in care decisions.

The following section describes the method of evaluating the impact of working with Positive Health and how it will be implemented for future health care professionals.

8.5   Positive Health: research and education

A sound scientific basis is a fundamental requirement for a further implementation of Positive Health in general medical practice, in policy and in medical training and education, as well as for the further development of the method. The Institute for Positive Health (iPH) is the catalyst for stimulating research on Positive Health around the Netherlands and to promote cooperation in this field between all stakeholders. iPH's research objectives are:

- Keeping track of any research being done both in the Netherlands and internationally with regard to Positive Health, and looking which subjects are still lacking from current research. An overview of studies can be accessed through the knowledge bank on iPH's website (▶ www.iph.nl);
- Stimulating and facilitating research on Positive Health;
- Cooperating with various universities and institutes.

iPH does not conduct any research itself, but does have an advisory role, in this respect. The institute monitors ongoing research and shares any resulting new knowledge and experience with parties on a national level. In this way, Positive Health can be further substantiated and anchored in science. The monitoring also shows whether investments are delivering the expected results. Experiences are shared, successful initiatives are scaled up and can be embedded. Where possible, research is ordered according to the four levels that are distinguished: personal level (nano; patient contact), organisational level (micro; general medical practice), community level (meso; neighbourhood, district, village, municipality) and provincial/national level (macro). New research results are continually added to the knowledge base at ▶ www.iph.nl. There, you will find articles by Jung, Huber and Van Vliet, amongst others. Research that has been receiving a great deal of attention from within the primary care community is, in part, described in ▶ Sect. 8.1 under 'catch-22'. In 2018, general practitioner and author Jung published an article in Huisarts & Wetenschap, the Dutch journal on primary care and science, about Positive Health's impact with more time for patients leading to fewer hospital referrals ('*Meer tijd voor de patiënt, minder verwijzingen*') (Jung et al., 2018). The article also describes that both patients and physicians felt more satisfied. This research, which was conducted in Afferden and surrounding areas, will continue on. In the practice from van den Brekel a report was published about following an alternative conversation (Oude Weernink, 2020). Another good example is the *hotspotters* project in the Dutch city of Zoetermeer (see case no. 8, ▶ Sect. 5.4), the first results of which seem to indicate that the *alternative dialogue* method of Positive Health reduces the number of hospital visits. The project, by general practitioner Ephraim, studies the impact of applying the Positive Health alternative dialogue in the case of frequent visitors ('hotspotters') to the general practice in Zoetermeer. Ephraim also pointed to an increase in job satisfaction amongst general practitioners who had been applying the Positive Health conversations when dealing with such complex patients. (Medisch Ondernemen, 2019).

Many more research projects are currently underway in the Netherlands – on process implementation and feasibility, as well as on particular target groups. Recently, new research has become available on measuring health. A cross-sectional survey was held amongst 708 Dutch respondents about the use of the Positive Health dialogue tool as a suitable measurement instrument. The results suggest that the current dialogue tool is reliable as a communication tool, but is not suitable as a measurement scale. The Institute for Positive Health, therefore, proposes a model with 17 questions with improved, acceptable psychometric properties that will serve as a basis for the further development of a measurement scale. (▶ https://tinyurl.com/health-measuring, ▶ www.iph.nl/evaluatiewijzer/). Further research will also be conducted on an international level, as in other countries other health-related questions may play a role, depending on the health topics for which they chose to implement the Positive Health concept.

There have also been some critical reactions, in the Netherlands, over the past years.

8.5.1 Criticism of Positive Health

The concept of Positive Health has also been receiving a fair amount of criticism. Critical articles describe Positive Health as a passing fashion and speak about confusion on the aspects of health and behaviour (Poiesz et al., 2016; Van der Stel, 2016). The word health is used for the state someone is in and for coping with that state. Depending on the perspective of the evaluator, someone can be called either healthy or unhealthy. Van der Stel et al. comment on the implication that people should adapt (active coping), which is seen as an obligation to work on one's health. The emphasis is on individual behaviour and self-care. There is also critical feedback on the six dimensions chosen; about them not being mutually exclusive. Quality of life is presented as one of the dimensions, while critics argue that physical and mental functioning are part of quality of life. Health is part of quality of life, but not the other way around, or so the critics claim.

In their publication of 2017, Arnoldus et al. claim to be amazed about the unquestioning embrace of the Positive Health concept in the Netherlands (Arnoldus et al., 2017). They describe how, under the concept, health appears to be perceived on the basis of cultural, social and political circumstances, and that, on this point, Positive Health also has a moral dimension. Arnoldus et al. consider that the tendency to see everything as health makes the desire for health boundless. Is there such a thing as negative health, they wonder? Are you only healthy if you do your best or adapt to the circumstances? Does the concept's definition of health pay sufficient attention to environmental factors? In traditional public health care, attention is actually paid to salutogenesis: to the environmental and individual factors that bring about health and well-being. The mobilising attention for opportunities under the Positive Health concept may be valuable, but too much emphasis on the positive could also result in suppressing disease and vulnerability, and lead to an accusatory discourse. Are you sick because you did not try hard enough? In this respect, according to the critics, disease and illness are viewed as an individual risk, whereas it would be better to clarify what people should address on a personal level and what should be considered a matter of public risk.

Another critical comment came from a study by Prinsen and Terwee. The study assesses whether Positive Health could serve as a measuring instrument for adults. Following both qualitative research of interview results and quantitative research on the developmental phase, a validation study was conducted. The conclusion of that study was that Positive Health questionnaires could not serve as a valid instrument for measuring health and that follow-up research would be needed (Prinsen & Terwee, 2019). In response to these results, iPH decided to use the spider web as a conversational tool rather than a measurement tool.

Questions are also being asked from a philosophical perspective, on both substantive, conceptual and practical grounds (Kingma 2019). Kingma's questions mainly focus on the aspect of adaptation. What could be considered 'normal', as people and circumstances vary, after all. There is insufficient elaboration on this subject, in order to formulate the term health, according to Kingma, who suggests changing the *ability to adapt* into being able to '*adapt well*'. Because there are also circumstances, such as in case of domestic violence, in which people should not make an effort to adapt. The Positive Health concept, furthermore, would also make insufficient distinction between, for example, a child, a depressed adult and an active wheelchair user. The focus is too largely on adaptability. Since Kingma's study in 2019, iPH has developed four different assessment tools for specific target groups: one for children, one for adolescents and one for adults, and a fourth tool that uses simplified language (see ▶ Chap. 4).

A study by Van Tol (2020), ethicist and medical sociologist, wonders whether health is not becoming a moral duty, from the viewpoint of Positive Health. This could jeopardise solidarity in health care. He also considers the possibility that Positive Health could have a medicalising effect.

In their article on Positive Health in *Bijblijven*, general practitioners Van Boven and Versteegde argue that health is becoming a catch-all term, whereas they are of the opinion that perception of health is a complex and individual affair. They [also] want more time and opportunity for talking to their patients about what the term health means to them, but that this is not dependent on a new concept. For them, Positive Health is one of many person-oriented models. Van Boven and Versteegde argue that all dimensions of Positive Health are already also part of the International Classification of Functioning, Disability and Health (ICF) (see text box, ▶ Sect. 8.4). However, ICF is a classification system that contains no elaboration of 'personal factors', whereas these factors are one of the main focal points of the Positive Health concept. ICF has recently published a questionnaire that applies to people with a chronic disease (Postma et al., 2018; Van Boven & Versteegde 2019).

8.5.2   Positive Health research agenda

Criticism and other feedback that iPH receives keeps the organisation on its toes and underlines the importance of scientific evidence in the continual development of the concept. For this purpose, iPH set up a scientific advisory board in 2019, which led to the research agenda described in the box.

The research agenda of iPH

A. *Make Positive Health measurable*. iPH supports researchers with the knowledge about suitable methods to measure health and changes in health, under the Positive Health concept, on four different levels (i.e., nano, micro, meso and macro). This enables comparison of research results, and includes:
   - Development of a new basic set of measuring instruments to measure Positive Health in a uniform way. A first guidance document (i.e., the Evaluation Tool, ► iph.nl) and underlying recommendations have been created, on the basis of an exploration of existing valid measuring instruments, with preferred instruments for measuring Positive Health. New studies are performed towards a new validated instrument to measure health in line with Positive Health (Van Vliet et al., 2021). New possibilities of data collection are considered, with data ownership remaining with the citizens concerned and where the data can also be used to gain insight into how health is experienced.
B. *The impact and effectiveness of Positive Health, in practice*. In addition to developing measuring instruments, iPH also stimulates research that provides insight into the measurable impact and benefits of working with Positive Health, in actual practice. This includes studying not only the concept as a whole, but also the separate components of the concept, by using:
   - quantitative impact studies to outline the added value of Positive Health on the following elements of the Quadruple Aim:
     1. Health of the population;
     2. The experienced quality of health care;
     3. Health care costs;
     4. Job satisfaction and well-being of care professionals.
   - qualitative process evaluations and best practices to increase the understanding of effective implementation strategies. What works well and how it is done will be studied during the implementation process, as well as what lessons could be learned from this. Subsequently, the possibilities of alternative methods of measuring and evaluating, in line with Positive Health, should also be explored. In this context, also see the trends described in a report by the Dutch Council of Public Health and Society (*Blijk van vertrouwen* [Trust Well Earned: a New Approach to Accountability for Better Healthcare]) (Meurs et al., 2021).

In addition to the substantiation that is important for follow-up implementation, it is also important that Positive Health is sufficiently included in inspiration (► https://tinyurl.com/iph-lectures), training and refresher courses for general practitioners. This can be done in training programmes in the context of person-oriented care and by following the training 'working with Positive Health' (► www.iph.nl/en/participate/training/) or the training for general practitioners by the National Association of General Practitioners (LHV) (scan the QR code at the end of this chapter for more information). This is a challenging aspect for the new generation of physicians, the health care professionals of the future, whose professional training currently takes place within a disease-oriented educational system.

8.5.3   Positive Health for future health care professionals

▶ Section 7.1 mentions how the book 'The Innovator's Prescription' by Christensen also describes the dilemmas and challenges in medical education, in the United States. Increasing numbers of medical students are being trained to become the type of health care professional that will not be needed, while there is also no coordinated policy to educate those students to become the physicians that society does need. In the United States, for example, the medical curriculum is over a hundred years old and focused on disease.

▬ *The focus of medical education*. Medical education in the United States is designed to train physicians as individuals who will be caring for their patients, in an autonomous manner. However, the complexity of care requires physicians to be part of health networks and to work together in teams, with citizens, other care institutions and welfare organisations. More and more patients are being treated and cared for outside hospitals, but most of the training is still taking place in a hospital setting. As a result, medical students are in less contact with the total cycle of disease, particularly when it comes to chronic conditions. There is too much emphasis on training super-specialists with a superior status and high income, and too little attention is paid to primary care, prevention and health. Such an educational system produces increasing numbers of health care professionals that society does not need.

▬ The United States is also training more and more nurses to perform the tasks of general practitioners. Meanwhile, over a quarter of graduated and practising general physicians have been trained outside the United States. They work mainly in inner cities and rural areas, where there is a growing number of vacancies for physicians. This situation of shortage will only get worse, and, as a result, nurses and practice assistants will see an increase in their medical responsibilities and will be taking over some of the tasks of general practitioners. At the same time, a huge shortage of nurses is expected to occur – in part, due to the ageing population, but also because young people are less likely to opt for a vocational training in health care. Instead, they will be choosing training programmes with greater career opportunities. Furthermore, Christensen also expects a disruption by technical solutions that will cause some nursing tasks to disappear altogether and others to be solved in a different way than they are today.

These circumstances are similar to those in the Netherlands, where the increase in the number of specialists since the 1950s is also evident (◼ fig. 8.7).

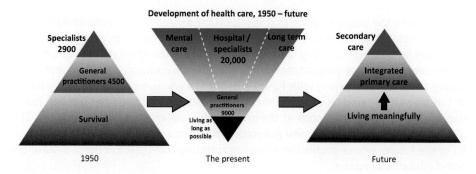

◼ **Figure 8.7**   The tilting of the pyramids, in relation to educational needs. Source: B. Leerink (formerly of Menzis; also see ◼ figs. 1.3 and 7.1)

Population ageing will certainly cause shortages of general practitioners and nurses in certain rural areas in the Netherlands. Because of the language barrier, these shortages in the Netherlands are less likely to be filled by care professionals trained in other countries, as is happening in the United States. This is an EU-wide problem, as ageing is an issue in all of the Member States. This means that in the Netherlands, too, disruptive solutions will be sought, with citizens taking over tasks from nurses, and nurses becoming responsible for the tasks currently performed by general practitioners. In turn, general practitioners will be doing more specialist work. Therefore, Dutch medical education will have to anticipate on this situation, to ensure that it will produce the types of health care professionals that are most needed in the future.

8.5.4 The promotion of health in basic medical training and general practitioner training

Education is the basis for the sustainable implementation of the Positive Health philosophy. This can be seen in the tilting of the pyramids in ◘ fig. 8.7 and the explanation of the T-shaped professional in ◘ fig. 2.4.

A commission on innovation in health care and medical education of the Dutch National Health Care Institute (▶ https://english.zorginstituutnederland.nl/) advises that care professionals need to develop different competences – thus, becoming the T-shaped professionals, with disease-oriented professional knowledge, with a person-oriented focus on a broader health approach. The focus should be on people's resilience, functioning and ability to self-manage, rather than on their diseases or disorders. The starting point should not be the existing way of providing care, the current professions or education programmes, but should rather be the future demand for care (Kaljouw and Van Vliet 2015).

It is essential for medical education to offer health care professionals sufficient knowledge and experience and pay adequate attention to Positive Health, lifestyle and prevention. The aim of iPH is for Positive Health to be included in medical curricula (i.e., at universities, higher secondary and intermediary vocational training) and as part of the programmes in primary and secondary schools. Recently, the new framework plan for the medical curriculum included ample attention for the Positive Health concept. It is also important that sufficient attention is being paid in training and raising awareness, to create skilled and resilient care professionals, on the level of general medical practices and within the community. In educational institutions, train-the-trainer programmes could be introduced to train teachers on the concept of Positive Health.

In the Netherlands, a study was conducted by medical students who wanted to call more attention to nutrition and lifestyle, after which, in 2020, a project was started about the promotion of health in basic medical training and general practitioner training ('*Gezondheidsbevordering in de basisopleiding geneeskunde en de huisartsopleiding*'), to ensure that physicians will be familiar with Positive Health, prevention and lifestyle, right from the time they graduate. Student lifestyle organisation, Student en leefstijl (2020) *Student en leefstijl*, association of lifestyle physicians *Arts en Leefstijl*, and the *Institute for Positive Health* formulated the joint objective that all medical students in the Netherlands, during their basic training, are provided with serious and thorough opportunities to develop a broader perspective of health and the skills to promote health. Not as an optional extra or voluntary course, but preferably interwoven with the entire medical study programme through one, and preferably several, study blocks or modules on lifestyle medicine and Positive Health. This addition to medical training is in line with the international development of health care professions towards the future 'T-shaped professional' (see ◘ fig. 2.4). Positive Health and lifestyle medicine share a broad view of health. Lifestyle medicine brings lifestyle therapeutic interventions into the consulting room with the aim of preventing, treating and/or favourably influencing chronic disorders, insofar as these are directly or indirectly related to lifestyle.

Knowledge and skills in all areas of non-acute medical problems, both preventive and curative, must be embedded in person-oriented communication, in order to achieve proper, customised care. It is important that this involves proven, scientific basic knowledge of lifestyle medicine and that future physicians should not become a new type of dietician. The vertical bar of the T-shaped professional also plays a role here. Professionals must be aware of their limitations and be able to cooperate with others. Learning about prevention is one of the 10 core tasks of the care professionals

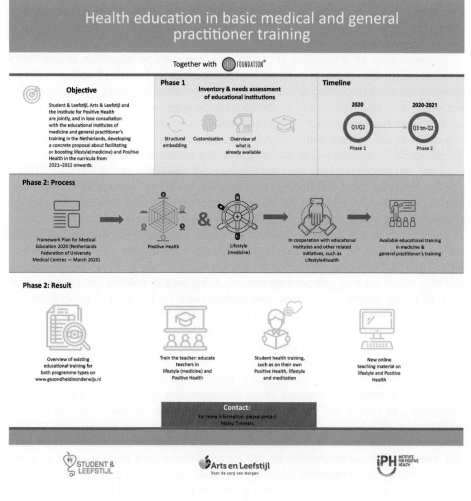

◘ **Figure 8.8**   Infographic of needs for more health education in basic medical and general practitioner training

of the future, although the 8 general practitioner educational courses in the Netherlands all address this in their own way. It is however clear that teacher–student joint learning programmes are desirable in learning about the application of Positive Health in medical practice. In 2020–2021, this project is being further developed with existing and new teaching material and substantiation, with courses for the further professionalisation of teachers and an inter-faculty sounding board group (□ fig. 8.8). Ideally, a broader health-oriented perspective should be started early on in medical training, and subsequent general practitioner training courses could include additional material about the promotion of health and Positive Health, in a more concrete way.

8.6 Conclusions

For care innovation and disruption, there are challenges along the way to achieving a real shift in health care. Implementation of Positive Health requires a number of preconditions, and it is important that Positive Health is included in the Dutch Government's National Policy Document on Public Health. The Institute for Positive Health (iPH) contributes to the further development of the Positive Health concept, in the areas of policy, practice, research and education, and looks at how Positive Health relates to other broad health concepts and working methods. The concept of Positive Health is also subject to criticism. Also from that perspective, there is ongoing attention for the further substantiation and scientific value of Positive Health. Further embedding Positive Health in general medical practices and beyond may also contribute to designing meaningful care. Positive Health, therefore, should become an essential element of the training and education of future care professionals.

> **Summary of the Dutch experiences with Positive Health**
> After having read this handbook about the situation in the Netherlands, you are ready to start working with Positive Health yourself. Many of you will ask themselves: but how, with what and where do I start? This depends on your situation and what is needed in your community.
> One of the reasons for writing this handbook was to provide scientific substantiation. Positive Health is a broad concept with health as its starting point. The concept is also a methodology, with the spider web as a tool that can be used, in various ways, when conducting the so-called *alternative dialogue* with patients. People are at the centre of this process and self-determination is stimulated. As a general practitioner, you could start working with the concept by practising the Positive Health *alternative dialogue* and experience the related benefits for yourself. Subsequent broader implementation can be done on various levels, from the consulting room and the medical practice, to the local community and even the region.
> Positive Health may contribute to a process of transformation in Dutch primary care.
> ▶ Chapter 8 outlines the challenges of innovation. In the Netherlands, attention has been focused, for some time, on more time for patients in primary care and general medical practices. And especially more time for what is called 'the *alternative* dialogue or conversation'. Insurance companies are stimulating care groups to pay more attention to person-oriented care, to organise care differently, to provide care at a distance

and to work more efficiently. This can be done, for example, through substitution, shifting tasks and differentiating between how single complaints and chronic care are approached. Self-care, e-health, prevention and community power are all necessary in order to ensure the continuity of care in the future. We hope that Positive Health will give you the tools you need to start working with the concept in your own professional environment.

Finally, Positive Health can also serve as an instrument of personal reflection. What do you value, and what do you need as a vital and healthy professional in primary care to work in this wonderful profession? To get you started, a number of tips and steps for working with Positive Health are provided below.

7 tips for Working with Positive Health

1. Ask yourself why you would like to start working with Positive Health?
2. Start working on your own Positive Health, in order to become an experience expert.
3. Find someone who also wants to work with the concept; start a coalition of the willing. Make sure your colleagues know about it and, if they are interested, invite them to join you.
4. Take your time to formulate a joint mission, vision and strategy.
5. Train yourself in conducting the *alternative dialogue* according to the Positive Health concept.
6. Look for broad cooperation within the local community. Everything relates to health; transcending health care and social domains.
7. Communicate often about your experiences and learn from them.

These tips are also shown in ◘ fig. 8.9. There are also a number of videos available; to view them, scan the QR code at the end of this chapter.

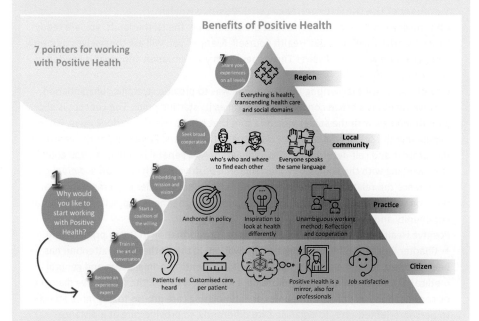

◘ **Figure 8.9**   Benefits and tips with regard to working with Positive Health

For more information, background or videos about this chapter scan the QR code.

SCAN ME

References

Arnoldus, R., et al. (2017). Hoe bruikbaar zijn de begrippen vitaliteit, veerkracht en positieve gezondheid voor interprofessioneel samenwerken in zorg en welzijn? *Tijdschrift Voor Gezondheidswetenschappen.* ▶ https://doi.org/10.1007/s12508-017-0052-7.

Bettery.nl (2020). *GG-app.* Accessed in October 2020 of ▶ https://www.bettery.nl/app/?utm_source=-Jleague.jp&utm_medium=PC&utm_campaign=PCsite&dlink=jLis.

Christensen, C. M., Grossman, J. H., & Hwang, J. (2017). *The innovator's prescription. A disruptive solution for health care.* McGraw Hill.

Heerkens, Y., De Weerd, M., Huber, M., et al. (2017). Reconsideration of the scheme of the international classification of functioning, disability and health: Incentives from the Netherlands for a global debate. *Disability and Rehabilitation.* ▶ https://doi.org/10.1080/09638288.2016.1277404.

Heerkens, Y. et al. (2021). *Functioneren als focus van zorg en welzijn. Met ICF-praktijkvoorbeelden.* Bohn Stafleu van Loghum.

Heller, H. (1961). *Catch 22: Simon en Schuster.*

InEen (2019). *Persoonsgerichte zorg.* Accessed in October 2020 of ▶ https://ineen.nl/wp-content/uploads/2020/02/InEen-Nhg-ZO-Infographic-Persoonsgerichte-zorg.pdf.

InEen (2020). *Visie regionale samenwerking en organisatievorming in de huisartsenzorg.* Accessed in October 2020 of ▶ https://ineen.nl/wp-content/uploads/2020/02/Visie_Organisatie_actief_def.pdf.

IPH Institute for Positive Health (2019a). *Paul Blokhuis over landelijke nota gezondheidsbeleid.* Accessed in October 2020 of ▶ https://iph.nl/staatssecretaris-paul-blokhuis-over-de-landelijke-nota-gezondheidsbeleid-2020-2024-met-positieve-gezondheid-kunnen-we-vraagstukken-in-onze-samenleving-in-een-anderlicht-bekijken/.

IPH Institute for Positive Health (2019b). *Positieve Gezondheid prominent in landelijke nota gezondheidsbeleid.* Accessed in October 2020 of ▶ https://iph.nl/positieve-gezondheid-prominent-in-landelijke-nota-gezondheidsbeleid.

IPH Institute for Positive Health (2019c). *Positieve Gezondheid – Leren van Limburg.* Accessed in October 2020 of ▶ https://www.iph.nl/kennisbank/pg-live-leren-van-limburg-bekijk-de-uitzending-terug/.

Iresearch (2018). *Positieve Gezondheid in Gemeentelijke beleidsnota.* Accessed in October 2020 of ▶ https://www.iresearch.nl/projecten/positief-gezonde-gemeenten-27-11-2018.

Jung, H. P. (2020). Overleven, zo lang mogelijk leven, betekenisvol leven. Kantelingen in de zorg aan de hand van de ervaringen van een plattelandsdokter. *Tijdschrift voor Geneeskunde en Ethiek, 30*(4), 118–122.

Jung, H. P., Jung, T., Liebrand, S., Huber, M., Stupar-Rutenfrans, S., & Wensing, M. (2018). Meer tijd voor patiënten, minder verwijzingen? *Huisarts En Wetenschap, 61*(3), 39–41. ▶ https://doi.org/10.1007/s12445-018-0062-y.

Jung, H. P. et al. (2019). Zinnige zorg dreigt utopie te worden. *Medisch Contact, 47*, 18–20.

Kaljouw, M., & Van Vliet K. (2015). *Naar nieuwe zorg en zorgberoepen: de contouren. Commissie Innovatie Zorgberoepen en Opleidingen.* Accessed in October 2020 of ▶ https://docplayer.nl/329738-Naar-nieuwe-zorg-en-zorgberoepen-de-contouren.html.

Kingma, E. (2019). Kritische vragen bij Positieve Gezondheid. *Bijblijven Positieve Gezondheid, 8*, P49–P54.

Laurant, M., & Vermeulen, H. (2018). *Gezondheid organiseren. Leerboek voor verpleegkundigen*. Bohn Stafleu van Loghum.

Lemmens, L., et al. (2019). *Factsheet. Het gebruik van brede gezondheidsconcepten, inspirerend en uitdagend voor praktijk*. Accessed in October 2020 of ▶ https://www.rivm.nl/documenten/gebruik-van-brede-gezondheidsconcepten-inspirerend-en-uitdagend-voor-praktijk-0.

Medisch Ondernemen (2019). Ephraim M. Positieve Gezondheidsgesprekken geven huisartsenzorg een boost. ▶ https://www.medischondernemen.nl/medisch-ondernemen/positieve-gezondheidsgesprekken-geven-huisartsenzorg-een-boost.

Meurs, P. L., et al. (2021). Accessed in Januar 2021 of ▶ https://www.raadrvs.nl/documenten/publicaties/2019/05/14/advies-blijk-van-vertrouwen-anders-verantwoorden-voor-goede-zorg.

NZa. (2020). Accessed in October 2020 of ▶ https://puc.overheid.nl/nza/doc/PUC_277025_22/1/.

Oude Weernink, T. (2020). *Een persoonsgericht gesprek in de Huisartsenpraktijk – Een Haalbaarheidsstudie*. Accessed in October 2020 of ▶ www.lrjg.nl/nieuws/ander-gesprek.

Poiesz, T., Caris, J., & Lapré, F. (2016). Gezondheid: Een definitie? *TSG, 94*, 252–255.

Porter, M. E. (2010). What is value in health care? *New England Journal of Medicine, 363*(26), 2477–2481.

Postma, S. A. E., Van Boven, K., et al. (2018). The development of an ICF-based questionnaire for patients with chronic conditions in primary care. *Journal of Clinical Epidemiology, 2018*, 92–100.

Prinsen, C. A. C., & Terwee, C. B. (2019). Measuring positive health: For now, a bridge too far. *Public Health, 170*, 70–77.

Rijksoverheid.nl (2020a). *Landelijke Nota Gezondheidsbeleid 2020–2024*. Accessed in October 2020 of ▶ https://www.rijksoverheid.nl/documenten/rapporten/2020/02/29/gezondheid-breed-op-de-agenda.

Rijksoverheid.nl (2020b). *Zorg goed voor jezelf*. Accessed in October 2020 of ▶ https://www.rijksoverheid.nl/onderwerpen/coronavirus-covid-19/documenten/publicaties/2020/07/15/poster-zorg-goed-voor-jezelf.

RIVM (2018). *Samenwerken aan gezondheid in de wijk loont, e-magazine*. Accessed in October 2020 of ▶ https://www.nhg.org/preventieindebuurt.

ROS-netwerk (2020). *Samenwerken aan zorg en gezondheid*. Accessed in October 2020 of ▶ https://www.ros-netwerk.nl/.

Studen ten leefstijl (2020). *Onderzoek implementatie voeding in onderwijs*. Accessed in October 2020 of ▶ https://www.studentenleefstijl.nl/implementatie/.

Juiste Zorg op de Juiste Plek (2019). ▶ https://www.rijksoverheid.nl/documenten/rapporten/2018/04/01/de-juiste-zorg-op-de-juiste-plek.

Van Boven, K., & Versteegde, T. (2019). Positieve Gezondheid een omsamenhangend concept. *Bijblijven Positieve Gezondheid, 8*, P55–P58.

Van der Stel, J. (2016). Definitie 'gezondheid' aan herziening toe. *MedContact, 71*, 18–19.

Van Stratum, L. (2019). *Requirements for implementing VBHC in primary care organizations. Thesis science, management and innovation*. Amsterdam: The Decision Group.

Van Tol, D. (2020). Van individuele naar gedeelde verantwoordelijkheid. *Tijdschrift Voor Gezondheidszorg En Ethiek, 30*, 123–124.

Van Vliet, M., et al. (2021). Development and psychometric evaluation of a Positive Health measurement scale: A factor analysis study based on a Dutch population. *BMJ*, ▶ https://bmjopen.bmj.com/content/11/2/e040816.

Whofic.nl (2020). *ICF*. Accessed in October 2020 of ▶ https://www.whofic.nl/familie-van-internationale-classificaties/referentie-classificaties/icf.

Zilveren kruis (2020). *Inkoopbeleid toekomstbestendige huisartsenzorg*. Accessed in October 2020 of ▶ https://www.zilverenkruis.nl/zorgaanbieders/zorgsoorten/huisartsenzorg/nieuws/inkoopbeleid-toekomstbestendige-huisartsenzorg.

I will maintain an open and verifiable attitude,
and I am aware of my responsibility towards society.
I will promote the availability and accessibility of
health care. I will not misuse my medical knowledge,
not even under pressure.

Thus, I will uphold the profession of physician.

This I promise

or
So help me God Almighty

Positive Health from an international perspective

© Bohn Stafleu van Loghum is an imprint of Springer Media B.V., part of Springer Nature 2022
M. Huber et al., *Handbook Positive Health in Primary Care*,
https://doi.org/10.1007/978-90-368-2729-4_9

▶ Main messages
   – There is increasing international interest in Positive Health.
   – Positive Health is a concept that has a proven track record on a small scale and
     seems to be an answer to global health problems.
   – The Positive Health movement has three phases: inspiration, implementation and
     embedment.
   – Start by formulating why you would like to begin working with Positive Health.
     Connect with culture- and country-specific local themes and initiatives.
   – The turning point of implementation in a new country or community is reached
     when key figures in leadership roles decide they want to work with the Positive
     Health concept.
   – The practical applicability of Positive Health in practice proves to be of added value
     for many professionals in the field of health and in the community.

The previous chapters describe the application of Positive Health in primary care – *The Dutch Example*. The application of the Positive Health concept supports the practical organisation of person-oriented care; in communication on an individual level as well as in the general medical practice and within the local community, as on regional and national levels.

Positive Health is seen as an innovative concept that will cause a transition from disease-oriented care to health-oriented and resilience care, with the focus on the whole person. This handbook describes many experiences and best practices. In ▶ Chap. 8 the role of Positive Health in policy, practice, research and education in the Netherlands is described. The transformation in health care also deals with challenges, related bottlenecks and preconditions that have not yet been sufficiently secured. Further substantiation and a larger support base are needed, so that the late majority will also be included and sufficient critical mass can be achieved (model by Rogers, ◻ fig. 6.7) for fully embedding the concept in the traditional methods of primary care in the Netherlands.

In the meantime, Positive Health is continually expanding into other domains, youth, schools, healthy workplaces, healthy living environments, and much more. Each time, a similar path appears to be followed whenever the concept is implemented in a new niche, new practice, local community or region. Like the tips described in ◻ fig. 8.9, the first question is: *why* are you interested in working with the Positive Health concept? What are your challenges in health care? What similar developments are taking place in your country, region or district? What are the needs with regard to health transformation and *how* could Positive Health contribute to that? These questions can be supportive towards a vision and strategy. The *what* question will focus more on the tactical (structure and network) and operational (routines and methods) steps to take, to learn to work with the concept of Positive Health, and implement this on the different levels. Sinek's '*why, how and what*' (Sinek, 2009) are also used as a leitmotiv to describe the experiences in the various countries where Positive Health has been introduced, so far (i.e., Belgium, Japan and Iceland). Case descriptions are provided as practical examples of how the concept of Positive Health is being implemented outside the Netherlands.

As the interest in Positive Health is increasing, also outside the Netherlands, we would like to take this opportunity to reflect on the lessons learned and the developments in Positive Health of recent years. In order to do so, we use an evaluation report by Johansen, PhD candidate at DRIFT (the Dutch Research Institute For Transitions), Erasmus University Rotterdam, on the rise of Positive Health

267   9

9.1 · Reflections on the success of Positive Health from a transition ...

(Johansen, 2021). ▶ Section 9.1 talks about the successes of Positive Health in the Netherlands, based on the theory of 'transformative social innovation': 'the process and methods by which new ways of thinking, working and organising spread and gradually become institutionalised.' We believe that the analysis, based on this strategy of transformative innovation (Loorbach, et al., 2020), can be inspiring for other countries in developing activities to strengthen Positive Health as a movement. With challenges in health care being linked to the changes in society, it is important to *uphold the profession of physician*: Health as the starting point, with people at the centre.

9.1 Reflections on the success of Positive Health from a transition management perspective

In the Netherlands, the dissemination and acceptance of Positive Health is considered a success. What are the characteristic elements that have led to its success? According to Johansen, transition management distinguishes various spheres of influence (strategic, tactical and operational). 'It is the actors' abilities that drive the development mechanisms of *growing, replicating, partnering, instrumentalising* and *embedding.*' (Johansen, 2021) These development mechanisms support the dissemination of Positive Health in the Netherlands (☐ tab. 9.1). Johansen has analysed the development of iPH and Positive Health, over the past years.

In the development and dissemination of Positive Health, iPH has the role of knowledge carrier. Instrumentalisation has been a key factor in the development of Positive Health in the Netherlands and builds on the mechanisms of replication and partnering. Central to these mechanisms is their connection with others, which is to experiment with Positive Health and its tools in a different context, to forge partnerships to pool resources and capacities, and to attract governance support to become more sustainable. The main result to date, in the Netherlands, has been the inclusion of Positive Health as part of the Dutch Government's vision of health in its National Policy Document on Public Health 2020–2024 (Rijksoverheid.nl, 2020). The incorporation of Positive Health in national public health policy is an important step towards the concept becoming mainstream or even the norm. In an ongoing process, the Institute for Positive Health (iPH) and its partners actively look for ways to embed Positive Health in regulation and regular funding schemes. As mentioned above, these development mechanisms, by themselves, are not enough to realise transformative innovation – it also requires the agency and network to create a shared discourse and identity to support a movement. A network can bring together individual or small initiatives that each address specific, persistent problems or that respond to opportunities in their specific context. These networks can also be used to exchange ideas on further development, experiences and practical applications to create transformative capacity. The Institute for Positive Health in the Netherlands aims to supports the exchange of lessons learned, experimentation, and the promotion of new practices, and lobbies to influence policy-making. ☐ Table 9.1 contains practical suggestions that would support the diffusion of Positive Health in the Netherlands, in local contexts, by applying the development mechanisms.

The development mechanisms of *growing, replicating, partnering, instrumentalising* and *embedding*, based on the theory of transformative innovation, are very similar to the three phases (i.e., inspiration, implementation and anchoring) that IPH has

◨ Table 9.1   Development mechanisms

development mechanism	suggestions for care professionals
growing (quantitative growth of an initiative or innovation)	Invest in **providing information** on the concept of Positive Health by giving presentations and interviews, writing articles and offering training opportunities
replicating (translation of ideas, models and practices into another context)	Look for ways to **translate the ideas** of Positive Health and its tools into other contexts. Connect with initiatives or institutions in other domains to explore how Positive Health would work in that context (i.e. in schools, voluntary organisations and local municipal projects)
partnering (pooling of resources, competences, and capacities between various initiatives)	Identify opportunities for cooperation and connect with others who are like-minded and have similar ideas, such as on a broad view of health, healthy living, sense of purpose in health care, and sustainability and continuity in health care. **Form a network** on the basis of like-mindedness to exchange experiences and best practices. Such a network may start locally, but also consider connecting to other networks around the country
instrumentalising (strengthening of an initiative by exploiting opportunities in a governance context)	Look for or create opportunities to connect with **influential others** by activating your own network (who knows who), to actively expand your network by being visible and easy to approach, trying to inspire others through your own personal experience or by addressing persistent problems. Try to connect with people who are familiar with navigating bureaucracy
embedment (institutionalisation of a transformative innovation through mainstreaming and structural anchoring)	Build **on existing connections and partnerships** to support mainstreaming Positive Health, such as in medical curricula, in vision and policy documents in specific areas of health care and care professions, in health care agreements between stakeholders, including government authorities and other parties
agency and capabilities	Search for intrinsically motivated actors who could be a role model (or take on this role yourself) by sharing an inspiring vision, personal experience, and/or connecting with influential actors in a specific field. Develop a narrative of change to help spread the concept of Positive Health. Connect with like-minded people (i.e. private citizens and entrepreneurs) and initiatives, as much as possible, to develop a strong network with a shared discourse on Positive Health. Use the network to adapt and learn and translate ideas into practice (small-scale action)

9

distinguished for expanding the movement of Positive Health to other contexts and locations. Informing and inspiring others and, thus, letting the movement grow is part of the first step. Subsequently, it is important that people join forces and cooperate. Starting with a coalition of the willing, to connect with partners in the medical practice or within the community, to broaden and expand (instrumentalising) to a larger network. This appears to be a universal process.

Why have Positive Health initiatives been started in the various countries, (*why*); why did early adaptors want to start Positive Health in their country? In which way is Positive Health an answer or solution to the health issues in those countries (*how*) and what has been done in this respect, so far (*what*)? The following section first outlines a broader perspective on universal health challenges. This is followed by a description of the first international experiences with Positive Health – in Belgium, Japan and Iceland – and their lessons learned with respect to the implementation of the Positive Health concept. We hope these stories will inspire readers to imagine what they would like to do with Positive Health within their own professional environment and what would be needed to achieve this.

9.2 Positive Health from an international perspective

Chapters 1 and 2 describe how an international conference, held in 2009 in the Netherlands, led to the formulation of a more dynamic description of health, namely '*as the ability to adapt and self-manage in the face of social, physical and emotional challenges*' (Huber et al., 2011). Meanwhile, the elaboration of this description into the Positive Health concept has become an increasingly well-known phenomenon, also on an international level.

> At the heart of working with Positive Health
> The most powerful force for building resilience is knowing what is meaningful to you. Becoming aware of this is the first objective, which isn't easy at all!
> It is expressed in what someone finds important, what is of value to them and what they would like to achieve. In the deepest sense, a person's will is linked to what is most important to them. Therefore, it is very important to feel what it is that you **want to do** – instead of what you **should do**. Quote: Machteld Huber (used in Positive Health training)

The challenges in health care in the Netherlands (see ▸ Chap. 1 on the various crises), with both an ageing population and an increase in chronic diseases, as well as pressure on the health care system due to costs and capacity, are also prevalent in other countries around the world. In many countries there is a similar shift from disease-oriented to health-oriented care. Person-oriented health care, prevention, lifestyle and self-determination also receive attention, internationally. De Maeseneer also addressed these themes in his book about the Family Medicine and Primary care, with the focus on societal change. (De Maeseneer, 2017) The need for change can be driven by a variety of forces, for example those related to financial, demographic, sustainable or organisational perspectives. Although countries all probably have to deal with the same international health challenges, it is also likely that there will be country- and culture-specifi aspects of how to deal with these challenges.

Author Karolien van den Brekel and Barbara Piper (Head of the iPH Academy) studied vision documents from several international organisations to find where Positive Health could contribute to international health challenges. Positive Health may contribute to some of the United Nations Sustainability Goals (SDGs) (see ◻ fig. 9.1). It especially connects to SDG 3: Ensure healthy lives and promote well-being for all at all ages (▸ https://sdgs.un.org/goals/goal3). Piper: 'With its holistic approach, Positive Health may

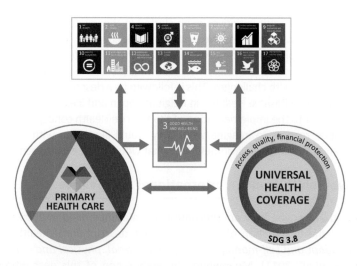

▣ Figure 9.1   Linking Primary Health Care (PHC), Universal Health Coverage (UHC) and Sustainability Development Goals (SDG). (Source: ▶ https://sdgs.un.org/#goal_section)

contribute to the world's health problems. Through the broad view of health and the focus on building resilience, with particular attention on personal sense of purpose, this concept not only broadens but also deepens people's thinking about their own health and health in general. At the same time, it is a framework of experience regarding implementation of the concept in health care, in various layers of society. In this way, the concept is embedded in personal experience and responsibility for one's own health as well as in overall organised health care within society.'

SDG 3: Good Health and Well-being

SDG 10: Reduced Inequalities

SDG 11: Sustainable Cities and Communities

SDG 17: Partnerships for the Goals

Looking at all sustainability goals, Positive Health may not only contribute to the goal of good health and well-being (SDG 3), but also to important other SDGs, such as SDGs 10,11 and 17. Positive health is a philosophy that has a connecting effect, encouraging cooperation and partnerships (i.e. the Positive Health networks, related to SDG 17). Furthermore, with its common language, stimulation of self-regulation and resilience, activation of active citizenship and community strength, Positive Health also contributes to sustainable communities, related to SDG 11 (see ▶ Chap. 7). If people are able to take better care of their health and award importance to it, this will also contribute to reducing health inequalities. ▣ Figure 9.1 shows how primary care and universal health coverage are also linked to SDG 3.

The focus on cooperation between public health and the social and medical domains is important to address health inequity and optimise health potential, and pay attention to a healthy living environment, which will promote good health and well-being. The views of various European organisations and partnerships also tend to focus on similar themes. For example, this international report from the WHO Regional Director for Europe: 'Rethink policy priorities in the light of pandemics', was recently published on behalf of the WHO's Pan-European Commission on Health and

Sustainable Development (Kluge, 2021). "The COVID-19 pandemic has reminded us of the vulnerability of societies, economies and health systems, and the weaknesses of our current systems of governance at national and global levels. Within a few weeks, a new strain of virus spread across the world, leaving a trail of human and economic devastation. Yet not everyone, or every nation, was affected to the same degree. The importance of a full implementation of the concept of One Health in all settings where health policies are developed is addressed in Kluge's report. It calls for a fundamental rethinking of policy priorities well beyond health policies, if the lessons from the pandemic are to be addressed proactively, with measures acting in the settings where the initial threats to sustainable health are most likely to occur." The 5 relevant elements in this WHO publication are:

- **Operationalise the concept of 'One Health' at all levels**
- Take action on all levels of society to fix the fractures that left so many people vulnerable to the pandemic
- Make changes to the global financial system
- Promote global public goods for sustainable improvements in health
- Support innovation in health systems

Sustainable societies cannot be achieved without resilient and universally accessible, high-quality health care and social systems. However, better governance, transparency and accountability, smart investment, and resilient health systems are only a means to an end. Several European organisations published a vision statements for 2030 and had done so before the COVID-19 outbreak, describing similar themes. For example, Eurohealthnet addresses the social determinants of health to help build fairer, healthier, and more sustainable communities for all (Eurohealthnet, 2021).

Other European primary care organisations include the European Forum for Primary Care (EFPC, 2021) the European Health Futures Forum (EHFF, 2021) and Europrev (Europrev, 2021), aim to make primary care providers able and willing to take responsibility for the health of the population under their care and stimulate preventive care. Barros and De Maeseneer et al. also publish about changes and disruptive innovation needed in European health care, in 'Considerations for health and health care in Europe'. The question is how to include this international context and the big picture of innovation in health transformation (Barros et al., 2016), and how to apply it in the general medical practice to provide more person-oriented care?

Positive Health turns out to be a refreshing new concept, with a broad perspective on health that connects well with several of the above-mentioned themes. The practical applicability proves to be of added value for many health care professionals (see sect. 8.5). The lessons learned in the Netherlands and the countries that have already started working with Positive Health provide the starting points for a further expansion of the concept.

Why did they want to start working with Positive Health? What problem were they addressing) and *how* did they do so using Positive Health? As mentioned in ▸ sect. 9.1, there are both strategic (discursive/cultural), tactical (network/structural) and operational (routine/methodical) pathways that could be taken. The experiences in the Netherlands as well as in the first three other countries where Positive Health has been applied in practice have shown that the process and the individual steps are reasonably similar.

9.2.1 The phases of learning how to work with Positive Health

The approach to introducing Positive Health in the Netherlands and the first three other countries, so far, has been similar, with early adaptors who became inspired when hearing about the concept. The experiences show the same three phases in introducing Positive Health in practice:

- Inspiration
- Implementation
- Embedment

The starting points for adopting a new initiative in a national health care system may vary per country. This is also true for Positive Health initiatives, which also must connect to and align with the existing programmes, structures and cultural settings in a specific area or country. But the most important question to begin with is the same for all countries and systems, namely:

- Why

Why do you wish to start working with Positive Health?
Why could Positive Health contribute to the particular health challenges of a certain country? What had been the original reason for one or two early adaptors to bring the concept of Positive Health to their country? What are the health themes in that specific region or country for which Positive Health was believed to offer a solution? All the implementation steps and lessons learned from the Netherlands regarding the implementation of Positive Health, and the way these has delivered person-oriented care are described in Chapters 5 to 8. The example of the Province of Limburg (see *Learning from Limburg* (see ▶ sect. 8.3.1)) is particularly useful to compare with implementation processes in the other countries where Positive Health has been introduced.

- How

How can Positive Health be an answer?
Positive Health appears to have been first introduced in a variety of domains, depending on the concept's ambassadors or early adaptors. It may begin first on a citizen level, with policymakers in public health care, or in a particular institute or organisation. Whatever the circumstances, in whichever domain, the 7 tips of working with Positive Health can always be used as starting points (see ◻ fig. 8.9).

- What

What steps to take?
The following section provides a number of practical examples to describe which steps have been taken. Following the three phases of inspiration, implementation and embedment the various examples in Belgium, Japan and Iceland are presented. **Inspiration** starts with early adaptors and ambassadors, inspirational lectures, workshops, presentations and training.

9.3 Reflection on the first international experiences with Positive Health in Belgium, Japan and Iceland

The following sections provide examples of experience with Positive Health in three countries. The why, how and what are described, providing examples and experiences from international colleagues who started to work with Positive Health. Why did they want to start working with Positive Health, and how could this be an answer to the health challenges in their countries? In 2017, Belgium and Japan showed interest in the concept, and, later in the year, so did Iceland.

9.3.1 Belgium

Positive Health Belgium was launched in 2018 during the Christelijke Mutualiteit (CM) symposium 'Together for Positive Health'. CM is Belgium's largest health insurance fund with 19 regional mutual health organisations and 4.5 million members. For Belgium, the concept was started, primarily, from the need for health promotion on the part of the Belgian health insurance fund, and it was decided to start with CM health consultants who conducted the Positive Health conversations. At the time of writing this book, further implementation was also planned in the field of health care (▶ www.mijnpositievegezondheid.be). The Belgian insurance company intends to stimulate the promotion of health; the starting points for Positive Health consisted of training the health consultants of the insurance companies. These consultants are in direct and daily contact with citizens (e.g., by telephone).

Luc van Gorp, CM Belgium, as early adaptor

▪ **Why**

Luc van Gorp, Chair of Christelijke Mutualiteit (CM), Belgium's largest health care fund (formerly public health insurance fund) with 4.5 million members, had an epiphany when he heard Machteld Huber speak at a conference in 2016. She was articulating what he had been thinking for years, and those thoughts had finally been given a name: Positive Health! Already, for a long time, he had been concerned about health insurance 'paying for the wrong things – reimbursing the costs of fixing medical complaints instead of preventing those complaints for arising in the first place'.

▪ **How**

Physicians are forced to earn money by performing services, while they should be involved in caring for their patients from a different perspective, and concern themselves with how their treatment contributes to improving their patients' health. Changes are called for, in health care, with a focus on health objectives. CM held a survey amongst its policyholders on the level of support for the broad concept of health and received a positive response from 90 % of respondents. Based on this knowledge, CM changed its name to 'Health Fund' in 2018 and subsequently launched *Positive Health Belgium* at the symposium 'Together for Positive Health' (▸ www.mijnpositievegezondheid.be/ ▸ www.masantépositive.be).

■ **What**

In Belgium, it was decided to start with health advisors from CM health care fund, who would conduct Positive Health-style conversations, and a number of physicians and other care professionals have also been trained by the Institute for Positive Health (iPH), on this subject. The implementation of the broad concept of health is progressing steadily, including the thinking about how hospitals could evolve into local health centres where citizens can go for advice. Luc van Gorp has successfully endeavoured to define health care policy on the basis of a broad vision of health, which was reflected in Belgium's federal coalition agreement of 2020.

Astrid Luypaert, project leader Positive Health Belgium: 'In Flanders, primary care transition is in full swing, with primary care zones being created, towards goal-oriented care (also see academievoordeeerstelijn.be). 'Positive Health Belgium wants to create a network of professionals, organisations, welfare workers, policymakers, municipalities and health insurance funds, with a broad view on health. To help people feel connected to life and society. The spider web of Positive Health relates to our motivational counselling and forms the ideal basis for doing this. Together, we can bring about a powerful movement in our society (▸ www.mijnpositievegezondheid.be). The concept of working with Positive Health can only expand when we learn from each other and by keeping the movement going together. That is why the Positive Health network was set up in Belgium. It is a learning network, with all the knowledge and experience gained along the way being shared within this network. Databases are created to refine and research the Positive Health approach.'

Anne Hoof has been working as a general practitioner in Belgium for 10 years now, in an immigrant community in Genk. She is also familiar with Dutch primary care, as she used to work as a substitute at the practice of Hans Peter Jung in Afferden: 'In my experience, health care in Belgium is more performance-oriented and based on the medical model. On both patient level and interprofessional level, equality is not a standard feature of the Belgian culture and system (which is reflected, for example, in credibility and remuneration differences). Belgian specialists often argue against general practitioners becoming gatekeepers to specialist care. In addition, psychological expertise and social work appear to be neglected when multidisciplinary consultations are organised. The health care system is fragmented. There are differences between community health centres and independent general medical practices.'

Hoof: 'My own experience is that Positive Health starts with the individual. In Belgium, we think it is important to embed the Positive Health model more broadly in existing health-promoting concepts and working frames, amongst other things, with the aim of achieving sustainable health goals and actively working to reduce health inequalities. In Belgium, we consider health a responsibility that is shared by individuals and society as a whole.' Next steps in Belgium besides the activities from CM are having more general practitioners follow the training working with Positive Health and start with research.

9.3 · Reflection on the first international experiences with Positive Health ...

275   9

9.3.2 Japan

In 2017, a delegation of 5 Japanese care professionals visited the Netherlands to be inspired in the field of elderly care and the Dutch health care system. Hiroyuki Beniya, Japanese physician at the Orange Home Care Clinic for the elderly in Fukui, became interested in the concept of Positive Health. The English-Japanese translator played a crucial role as ambassador in the start of Positive Health in Japan (see text box). The support base of Positive Health in Japan is still small, but with innovativeness and enthusiasm they expect to stay inspired to work with Positive Health. The implementation of the concept started in elderly care, but has since also expanded to the domain of youth care, in a unique Japanese project (see text box).

- ▪ **Why**

The *why* element, for the early adaptors in Japan, stems from the ageing population, financial burden of health care, scepticism concerning over-medicalisation and a growing interest in an individualistic approach, as is also the case in most developed countries. People in Japan, at birth, have the longest life expectancy in the world (84.43 years, in 2020). The challenges are also similar: resistance to change (particularly by those who benefit from the current system), the treatment remuneration system which encourages over-medicalisation, and a non-holistic approach in the education of care professionals and citizens, in general.

- ▪ **How**

Ambassador of Positive Health in Japan (Jeanette Chabot, Japanese–English/Dutch interpreter)
    'Over the past decade, much of my work was related to elderly care and health care in the Netherlands. Through these assignments, as writer and interpreter, I encountered Positive Health and I became totally fascinated by it. When the Japanese physician Hiroyuki Beniya asked me to come up with 'an interesting programme for their visit to the Netherlands', I included an interview with Machteld Huber. That was the first of many visits by Japanese delegations to the Netherlands. In a similar way, I introduced Machteld to Mr Matsumoto, Chairman of Sakura Global Holding and founder of the Matsumoto Foundation. As a member of this foundation, Fujiko Hasegawa eagerly began her research on Positive Health. In the meantime, I wrote a book about it, so, in 2018, there was already a book on Positive Health in Japanese.'
    In 2019, Machteld gave a training course in Fukui (see ◻ fig. 9.2). The first group of participants in the Positive Health training in Fukui included early adaptors Dr Hiroyuki Beniya and Fujiko Hasegawa and several others who are currently also involved in Japan's first Positive Health clinic. A second training is scheduled for early 2022 to be held in Japan and is to be led by Karolien van den Brekel. As was also the case in the Netherlands, the individuals and organisations in Japan who have embraced Positive

で管理する能力としての健康（Health as the ability to adapt and to self-manage, in face of social, physical and emotional challenges)」というものである。

つまりヒューバー氏は健康を「適応してセルフマネジメントをする力」として見ることを提案している。これは、健康を静止した「状態」とするのではなく、それが個人や社会で変化させられる"動的"なものであり、健康を「能力」として捉え直したものである。「疾患や障害があっても、周りの力などを支えにして、気落ちすることなく人生を前向きに歩いて行けること、その力こそが健康！」とする捉え方である。

そしてヒューバー氏は、これを定義ではなく"コンセプト"とし、「ポジティヴヘルス」とネー

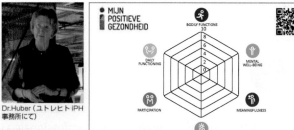

Dr.Huber (ユトレヒト iPH 事務所にて)

くもの巣ツール:成人用、8〜16歳（小児）用、16〜25歳（思春期）用があり、iPH のホームページで閲覧・ダウンロードできる

以下の3要素によってポジティヴヘルスは構成されている。

①このツールを通じて患者は人生の振り返りを行う。

②医療従事者は患者にとって大切なものは何か、またそれを得るためには何を変えていかなければならないか、本人と共に探る。

■ **Figure 9.2** Machteld Huber teaching the Training 'Working with Positive Health' in Japan. (Source: Hasegawa 2020)

Health have been already practicing working with a broad perspective on health. However, they were lacking substantiation and the tools to do what they were trying to do. Becoming acquainted with the Positive Health concept and benefiting from using its tools, gave them important insights that enabled them to grow further.

■ What

Two examples are described of the implementation of Positive Health in Japan among elderly in de Orange Home Care Clinic and among kids in de kidslab.

■ Orange Home Care Clinic, Fukui City

Orange Home Care Clinic was established in 2011 by Hiroyuki Beniya. It specialises in primary care, with emphasis on making house calls, but there is also a large amount of other medical care and welfare. What this clinic offers is rather unique to Japan, which does not have a primary care system, as such. Although the outpatient department of Orange Home Care Clinic can be visited by anybody, the main service of this department is to enable those who would otherwise be hospitalised to receive care as outpatients, at home. The department has a team of cooperating care providers that includes a nurse, physiotherapist, speech therapist, occupational therapist, dietician, early childhood education specialist, social worker and care manager. Some of the social workers used to be musicians, one other is a Buddhist monk. Amongst the physicians is an oncologist, nutrition specialist and palliative care specialist. Some of the care professionals have followed the Positive Health training. They all believe that by making house calls, and by using Positive Health to they get to know their patients in a more holistic way and within the context of their community.

9.3 · Reflection on the first international experiences with Positive Health ...

277

9

■   Kids Lab

When he started the home care clinic, Hiroyuki Beniya initiated an other innovation in Japan: the Kids Lab day care, based on the six dimensions of Positive Health, for children who require a large amount of medical attention. These are children who, if they were in the Netherlands, would be admitted to a *children's hospice* (inspired on nikutrecht.nl). Hiroyuki Beniya's concept is not only to give such children a place to stay other than in a hospital or their own home, but also to enable their parents to go back to work, if they so wished. Kids Lab was first started as a summer holiday programme in Karuizawa, one of the oldest summer resorts of Japan. The area is surrounded by woods and close to mountains, and the children, some of whom in wheelchairs, with ventilators and other heavy equipment, were very happy in the summer programme. In April of 2020, the Hotch Lodge at Karuizawa was founded. This day care and cultural centre is based on the concept of Positive Health. It combines medical care (outpatient medical care, house calls, day care for children with medical needs), welfare (day centre for the elderly), culture (original theatre performances and art shows by interns), food (home-grown and prepared on location) and education (cooperation with kindergarten/elementary school Kazakoshi Gakuen). Across the street from the Hotch Lodge is Kazakoshi Gakuen School, which officially opened its doors in April 2020, in the middle of the COVID-19 pandemic. It is probably the most innovative school in Japan, at this moment, focusing on individual students, rather than forcing a system on them. The Positive Health spider web Children's tool was used to perform a health check on the elementary schoolchildren, and care providers had a lengthy talk with each of the children. Later, while they were taking body measurements, one child said 'While I was filling out the spiderweb, I realised that I'm a pretty happy kid!' Another said: 'My foot hurts, but I can do everything I want to do, so it's all right.' One did say: 'Something sad has happened. Would you listen to my story another time?'

In this way, what would normally be a passive mandatory school health check-up for these children, now became a lively occasion that excited curiosity about their body and its inner workings.

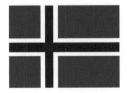

9.3.3 Iceland

Why, how, what on Positive Health in Iceland – so far ...

Over the past two years, the Institute for Positive Health (iPH) has been actively inspiring professionals and training participants to implement Positive Health in Iceland. The implementation of Positive Health is taking place in the local community, starting with the social and medical domains. Work is being done simultaneously on the level of the consulting room, practice organisation and the local community. Social workers and two groups of nurses and general practitioners in Reykjavík have already been trained, and who are also interested in starting with courses for the general practitioner's training.

■ **Why**

Why start with Positive Health in Iceland? The need to move from disease-oriented care to the type of care that is focused on health seems the biggest driving force behind the implementation in Iceland. *GP trainee Martijn Veenman* is quoted as saying: 'I think that it is a good tool for obtaining more clarity on the issues and needs of patients. It is easy to prescribe medication or refer to another specialist but certain issues will not be resolved without revealing and addressing the underlying causes. Knowing what the actual underlying subjective and objective issues are will make it possible to find a solution for those issues.' The main health themes Martijn encounters on a daily basis are complaints of anxiety, depression and pain. Chronic diseases, such as obesity, hypertension, diabetes as well as psychological issues and pain management tend to be the main topics.

Martijn: 'As time and resources are limited, too often, we tend to prescribe medication to ease the pain of mental and physical suffering, which then creates a dependency on substances that often are addictive and as such create a new problem.' The motivation, in Icelandic primary care, for shifting from disease- to health-oriented care consists of the fact that diseases often result from problems related to an unhealthy lifestyle. Managing to change people's mindset to lead a healthier lifestyle will have a positive impact on physical and mental well-being. Psychologist Linda Bára Lýðsdóttir recognises the same health themes, including long-term care and chronic diseases: 'The Icelandic health care system focuses on diagnoses and how to treat and cure these. That is important but can be overly simplifying and may miss the opportunity to find the answers by looking at the whole person, from a broader perspective.'

■ **How**

Positive Health can support the shift from disease- to health-oriented care.

Martijn Veenman: 'Using the Positive Health tool offers patients the possibility to explore, discover and realise the main issues and problems they are struggling with. It enables them to either work on the issues themselves or helps them to express what help they need.' Linda Bára Lýðsdóttir: 'Positive Health can help to empower people.' She notices an increase in medical diagnoses, and treatments among children in Iceland such as of ADHD, with more and more children on sleep medication. Another example is that people describe themselves as: 'I am a depressed person', instead of 'I suffer from depression, and would like to find out how to deal with it, and to learn what is possible'. Linda thinks that Positive Health can contribute to more resilient care. Focusing on what makes a person healthy rather than looking at what makes them sick.

Elínborg Bárðardóttir is general practitioner and programme director for the primary care training programme at the Development Centre for Primary Healthcare in Iceland (DCPHI): 'We are working towards high-quality training and new knowledge in primary care and we need new and different views and methods with respect to the future health of our patients as well as our workforce, in order to serve the

9.3 · Reflection on the first international experiences with Positive Health ...

279

9

community. One of the biggest challenges we face is a growing number of people with chronic and complex problems and we need to further promote and support self care and self management by patients. When I heard about Positive Health and the spider web, I felt that it gave us a much-wanted tool to empower our patients and the community.'

- ▪ **What**

Following inspirational and training sessions in 2019, a partnership was forged at the beginning of 2020. The coronavirus measures that were put in place in March 2020 meant that the start of the project had to be postponed, but after the summer, it was off to a good start. To date, there have been multiple inspirational webinars, An online training working with Positive Health in East Iceland and two Positive Health Ambassador sessions, with the last one in January 2021. A sustainable next step towards embedment is the 'Train the Trainer' programme for the ambassadors to support and embed Positive Health. With local certified Positive Health trainers in Iceland, it is much easier to connect to the local community and existing infrastructure.

Elínborg sees good possibilities to connect Positive Health ideas to existing activities and initiatives in Iceland: 'We are implementing wellness clinics to promote salutogenesis and empowering primary care and Positive Health. The spider web fits right in there as one of our new methods and is supported at all levels by our governing institutions. I also believe we will introduce and implement Positive Health in schools as well as in social services and occupational rehabilitation in the nearest future. Positive Health and the spider web make me optimistic that we are moving into the right direction in primary care, with increased sensitivity to finding the right balance between the needs of our patients and the health system that serves them.'

- ▪ **The leading role of ambassadors/early adaptors in Iceland**

In 2017, **Linda Bára Lýðsdóttir**, psychologist, (working for VIRK in vocational rehabilitation), heard Machteld Huber speaking at a conference in Amsterdam. Linda was inspired by Machteld's presentation about the broad perspective on health and the importance of meaningfulness. The concept of Positive Health could be helpful for vocational rehabilitation in Iceland, where an increasing number of people are getting sick, many with burnout symptoms, who are not getting back to work. Linda notices that it is not the affliction itself, but the state of mind that causes these people to not go back to work and participate in the workplace. People are also diagnosed with mental disorders at increasingly younger ages.

Machteld invited Linda to join the conference, 'Learning from Limburg' (▶ sect. 8.3), where more speakers talked about experiences and implementation of Positive Health in the community. Once back in Iceland, Linda introduced Positive Health to her colleagues from Virk and to Alma Möller, the Director of Health of the Icelandic Medical Association. The implementation of the concept, from then on, was in the hands of Elínborg Bárðardóttir, general practitioner and Doorgehaalde tekst vervangen door: program director of the Icelandic GP residency program.

Elínborg Bárðardóttir played a key role as early adaptor to inspire other general practitioners in Iceland. A group of ambassadors of Positive Health in Iceland was formed, with Linda from Virk, general practitioner Pétur Heimisson and Guðjón

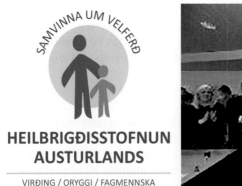

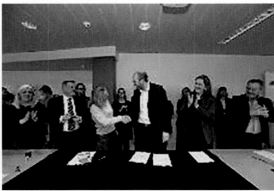

■ Figure 9.3   HSA Health care institute of East Iceland; signing of the partnership between iPH and HSA East Iceland. The picture shows iPH Director Angelique Schuitemaker and HSA Director Guðjón Hauksson

Hauksson from East Iceland (from HSA) and a representative of the Directorate of Health and Elinborg Bardadottir from The Development Centre for Primary Health-care in Iceland). In 2019, Karolien van den Brekel and Machteld Huber came to Ice-land for a few inspirational sessions, such as the annual Icelandic Medical Association conference and the first training working with Positive Health. The spider web was also translated in Icelandic. Pétur Heimisson CEO toevoegen voor Gudjon Hauksson (met and Guðjón Hauksson involved the HSA, came to visit the Netherlands and the contract with iPH was signed in February 2020.

Guðjón Hauksson, from HSA, worked on the implementation of Positive Health in East Iceland. He said: 'The knowledge of Positive Health reached the shores of Ice-land in 2018 and sparked the interest of a small number of health care professionals. Since then, the interest has been growing with a number of lectures and inspirational sessions. After the formal contract between iPH and the Health care institute of East Iceland was signed, the interest and use of the Positive Health method has further increased. We are now at the point of educating trainers so that the movement in Iceland becomes sustainable. It is important to have the knowledge and understand-ing of the method of Positive Health, but it is as important to be able to pass on the knowledge, in order to shift from pure *disease care* to more *health care*. Along with education for both citizens and care professionals, it is critical to implement digital solutions to simplify communication, recording and visualisation of Positive Health. I think it is safe to say that the idea of Positive Health has laid down strong roots in Iceland, and now it is time to nurture these roots to build a strong and stable Positive Health tree.' (■ fig. 9.3)

■   The implementation process in Iceland

Following the implementation process in Iceland, first an ambassador and early adaptors became inspired about Positive Health; then came the phase of training, obtaining experience and creating a coalition of the willing.

It is not so easy to organise Positive Health, centrally. As in the Netherlands, implementation seems to be a stepwise process. It is interesting to see the imple-mentation in the community of East Iceland evolve, and hopefully, with these learning experiences, the next steps towards further implementation will also be made in the Reykjavík region. Both movements are needed: top down to facilitate implementation and create good conditions, and bottom up for the Positive Health movement to evolve and grow through awareness, preferably organically from within the community. Connecting to existing programmes, such as the use of the Positive Health children's tool, may provide synergy with the already successful prevention programme for the Icelandic youth (Planet Youth, 2021). The same empowering language is needed. It would be good to stimulate this focus on health and role models.

- **Challenges to overcome**

General practitioner Veenman: 'One of the biggest challenges is the fact that, for instance, social services often are not in direct contact with general practitioners. Frequently, I get questions from patients about what social services have advised or demanded from a patient. Patients often cannot express these needs or demands, which frustrates them as well as the health care workers.' Veenman continues: 'Implementing a new approach to health care will take some time. Certain issues are the same as those experienced in the Netherlands, such as lack of time and funding, which make implementation of Positive Health difficult in de daily general medical practice. Various physicians in East Iceland have indicated that the discontinuity of care (no patient registration system) is a barrier to the implementation of Positive Health. Positive Health will initially be limited to those who prefer to stay with the same general practitioner.

Elinborg: 'Since the coronavirus crisis, we have established a new ambassador group, and a train-the-trainer programme will start soon. In this way, the next steps towards embedment can be made'.

9.3.4 Research of Positive Health in Belgium and Japan

It is interesting that people from all cultures are able to say what health means to them, recognise the six dimensions and are able to apply them in the various countries.

In Belgium, soon after becoming aware of the Positive Health concept, insurance company CM surveyed almost 10,000 policyholders on whether they were able to identify themselves with the six dimensions of Positive Health (see ▸ sect. 9.3.1). The support turned out to be more than 90 %, upon which the management decided to turn CM into a health fund. This is currently being worked on, step by step. In Belgium, the Positive Health Belgium network was subsequently set up. Anne van Hoof, Belgian general practitioner: 'Quality of life is included in the spider web model as part of Positive Health. We see health, in the broadest sense of the word, as a way to live life to the fullest. Quality of life, therefore, transcends health, because we do not want to fall into the trap of health imperialism.' In Flanders, primary care is in transition and so-called primary care zones have been created: (academievoordeeerstelijn.be).

In 2020, Fujiko Hasegawa, one of the early adaptors in Japan, conducted an online survey at the Tokyo Healthcare University, Institute for Future Initiatives (Hasegawa 2020). The 2,400 respondents evenly represented the age groups between people in their twenties to those in their seventies. The survey was nationwide. Since the concept of Positive Health is not yet widely known in Japan, a brief explanation about

Positive Health preceded the questionnaire. The respondents all had a high degree of interest in internet research. As such, they may not be representative of typical Japanese people.

The survey was limited to people's sense of health based on the six dimensions of Positive Health. Although the spider web is often used for people to rate their own level of health according to the six dimensions, this survey did not use the spider web tool. Nevertheless, this was the first significant survey in Japan that focused on the concept of Positive Health. The total affirmative response to the question of whether the six dimensions of Positive Health reflected people's sense of health was 76.5 %. The survey will be extended to include a wider range of stakeholders, including health care providers, policymakers, patients and researchers.

9.3.5 Culture- and country-specific differences

In our experience, thus far, the approach to introducing Positive Health and the domains involved differ per country. This is also true for where Positive Health *inspiration* starts. The most effective entry point to embed a new initiative has therefore also been country-specific and different, each time. Where the Positive Health *inspiration* starts, differs per country. The most effective entry point for embedding a new initiative, therefore, has also differed between countries.

▶ Chapter 8, under 'Learning from Limburg' describes how the process itself is the result. Positive Health is a catalyst for transformation and that is universal. The themes of implementation can be recognised everywhere. After inspiration follows a phase of meetings, workshops, presentations, training courses and first a large amount of training before applying the concept in practice. The way in which this is implemented in practice differs per region or country; partly, because of cross-cultural differences, but also due to different starting points, sometimes, depending on which domain the ambassador or early adaptor comes from.

The Belgian insurance company intends to stimulate the promotion of health; the starting points for Positive Health consisted of training the health consultants of the insurance companies. These consultants are in direct and daily contact with citizens (e.g., by telephone). Belgium was eager to start as soon as possible with the health consultants and share experiences.

In Iceland, Positive Health started with a combination of community approach and integrated implementation through primary health care locations. In Japan, it started locally and was oriented more on target groups where Positive Health started in a home clinic for the elderly and, later on, a new project was started for children who needed extensive medical care.

Which training method is the most appropriate for which country, within which timeframe? In Belgium, the training courses were from week to week, which had the advantage that the lessons learned were still fresh on everyone's mind, but sometimes there was too little time for practicing the newly learned material in the time in-between courses. In Iceland, there was a longer gap between training courses, due to the coronavirus outbreak. However, this time appeared to have been well spent, with people working by themselves with a group of ambassadors who were interested in promoting Positive Health locally. In the intervening time, the power of working with

Positive Health emerged bottom-up, from the inside. During the ambassador meetings in Iceland, it became clear which steps they could take themselves before the start of the iPH training. Piper: 'It is about taking your responsibility versus waiting until someone else will implement it for you.'

Cultural differences became evident, for example, during training sessions. In Japan, for instance, it is not customary to reflect on what you as an individual consider important, let alone to talk about it with each other. The Japanese are not used to this, it is not part of their culture; group interests are paramount. There are also differences in terms of organisation and cooperation, between general practitioners, with the local community and with hospitals. In Iceland, the expectations of patients are still very much focused on disease. Care in Belgium is also performance-oriented and based on the medical model.

The iPH trainer (Stephan Hermsen) in Belgium said: 'I take cultural differences and needs into account; for example, by asking how this is done in their setting or culture and then responding to that. By asking how people are really doing, how things are going, and what they may need. In Belgium, for example, hierarchy is taken into account. Forcing a young employee to speak up, just because he is rather quiet, is not appropriate here. That is not how it works here, there may be 'unconscious' social behaviour. The Dutch culture is much more direct and we must be careful not to apply this approach in Belgium.

Piper: 'The iPH Academy connects individual people and organisations, also on an international level, who are interested in working with Positive Health principles. We are aware of the differences in needs and on regional, national and cultural levels. We train trainers to pass on the essence of working with Positive Health. We want to support the movement towards a meaningful life, living from resilience, from self-determination and personal well-being.

9.4 Conclusions

Positive Health is a concept with a proven track record, on a small scale, and may be an answer to global health problems. Based on experiences in Positive Health in the Netherlands and with respect to transition management, three phases can be identified: inspiration, implementation and embedment. The tips included in this handbook appear universally applicable, looking at best practices and experiences in the Netherlands and, on a smaller scale, also in Belgium, Japan and Iceland (fig. 8.9). There are similarities in relation to the process and differences in the method of implementation. The culture- and country-specific themes vary, such as the organisation and infrastructure of care per country, business organisation culture (bottom up/top down), and having a group-oriented or individual focus. In the various countries where experience has been gained with Positive Health, there are differences as to for which target group Positive Health was first implemented. It is important that the concept can be aligned with existing initiatives and level of urgency, and that people in a leadership role embrace Positive Health to further the implementation in their country. We are working hard on further implementation research and effect. In the Netherlands, we started with primary care, but, over the course of time, the Positive Health method has been widely disseminated (e.g., to youth, social domain, mental care, public health, sustainable employability, hospital care and elderly care). Although, within Europe and beyond, primary care takes on many different forms, at its core, primary care is for care providers to assess what their patients need, and that always starts with a good conversation (i.e., the *alternative dialogue*). If reading this book has inspired you, and you would also like to start working according to the Positive Health concept, think of which health issues Positive Health could help to solve, and start with gaining experience in applying the *alternative dialogue* model. Forming coalitions of the willing will further develop cooperation, within the general medical practice as well as the local community, region and country.

References

Academie voordeeerstelijn (2021). Accessed in June 2021 of ► https://academievoordeeerstelijn.be/.

Barros, et al. (2016). *EXPH disruptive innovation considerations for health and health care in Europe.* Affiliation: European Commission Accessed in June 2021 of ► https://ec.europa.eu/health/sites/default/files/expert_panel/docs/012_disruptive_innovation_en.pdf. ► https://doi.org/10.13140/RG.2.2.22264.80642.

De Maeseneer, J. (2017). *Family medicine and primary care: At the crossroads of societal change.*

EFPC (2021). European Forum for Primary Care. Accessed in June 2021 of ► http://euprimarycare.org/.

EHFF (2021). European Health Futures Forum. Accessed in August 2021 of ► https://ehff.eu/.

Eurohealtnet (2021). Accessed in June 2021 of ► https://eurohealthnet.eu/about-us/who-we-are.

Europrev (2021). *European network for prevention and health promotion in family medicine and general practice.* Accessed in June 2021 of ► https://europrev.woncaeurope.org/.

Hasegawa, F. (2020). You can be healthy, even with sicknesses! Origin Holland: 'Positive Health' From 'restoring to normal' to 'support ability to adapt'; JMCC [Japan Association of Healthcare Management Consultants]; Japans verslag opgehaald op augustus 2020 van ► www.iph.nl; ► https://www.1limburg.nl/japanners-onder-de-indruk-van-limburgs-zorgconcept.

Huber, M., Knottnerus, J. A., Green, L., et al. (2011). How should we define health? *BMJ, 343*(4163), 235–237.

Johansen, F. (2021). *Positieve gezondheid: van niche-discours tot overheidsjargon* (unpublished manuscript). PhD candidate at DRIFT (the Dutch Research Institute For Transitions). Erasmus University.

Kluge, H. H. P. (2021). *Rethinking policy priorities in the light of pandemics.* Pan-European commission on health and sustainable development. Accessed in June 2021 of ► https://www.euro.who.int/en/health-topics/health-policy/european-programme-of-work/pan-european-commission-on-health-and-sustainable-development.

Loorbach, D., et al. (2020). Transformative innovation and translocal diffusion. *Environmental innovation and societal transitions, 35*, 251–260; ► https://doi.org/10.1016/j.eist.2020.01.009.

Nikutrecht.nl (2021). Accessed in June 2021 of ► https://www.nikutrecht.nl/nieuws/delegatie-van-de-japanse-orange-home-care-clinic-op-bezoek-bij-kinderhospice-zonnacare.

Planet, Y. (2021). The Icelandic Prevention model, accessed in August 2021 of ► https://planetyouth.org/the-method/.

Rijksoverheid.nl (2020). *Landelijke Nota Gezondheidsbeleid 2020–2024.* Accessed in October 2020 of ► https://www.rijksoverheid.nl/documenten/rapporten/2020/02/29/gezondheid-breed-op-de-agenda.

Rogers, E. (2003). *Diffusion of innovations.* Free Press.

Sinek, S. (2009). *Start with why.* Penguin Books Ltd.

Supplementary Information

© Bohn Stafleu van Loghum is an imprint of Springer Media B.V., part of Springer Nature 2022
M. Huber et al., *Handbook Positive Health in Primary Care*,
https://doi.org/10.1007/978-90-368-2729-4

Words of thanks

A first word of thanks is to the northern Meuse valley network. This initially small, but ever-growing group of dedicated people were the first to start working with Positive Health as an answer to the health issues that arose in Limburg. They were the first to put the ideas into practice. The newly established Institute for Positive Health (iPH) was also able to make grateful use of their experiences.

Our thanks go to experienced writer Cecile Vossen, who, even before the writing process of the Dutch handbook started, pointed out important choices and sketched clear outlines. Once the Dutch text was in place, the fresh and professional eye of editor Tirza van Hengstum helped to make it more accessible. For this English version of the handbook, Annemieke Righart's careful translation was invaluable to the process.

The ultimate form and layout of the book were partly determined by the enthusiastic contribution of all who participated in focal group meetings and interviews. Our particular thanks go to Pim Assendelft, Saskia Benthem, Simone Dekker, Hylke de Waart, Kees Jan Dijkstra, Marco Ephraïm, Neelke Groen, Simone Helmer, Theo Hermsen, Frederik Jaspers Faijen, Selma Jonkers, Lili Jung, Robin Jung, poet J.K., Karlijn Marissink, Dante Mulder, Carola Penninx, Jessie Roelofs, Estelle Schatorié, Thomas Steensma, Janneke van den Berg, Paul van den Brekel, Naomie van der Ven, Martijn van der Waart, Luz-Anne van Diest, Wim Venhuis, Chantal Walg and Rene Wolters. For the English version, we would like to thank Barbara Piper for her contribution to the chapter on the Positive Health international perspective and all other international colleagues who contributed by sharing their experiences with Positive Health: Elínborg Bárðardóttir, Hiroyuki Beniya, Jeanette Chabot, Luc van Gorp, Linda Bára Lýðsdóttir, Guðjón Hauksson, Fujiko Hasegawa, Pétur Heimisson, Anne van Hoof, Francoise Johansen, Astrid Luypaert, Niels Rogger, Viktoria Schmidt en Martijn Veenman.

Our thanks also go to Gideon van Voornveld for the photographs of the Hippocratic Oath and Thomas Jung for the author photograph.

Thanks to Anouk Middelkamp and Ronald Bakvis of Bohn Stafleu van Loghum publishers for their pleasant cooperation and trust; to the Institute for Positive Health; to our colleagues with their sharp eye; and to All about Health, who provided us with the opportunity and space to work on this book.

Thanks to the Dutch island of Vlieland, where the three of us retreated to work on this book.

Thanks also to all the people we had the privilege of meeting in our consulting rooms during our careers as general practitioner – some of whom feature in the cases in this book. Calling you 'patients' in this word of thanks would not do justice to what we have learned from you and what we aim to achieve with this book. Without you, this book would never have come about.

And our final thanks go to you, our readers – for your early interest in Positive Health.

We hope it will benefit you as much as it did us!

Abbreviations

CPB - CPB Netherlands Bureau for Economic Policy Analysis

GDPR - General Data Protection Regulation

IPC - Integrated primary care

GGD - Community Health Services

GGZ - Dutch Association of Mental Health and Addiction Care

HRMO - Manifest of concerned general practitioners 'Het roer moet om' (*things need to change*)

ICPC - International Classification of Primary Care

InEen - Association of primary care organisations

IOH - Interfaculty consultative body for general medical practice

iPH - Institute for Positive Health

LSA - National alliance of active residents

LOVAH - National organisation of general practitioners in training

LHOV - National association of general practitioner trainers

LHV - National Association of General Practitioners

NZa - Dutch Healthcare Authority

NHG - Dutch College of General Practitioners

NPF - Netherlands Patients Federation

NWO - Dutch Research Council

O&I - Organisation and Infrastructure

PGZ - Personalised Care

SER - The Social and Economic Council of the Netherlands

SPV - Advanced practice nurse

RIVM - National Institute for Public Health and the Environment

ROS - Regional support structure primary care

RVS - Council for Public Health and Society

RVZ - Council of public health and health care (Raad voor Volksgezondheid en Zorg)

SROI - Social Return on Investment

VNG - Association of Netherlands Municipalities

VPHuisartsen - Association of general practitioners who are also practice owners

VWS - Ministry of Public Health, welfare and Sport

WMO - Social Support Act

Wpg - Public Health Act

ZonMw - The Netherlands Organisation for Health Research and Development

Zvw - Health Insurance Act

Index